Current Clinical Practice

Series editor
Neil S. Skolnik

More information about this series at http://www.springer.com/series/7633

Pamela A. Fenstemacher • Peter Winn
Editors

Post-Acute and Long-Term Medicine

A Pocket Guide

Second Edition

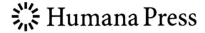 Humana Press

Editors

Pamela A. Fenstemacher, MD, CMD,
  FAAFP
Chief Medical Officer
Living Independently for Elders (LIFE)
University of Pennsylvania School
  of Nursing
Philadelphia, PA, USA

Peter Winn, MD, CMD
Department of Family and Preventive
  Medicine
Geriatric Assessment Clinic
University of Oklahoma
OUHSC Family Medicine Center
Oklahoma City, OK, USA

Current Clinical Practice
ISBN 978-3-319-16978-1   ISBN 978-3-319-16979-8   (eBook)
DOI 10.1007/978-3-319-16979-8

Library of Congress Control Number: 2015953500

Springer Cham Heidelberg New York Dordrecht London

Humana Press is a brand of Springer
Springer International Publishing AG Switzerland is part of Springer Science+Business Media
(www.springer.com)

Preface

Whether practitioners are still in training, recently graduated, or deciding to change the direction or focus of their career paths, either by choice or necessity, they can find themselves immersed in the long-term care (LTC) arena. Any practitioner of LTC can be overwhelmed when confronted by an LTC system that is both complex and highly regulated, let alone taking care of patients that are challenging even to the most experienced among us. These patients are challenging not only because they have numerous chronic medical conditions and extensive and complicated medication regimens but also because of advanced age and frailty. As experienced clinicians, educators, and medical directors in LTC, we have written this guide for practitioners in hopes of continuing to improve the quality of care provided throughout the LTC continuum by imparting to practitioners the current knowledge in this field as well as the experience our chapter authors have acquired over many years working in LTC.

Both The Society for Post-Acute and Long-Term Care Medicine (AMDA) and its state chapters continue to work tirelessly to meet the LTC practitioner's needs. Even the most experienced practitioners who have taken AMDA's course on medical direction have commented on how much of the information on LTC care presented in the course is neither readily available nor frequently taught. The content of this guide for practitioners is aimed at filling this void. The chapters of this guide address the varied components of the LTC system as well as how to take care of the patients and residents living within it.

Since the first edition of the guide was written, the LTC system has continued to evolve. The Center for Medicare and Medicaid Services (CMS) is promoting high-quality cost-effective care through initiatives that encourage the use of innovation, technology, and collaboration to improve quality. Accountable Care Organizations (ACOs) and Population Health Management are two examples of CMS innovation, focusing on prevention and early treatment of chronic medical illness. Chapters on PACE, Nurse Practitioners, Clinical Nurse Specialists and Physician Assistants, and the Department of Veteran Affairs Options were added to reflect the increase in community-based care that is being offered to our elders. The focus of some chapters was shifted as well. The first edition's chapter on Acute Change in Condition was changed to reflect the increasing focus on Preventing Hospital Admissions and Readmissions that is seen in LTC today. All of the chapters were updated to include the latest innovations such as INTERACT II.

As practitioners, we are all challenged by an ever-changing healthcare environment that entails bundling of healthcare services, value-based purchasing, transitions in care, medication reconciliation (including the recent CMS Quality Prescribing Initiative), PQRS reporting, HIPAA compliance (and possible audits), different electronic medical records at different healthcare settings, and EMR meaningful use. As editors of this guide, we hope these challenges will be less daunting with the information provided in this guide.

The contributors to this guide are passionate about LTC and many have worked within AMDA to create and disseminate a knowledge base for practitioners through varied means such as AMDA's clinical practice guidelines, conferences, and white papers, all of which have served as resources to this guide. We hope that you find *Post-Acute and Long-Term Care Medicine* an invaluable resource to complement your quest to optimize the care and living experience of your patients in LTC that supports patient-centered care as well as patient choice, well-being, dignity, and an improved quality of life.

This guide is dedicated to Chris Laxton and the AMDA staff, and all our AMDA colleagues who have mentored both of us over the years, many of whom have written chapters for this guide.

Philadelphia, PA   Pamela A. Fenstemacher
Oklahoma City, OK   Peter Winn

Series Editor Introduction

There is no better time for an update of *Long-Term Care Medicine*. Individuals over 65 represent the fastest-growing portion of the population in the United States, consume the highest proportion of the country's healthcare dollars, and often live in long-term care facilities or receive intensive outpatient home-based management for the latter portion of their lives. The editors, Drs. Fenstemacher and Winn, have extensive academic and practical experience in long-term care and have been involved in leadership positions with the American Medical Directors Association, which is the professional association for long-term care physicians. From this vantage point, they have selected authors who have both an academic and practical perspective on issues most relevant to the patients we take care of in long-term care facilities. The book's emphasis is on giving the practicing physician an accessible guide to understand and better manage the issues that come up in taking care of frail elderly patients. The book goes over the changing environment and regulations of long-term care. It does so by providing an expansive general overview of places and processes of care as well as details of care including chapters on wound care, dementia, delirium, rehabilitation, and many more.

The book is readable, practical, interesting, and relevant. For this the editors and authors are owed our thanks.

Neil Skolnik, MD
Professor of Family and Community Medicine
Temple University School of Medicine

Associate Director
Family Medicine Residency Program
Abington Memorial Hospital

Contents

Contributors

Alva S. Baker CMDR, HMDC, Hagerstown, MD, USA

David Brechtelsbauer Department of Family Medicine, University of South Dakota Sanford School of Medicine, Sioux Falls, SD, USA

George Brown Director of Clinical Services, The Access Group, Berkeley Heights, NJ, USA

J. Kenneth Brubaker Masonic Villages, Elizabethtown, PA, USA

Geriatric Associates, Suburban Outpatient Pavilion, Lancaster General Health, Lancaster, PA, USA

Pamela Z. Cacchione Department of Family and Community Health, University of Pennsylvania, Philadelphia, PA, USA

Andrew Neal Dentino Donald W. Reynolds Department of Geriatric Medicine, University of Oklahoma Health Sciences Center, Oklahoma City, OK, USA

Leonard Gelman Capital Care Family Medicine, Ballston Spa, NY, USA

Todd H. Goldberg Department of Internal Medicine, West Virginia University Health Sciences Center, Charleston, WV, USA

Daniel Haimowitz Multi-facility Medical Director, Levittown, PA, USA

Kourtney Harrington Donald W. Reynolds Department of Geriatric Medicine, University of Oklahoma Health Sciences Center, Oklahoma, OK, USA

Randall D. Huss Department of Family Medicine and Geriatrics, Mercy Clinic, Rolla, MO, USA

Cynthia Kuttner Department Chair and Assistant Professor, Department of Geriatrics and Gerontology, Ohio University Heritage College of Osteopathic Medicine, Ohio, USA

Thomas Lawrence Department of Geriatric Medicine and Long Term Care, Main Line Health System, Main Line Health Center, Newtown Square, PA, USA

Steven A. Levenson Genesis Healthcare, Baltimore, MD, USA

Joel A. Levien Department of Gastroenterology, Jackson Madison County General Hospital, Jackson, TN, USA

Stefani D. Madison Donald W. Reynolds Department of Geriatric Medicine, Hospice and Palliative Care Fellow, Oklahoma University Medicine Senior Health Center, Oklahoma City, OK, USA

Susan T. Marcolina Public Health Seattle and King County, Seattle, WA, USA

Eastgate Public Health Center, Bellevue, WA, USA

Ganesh Merugu Department of Geriatric Medicine, Albert Einstein Medical Center, Philadelphia, PA, USA

Naushira Pandya Department of Geriatrics, Nova Southeastern University College of Osteopathic Medicine, Fort Lauderdale, FL, USA

Shelley Reich The Access Group, Berkeley Heights, NJ, USA

Andrew Rosenzweig Department of Geriatric Medicine, Albert Einstein Medical Center, Philadelphia, PA, USA

Robert C. Salinas Family and Preventive Medicine, OU Medical Center, Oklahoma City, OK, USA

Reshma Shah Living Independently For Elders (LIFE), University of Pennsylvania, Philadelphia, PA, USA

David A. Smith Geriatric Consultants of Central Texas, Brownwood TX, USA

Richard G. Stefanacci Chief Medical Office, The Access Group, Berkeley Heights, NJ, USA

Thomas Jefferson University, College of Population Health, MercyLIFE Philadelphia, PA, USA

Laura Trice Physician Hospital Organization, TriHealth, Cincinnati, OH, USA

Deborah Way Department of Palliative Care, Corporal Michael J. Crescenz VA Medical Center, Philadelphia, PA, USA

Pamela A. Fenstmacher Living Independently for Elders (LIFE), University of Pennsylvania School of Nursing, Philadelphia, PA, USA

Peter Winn Department of Family and Preventive Medicine, Geriatric Assessment Clinic, OUHSC Family Medicine Center, University of Oklahoma, Oklahoma, OK, USA

Home Health Care

Robert C. Salinas and Stefani D. Madison

Introduction

It is estimated that by the year 2030, the number of people age 65 and over in the USA will increase from 39.6 million to 72 million, representing the fastest growing segment of our population. Although this age group makes up 13 % of the current population, it disproportionately accounts for approximately 36 % of all health care-related expenditures in the USA [1]. As older Americans have a strong desire to remain in their homes and age in place, this trend will increase the need for community-based home care services in the coming years. Many older Americans are afflicted with multiple chronic conditions (multi-morbidities), homebound, and experience difficulty in accessing timely and needed healthcare services. As a result, many "high-risk" elderly are isolated at home and receive fragmented and inadequate medical care.

With hospital-based care shifting to community-based care, a dramatic paradigm shift is occurring [2]. Hospital at home programs are being developed that enable patients to receive acute care at home. They have proven effective in reducing complications while cutting the cost of care by 30 % or more, leading to entrepreneurial efforts to promote their use. But widespread adoption of the model in the USA has been hampered by physicians' concerns about patient safety, as well as legal risk, and by the reluctance of payers, including Medicare, to reimburse providers for delivering services in home settings [3].

R.C. Salinas, MD (CAQ-G, HPM) (✉)
Family and Preventive Medicine, OU Medical Center,
900 NE 10th Street, Oklahoma City, OK 73013, USA
e-mail: robert-salinas@ouhsc.edu

S.D. Madison, MD
Donald W. Reynolds Department of Geriatric Medicine, Hospice and Palliative Care Fellow, Oklahoma University Medicine Senior Health Center,
1177, NE 13th street, Oklahoma City, OK 73117, USA

© Springer International Publishing Switzerland 2016
P.A. Fenstemacher, P. Winn (eds.), *Post-Acute and Long-Term Medicine*, Current Clinical Practice, DOI 10.1007/978-3-319-16979-8_1

The elderly often require emergency room evaluation for acute medical problems, unintended injuries, and exacerbation of chronic conditions such as congestive heart failure, chronic obstructive pulmonary disease, and diabetes [4]. These patients are experiencing shorter lengths of stay in the hospital setting [5]. Many elderly need post-acute care to regain their pre-morbid functional status and remain safely in the community [6]. With distant monitoring technology, changes in clinician reimbursement and more inter-system communication to prevent hospital admissions and readmissions, home care has become a vital part of the health care system. Further expansion and integration of home care can help meet the needs of an overstressed health care system and homebound patients [7]. This chapter reviews the delivery of medical care in the home, practitioner home visits and services provided by home health care agencies.

Home Care

Home care is defined as the provision of healthcare-related services and equipment to patients in the home for the purpose of restoring and maintaining his or her maximal level of function, comfort, and health [7, 8]. It entails an interdisciplinary approach and the use of therapeutic, diagnostic, and social support services. Generally, the goals of care determine the plan of care and the level of services needed. This can include house calls by a physician, nurse practitioner, or physician assistant in collaboration with the services provided by the home health care agency.

Generally, home care services are available to patients who have intermittent skilled needs subsequent to a decline in functional status due to an exacerbation of a chronic condition, acute illness, or injury, or who transition to home upon hospital discharge after surgery or acute illness.

The Physician House Call

Despite wanting to "age in place" in their traditional home setting, some older adults have opted to move to an assisted living facility (ALF) or an independent living facility (ILF). *Contrary to a common belief, patients are not required to be homebound in order for a physician to provide a house call and to be reimbursed for their medical services.* However, there *are* homebound requirements for those patients who require health care services delivered by a home health agency and this will be more thoroughly discussed later in this chapter. There are several situations for a practitioner to visit a patient at home. These include:

- An acute care visit when the patient is unable to come to the outpatient clinic setting.
- Ongoing management of a progressive chronic condition.

- Need to gather more information about the environmental conditions of a patient who continues to experience recurrent falls and injuries.
- Provision of palliative care and discussion end-of-life care preferences, including hospice care [9].

Some physicians have established a practice exclusively in home care. Home-based primary care (HBPC) can be a viable alternative for some practices, and can reduce overall cost of care for patients with serious illness [10].

Preparing for the House Call

When making a home visit, it is important to determine the purpose and goals of the visit. This requires advance notice to the patient, family members or caregivers, and the home health agency, hospice and/or community-based caseworker responsible for coordination of the patient's care. Planning ahead can determine what procedural instruments may be required such as toenail clippers or supplies for injections (Table 1).

During the home visit, address the patient's medical condition, review all medications, assess the patient's functional status, memory and cognitive ability, and level of independence (ADLs and Instrumental ADLs). For patients with physical limitations, assessment of functional status can identify the need for adaptive equipment. Assistive devices and durable medical equipment such as a walker or bedside commode can aide a person in remaining independent in the home and delay institutionalization.

A house call may also identify the need for home adaptation, remodeling, or retrofitting that can improve home access, safety, and mobility. *Caregiver assessment* is also important in determining a plan of care that can be successfully implemented in the home (Table 2 lists some important aspects of a home assessment). Monitoring for caregiver burnout is essential.

Table 1 The Doctors Bag

Stethoscope
Blood pressure cuff
Thermometer
Pen light
Prescription pad
Pharmacopeia
Toe nail clippers
Examination gloves
Syringes and needles
Sharp containing box
Scissors
Street map or GPS

Table 2 Assessment in the Home

Patient assessment
Functional assessment
Mental/cognitive assessment
Nutritional assessment
Medication use and compliance
Advance care planning
Caregiver assessment
Assessment of burden of caregiving
Assessment of caregiver
Environmental assessment
Safety in the home
Needs for durable medical equipment
Community assessment
Safety of neighborhood for health care providers
Availability of community resources

Table 3 Medicare part B reimbursement 2015[a]

New patients		Established patients	
Code	Reimbursement	Code	Reimbursement
99341	$52.58	99347	$53.16
99342	$76.69	99348	$80.62
99343	$125.21	99349	$122.76
99344	$174.89	99359	$170.08

[a]Reimbursement will vary from state to state

Billing for Services

Under current Medicare rules, any licensed physician, nurse practitioner, or physician assistant, can make a house call and bill for services rendered. Practitioners use CPT codes for the level of service provided [8]. Most third party payers follow the rates and guidelines for billing set forth by Medicare and Medicaid. Physicians are also allowed to bill based on the amount of time directly spent with or in counseling the patient. It is important that each component of the patient encounter be appropriately documented for the level of service coded (see Table 3). Note that practitioners are not allowed to bill for travel time associated with making a house call. Numerous versions of mobile-capable electronic health records (EHR) have the ability to document and to coordinate the exchange of patient information such as medication reconciliation, laboratory results, and diagnostic studies.

Agency Home Health Care

Under current Medicare guidelines beneficiaries who have a documented need for episodic care may be eligible for home health care. The purpose of home health care is to have an interdisciplinary team of qualified health care providers (see Table 4) to provide assistance in the home for a person who requires skilled nursing care, physical therapy, speech therapy, and other services. Often a referral is made when the physician notes a patient decline in health and level of function that places the patient at risk for hospitalization or institutionalization [7]. At other times, home health care can assist in delivery of palliative care in seriously ill patients who are ineligible for hospice or have chosen not to enroll in hospice [11].

Requirements for Agency Home Health Care

There are important requirements that must be met before a physician can order home health care for a Medicare beneficiary. First, a physician must determine that the patient meets the requirement for "homebound" status and secondly has a need for episodic skilled nursing care, physical therapy, or speech therapy. The interpretation of homebound status often leads to confusion. Its definition is explained in Table 5.

Table 4 Members of the Home Health Care Team

Skilled nurse
Physical therapist
Speech therapist
Occupational therapist
Home health care aide
Social worker
Case manager
Wound care nurse

Table 5 Definition of Homebound Status

A patient is considered home bound if "leaving the home would require a considerable and taxing effort" and if the patient "has a condition due to illness or injury which restricts ability to leave the residence except with the aid of supportive devices, the use of special transportation, or the assistance of another person, or if the patient has a condition such that leaving the home is medically contraindicated." Homebound patients may leave the home "if absences are infrequent or for periods of relatively short duration … or for the purpose of receiving medical treatment"

For the *initial Home Health certification*, the Affordable Care Act (ACA) now requires that the certifying physician document that the physician himself or herself, a resident physician, or a non-physician practitioner (NPP) working with the physician has had a *face-to-face encounter* with the patient. This encounter *must have addressed the medical condition for which this episode of home health care is being ordered. The documentation of a face-to-face encounter must occur within 90 days prior to the start date of home health care or within 30 days after the start of care. This encounter is only required for the initial certification period and not recertification.* The documentation for necessity includes the name of the certifying physician, date of the face-to face encounter, the patient's homebound status, the need for skilled services, and a signature and date from the ordering physician. The face-to-face encounter can be performed by a resident physician in training under the supervision of the teaching physician, or a nurse practitioner, clinical nurse specialist, certified midwife, and physician assistant (all must be under the supervision of the certifying/signing physician). The face-to-face documentation can be included in the certification document, a separate standardized form or via telehealth [12].

At times, the home setting may not be the best venue to provide and coordinate complex care, especially for very frail patients with multiple health care needs. In such cases, options may include admission to a rehabilitation center, a long-term acute care hospital (LTAC) or a skilled nursing facility. Any physician involved with the patient's care may order home health. *Many patients now leave the hospital with a referral for home health care services in an attempt to reduce readmission to the hospital within 30 days and to avoid financial penalties to the hospital.*

Home health care can improve transitions in care through medication reconciliation, patient and caregiver education related to the recent hospitalization, symptoms that warrant medical attention, and ensuring practitioner follow-up [13]. Multiple medical providers are often involved in patient care as the patient transitions to another health care setting. Effective communication among providers during these "transitions in care" is paramount to ensuring that providers are aware of any changes in the patient's needs and plan of care [14–16].

A physician can provide a written or verbal order to the home health agency to begin services. The referral should include information on the patient's overall functional status as well as the primary reason for the referral while keeping the patient's goals and purposes in mind. Background information regarding the caregivers in the home and any concerns should be shared with the home health agency. This information can help identify potential barriers that can affect patient outcomes.

Members of the Team

Delivering effective home health care depends on each member of the health care team using their skill set aimed at restoring health according to patient needs [17], while negotiating health care goals with the patient and family and then developing a plan of care that can sustain efforts to reach these goals. The home health team has regular contact with the patient's family and is in a position to ascertain whether a plan of care can be successfully implemented in the home (or elsewhere).

Skilled Nursing

A licensed practice nurse (LPN) or registered nurse (RN) can provide skilled-level care to patients in the home that may include:

- Educating patients and caregivers on acute and chronic medical conditions.
- Instructing on how/when to administer medication.
- Obtaining laboratory specimens and reporting results.
- Coordinating home X-ray studies, home infusion, and IV therapy.
- Providing wound care.

The nurse's admission assessment includes functional, memory and cognitive status, and medication reconciliation of prescribed and all over-the-counter medications [18–21]. Most home health care agencies now use a software program to screen for potential drug-drug interactions with this report then sent to the patient's physician for review.

Nurses usually provide services two to three times a week, but can be more frequent at the start of care (front loaded visits) in order to meet patient needs. Nurses may identify other medical problems that need to be brought to the attention of the practitioner and recognize barriers to the delivery of care, such as caregiver stress or financial burdens. The role of the home health nurse continues to expand and can include the promotion, monitoring, and maintenance of health in homebound persons [22].

Physical Therapist

Home health physical therapists provide therapy to improve lower extremity strength and conditioning. Patients often have a history of falls or have become deconditioned following hospitalization. Referrals for home physical therapy frequently are for patients who have suffered a stroke or had lower extremity orthopedic surgery [23, 24]. Physical therapists assist in educating the patient's caregivers on how to improve patient function, safety, and independence and provide recommendations for durable medical equipment (DME) such as canes, walkers, shower chairs, and suggestions for retrofitting bathrooms.

Speech Therapist

Under the current Medicare home health care guidelines, a physician can request a referral for home health care solely for the purpose of providing speech therapy in the home. The speech therapist can also perform an initial screen for swallowing that may subsequently necessitate a formal swallowing study in order to more adequately assess dysphagia and make recommendations as to diet consistency.

Occupational Therapist

Home health occupational therapists often work in tandem with physical therapists to promote better function of the upper extremities and self-care ADLs. The occupational therapist may also recommend adaptive equipment or DME that will assist the patient.

Social Worker

Most home health care agencies have medical social workers or will contract this service out. Medical social workers can play an important role in the care of patients who have complex psychosocial needs. This may include helping to identify caregivers (paid and informal), to address caregiver stress, and to make inquiries and suggestions to alleviate financial hardship.

Home Care Aide

Based on necessity, home health care agencies can provide nurse aides to assist patients in their ADLs such as bathing and to provide light housework if a patient is too weak to do so. They supplement the personal care provided by family members and other caregivers.

Physician Reimbursement for Home Health Care Services

Certification/Recertification Codes

Physicians who order home health care from a qualified Medicare agency are eligible to receive payment for reviewing the home health care agency plan of care. Once a referral to home health has been made, the physician will receive an *initial certification form (Form 485)*, which the physician will review, agree with the plan of care, and return the signed and dated form to the home health care agency. The face-to-face necessity documentation is only required for the initial certification. Upon review and completion of the Form 485, *the physician can bill for the initial certification period/initial plan of care (G01800), as well as subsequent recertification (G0179)*. Note that each certification period is for 60 days.

Table 6 Billing for home health care services

	Initial certification	Recertification	CPO
Licensed doctor (M.D./D.O.)	Yes	Yes	Yes
Resident doctor (in-training)	No	No	No
Non-physician practitioner (NP/PA)	No	No	Yes

Table 7 Certification, recertification, CPO codes

Code	Description
G0180-certification	Initial home health certification, also known as reviewing and signing the initial plan of care (Form 485)
G0179-recertification	Recertification of the plan of care: if the patient's care continues for an additional 60 day, the physician must review and sign recertification plan of care (Form 485)
G0181-care plan oversight	Indicated for the supervision of a patient under the care of a Medicare-certified home health care agency (patient not present). Oversight is indicated for the patient whose care is complex and involves multiple disciplines, therapy that requires regular physician/NP/PA contact

Care Plan Oversight Code

If a physician spends a minimum of 30 min in a 30-day period providing oversight and directing services during an episode of home health, he or she is allowed to bill for Care Plan Oversight (CPO) using code (G0181). When billing for CPO the time involved must be documented throughout the 30-day period. In contrast to billing requirements for certification and recertification, nurse practitioners or physician assistants *are* allowed to bill for CPO (Table 6). One important caveat is that surgeons are not allowed to bill for CPO as it is already bundled into the fee for postoperative care. Table 7 lists the G codes for home health care. Physicians are encouraged to document and bill for CPO, however physicians *are not allowed to concurrently bill for Transitional Care Management Services* or *Chronic Care Coordination* during a CPO 30-day period unless they decide not to bill for CPO.

Summary: The Future of Home Health Care

Due to the sustained growth in the number of people living with chronic illness and escalating medical expenditures, the provision of medical care in the home continues to evolve as a viable means of curtailing costs. It is alarming that approximately two million people, or 5 % of the Medicare population, account for nearly half on the Medicare budget [1]. As such, the US Government and Medicare are exploring innovative cost-effective alternative healthcare delivery models in an attempt to contain future costs. For example, new technological advances that allow monitoring of vital signs in the home of heart failure patients in order to identify exacerbations early and to prevent costly hospitalization [25]. Telemedicine technology not only allows home health nurses to monitor a patient's vital signs and daily weight from a distance, but also to share this information with the physician. Other models of care such as the "hospital at home" program can serve to reduce the high costs associated with hospitalization while still obtaining good health outcomes for patients who opt for treatment at home [3, 26].

Pearls for the Practitioner

- Many frail elderly are homebound and experience great difficulty in accessing timely and needed healthcare services, including regular visits to a physician's office.
- Home care is defined as the provision of health care-related services and equipment to patients in the home for the purpose of restoring and maintaining his or her maximal level of function, comfort, and health.
- Home health care provides an interdisciplinary team of qualified professionals that maximizes outcomes for patients.
- Home health care services are best delivered by determining health care goals with the patient and family and then developing a plan of care that can sustain the efforts in reaching those goals.
- Only licensed physicians working with a qualified Medicare agency are eligible to receive payment for reviewing the home health care agency plan of care. But, physicians, physician assistants, and advanced practice nurses are allowed to bill for Care Plan Oversight.
- During a home visit clinicians should not only assess the patient's medical conditions, but also assess the patient's functional status, cognitive ability, and level of independence/dependence.
- Patients are not required to be homebound in order for a physician to submit billing for a house call.
- The documentation of a face-to-face encounter must occur within 90 days prior to the start date of home health care or within 30 days after the start of care and is only required for initial certification and not recertification. Each certification period is 60 days.
- The face-to face encounter form should include the name of the certifying physician, date of encounter, the patient's homebound status, the need for skilled services, signature, and date of the ordering physician.

References

1. Census Bureau releases comprehensive analysis of fast-growing 90-and-older population. https://www.census.gov/newsroom/releases/archives/aging_population/cb11-194.html. Accessed 16 Jun 2015.
2. Holtz-Eakin D. High-cost medicare beneficiaries. Congressional Budget Office. 2005. pp. 1–12. http://www.cbo.gov/ftpdocs/63xx/doc6332/05-03-MediSpending.pdf.

3. Leff B, Burton L, Mader SL, et al. Hospital at home: feasibility and outcomes of a program to provide hospital-level care at home for acutely ill older patients. Ann Intern Med. 2005;143(11):798–808.

4. Roberts DC, McKay MP, Shaffer A. Increasing rates of emergency department visits for elderly patients in the United States, 1993 to 2003. Ann Emerg Med. 2008;51(6):769–74.

5. Baker DW, Einstadter D, Husak SS, Cebul RD. Trends in postdischarge mortality and readmissions: has length of stay declined too far? Arch Intern Med. 2004;164(5):538–44.

6. Kane RL. Finding the right level of posthospital care: "we didn't realize there was any other option for him". JAMA. 2011;305(3):284–93.

7. Murkofsky RL, Alston K. The past, present, and future of skilled home health agency care. Clin Geriatr Med. 2009;25(1):1–17.

8. Levine SA, Boal J, Boling PA. Home care. JAMA. 2003;290(9):1203–7.

9. Lukas L, Foltz C, Paxton H. Hospital outcomes for a home-based palliative medicine consulting service. J Palliat Med. 2013;16(2):179–84.

10. De Jonge KE, Jamshed N, Gilden D, Kubisiak J, Bruce SR, Taler G. Effects of home-based primary care on Medicare costs in high-risk elders. J Am Geriatr Soc. 2014;62(10):1825–31.

11. Labson MC, Sacco MM, Weissman DE, Gornet B, Stuart B. Innovative models of home-based palliative care. Cleve Clin J Med. 2013;80(Electronic Suppl 1):eS30.

12. Medicare Benefit Policy Manual. Chapter 7 home health service. http://www.cms.gov/Regulations-and-Guidance/Guidance/Manuals/downloads/bp102c07.pdf. Accessed 16 Jun 2015.

13. Gorodeski EZ, Chlad S, Vilensky S. Home-based care for heart failure: Cleveland Clinic's "Heart Care at Home" transitional care program. Cleve Clin J Med. 2013;80(Electronic Suppl 1):eS20–6.

14. Coleman EA, Berenson RA. Lost in transition: challenges and opportunities for improving the quality of transitional care. Ann Intern Med. 2004;141(7):533–6.

15. Kripalani S, LeFevre F, Phillips CO, Williams MV, Basaviah P, Baker DW. Deficits in communication and information transfer between hospital-based and primary care physicians: implications for patient safety and continuity of care. JAMA. 2007;297(8):831–41.

16. Kuo YF, Sharma G, Freeman JL, Goodwin JS. Growth in the care of older patients by hospitalists in the United States. N Engl J Med. 2009;360(11):1102–12.

17. Toto P. Success through teamwork in the home health setting: the role of occupational therapy. Home Health Care Manag Pract. 2006;19(1):31–7.

18. Mager DR. Medication errors and the home care patient. Home Healthc Nurse. 2007;25(3):151–5.

19. Forster AJ, Murff HJ, Peterson JF, Gandhi TK, Bates DW. The incidence and severity of adverse events affecting patients after discharge from the hospital. Ann Intern Med. 2003;138(3):161–7.

20. Meredith S, Feldman P, Frey D, Giammarco L, Hall K, Arnold K, et al. Improving medication use in newly admitted home healthcare patients: a randomized controlled trial. J Am Geriatr Soc. 2002;50(9):1484–91.

21. Coleman EA, Smith JD, Raha D, Min SJ. Posthospital medication discrepancies: prevalence and contributing factors. Arch Intern Med. 2005;165(16):1842–7.

22. Boult C, Reider L, Frey K, et al. Early effects of "guided care" on the quality of health care for multimorbid older persons: a cluster randomized control trial. J Gerontol A Biol Sci Med Sci. 2008;63A(3):321–32.

23. Stevens JA, Thomas K, Teh L, Greenspan AI. Unintentional fall injuries associated with walkers and canes in older adults treated in U.S. emergency departments. J Am Geriatr Soc. 2009;57(8):1464–9.

24. Fortinsky RH, Baker D, Gottschalk M, King M, Trella P, Tinetti ME. Extent of implementation of evidence-based fall prevention practices for older patients in home health care. J Am Geriatr Soc. 2008;56(4):737–43.

25. Boling PA, Chandekar RV, Hungate B, Purvis M, Selby-Penczak R, Abbey LJ. Improving outcomes and lowering costs by applying advanced models of in-home care. Cleve Clin J Med. 2013;80(Electronic Suppl 1):eS7–14.

26. Sheppard S, Doll H, Angus R, et al. Avoiding hospital admission through provision of hospital care at home: a systematic review and meta-analysis of individual patient data. Can Med Assoc J. 2009;80(2):175–82.

Assisted Living and Residential Care

Daniel Haimowitz

Introduction

Assisted living (AL) is becoming an increasingly important component of the long-term care continuum especially for those who do not require or choose not to avail themselves of nursing home services in preference for a less medicalized environment. There is a continued trend for greater numbers of people who choose to reside in assisted living communities (ALC) or residential care communities. As of 2012 in the USA, there were an estimated 22,200 residential care communities with 851,400 licensed beds [1].

AL is usually significantly less expensive than nursing home care, and can offer more autonomy and privacy. Due to a variety of factors including patients' desires to age in place, remain independent as long as possible, and avoid nursing home placement, AL residents have experienced an overall increase in frailty and ADL dependence. Many in healthcare have commented that residents in AL today have characteristics similar to nursing home residents of several decades ago. The increased number of AL beds, along with some publicity about poor care, has caused intermittent scrutiny of the AL industry from state legislators, regulatory agencies, and federal lawmakers. As such, state regulations are being changed with attention to improving staff education and oversight. New concepts related to affordability and community design in AL are being developed. AL can serve as a bridge for persons between independent living and the nursing home, but there are important differences between the two.

D. Haimowitz, MD, FACP, CMD (✉)
Multi-community Medical Director, 1 Gardenia Road, Levittown, PA 19057, USA
e-mail: geridoc1@comcast.net

© Springer International Publishing Switzerland 2016
P.A. Fenstemacher, P. Winn (eds.), *Post-Acute and Long-Term Medicine*,
Current Clinical Practice, DOI 10.1007/978-3-319-16979-8_2

Assisted Living History

AL has experienced rapid growth over the past several decades. AL Communities (ALCs) were opened initially to respond to consumer need that occurred when patients could no longer be cared for at home, yet did not require nursing home services. Core values of ALCs include autonomy, choice, privacy, dignity, and the ability to age in place in a homelike environment that differs from more formal institutional settings. These values increased the use of AL over the past 15 years, in contrast to a much smaller rise in nursing home bed utilization. A wide variety of ALCs have developed over this time, ranging from small "mom and pop" 4–8 resident homes to large ALCs housing several hundred residents, most of which are for-profit. There are a multitude of names for AL nationally (Table 1), which will be hereafter referred to as ALCs. The needs of consumers and the variety of options drive the AL market.

There has been conflict in the past between community owners/providers and consumers groups. Providers have vigorously defended a "social" model for ALCs, due to a wish to keep communities as homelike as possible, and to not have requirements that would entail costly and time-consuming paperwork. Unfortunately, there have been multiple instances of elder abuse, poor care, and malpractice, which have led consumer advocates to favor a more "medical" regulatory model. This underscores the increasing medical needs of AL residents. The trend has been toward a more conciliatory attitude between these two positions, moving toward a *medical model with a social conscience.* Recent initiatives have focused on the provision of person-centered care and research geared specifically toward AL.

There are multiple provider, consumer, profit and non-profit groups currently focusing on AL. National organizations are coming to agreement on how to improve care in AL. In 2003, the national Assisted Living Workgroup (ALW) was established at the request of the U.S. Senate Special Committee on Aging, and subsequently provided 110 recommendations aimed at assuring quality in AL. While this report was published over ten years ago, many of the recommendations are still pertinent today. The Center for Excellence in Assisted Living (CEAL) is an outgrowth of the ALW. CEAL is an ongoing effort at the national level to promote

Table 1 Various names for assisted living communities

Adult congregate living care, adult foster care, adult homes, adult living communities, basic care communities, board and care, catered living services, community based retirement communities, community residence communities, community residential care communities, congregate care, domiciliary care, elder care homes, enhanced care, enhanced living, home for the aged, old-age homes, personal care, residential care communities for the elderly, residential communities for groups, retirement residences, service-enriched housing, shared housing establishments, sheltered housing, supportive care, and supported living high-quality AL. CEAL serves as an informational clearinghouse, bringing together research, best practices, and policy. Data collection, person-centered care, and disclosure collaboratives in AL are some of the projects that have been developed and disseminated by CEAL.

Definition of Assisted Living

The variation among the different communities makes it difficult to establish a uniform definition of AL. The ALW developed the following definition:

> Assisted living is a state regulated and monitored residential long-term care option. Assisted living provides or coordinates oversight and services to meet the residents' individualized scheduled needs, based on the residents' assessments and service plans, and their unscheduled needs as they arise [2].

Services required by state law and regulation must include but are not limited to:

- 24-h awake staff to provide oversight and meet scheduled and unscheduled needs.
- Provision and oversight of personal and supportive services (assistance with activities of daily living and instrumental activities of daily living).
- Health related services (e.g., medication management).
- Social services.
- Recreational activities.
- Meals.
- Housekeeping and laundry.
- Transportation.

A resident has the right to choose and receive services in a way that will promote the resident's dignity, autonomy, independence, and quality of life. These services must be disclosed and agreed upon in the contract between the ALC and resident. AL does not generally provide ongoing, 24-h skilled nursing. However, residents are eligible to receive home health services on an intermittent basis to fulfill skilled nursing needs when these are unable to be provided by the AL staff. Residents are also entitled to receive *hospice services in place* if a revised plan of care is able to meet the needs of the resident and the community.

Community Characteristics

One of the key differences between nursing communities and AL is that there are no federal regulations for AL. Each state has developed its own specific regulations, thereby avoiding onerous federal regulations that would likely lead to increased cost to both communities and residents. Some advocate that there would be potential benefit to federal oversight that establishes clearer and more uniform enforceable standards in order to maintain quality patient care and safety.

ALCs differ widely in size, capabilities of care, and philosophy. The adage "if you've seen one assisted living facility you've seen one assisted living facility" applies. Many are freestanding communities, while others may be part of a continuing care retirement community (CCRC). Rooms are typically a private or semi-private studio and one- or two-bedroom apartments. As part of resident rights, recent proposals admonish private rooms for all AL residents. There are many corporate AL chains, with 78 % being for-profit, 20 % nonprofit, and 1 % government/other [1]. Sixty percent of ALCs serve 1–25 residents, 35 % have 25–100, and only 5.5 % have greater than 101; however, 71 % of all residents dwell in communities with more than 50 beds. Smaller communities tend to be newer than larger communities. In 2014, the largest chains were Brookdale Senior Living, Sunrise Senior Living, Evangelical Lutheran Good Samaritan Society, Emeritus Corporation, Five Star Quality Care, and Assisted Living Concepts. Most states in the West and Midwest, as well as a few northeast states (ME, PA, VI and VT) had higher use of residential care communities than the national average. Only in the West is there a comparable supply of residential care beds and nursing home beds per 1000 persons aged 65 and over, whereas nursing home beds far outnumber residential care beds in all other regions of the country [1].

Staffing in ALCs varies widely. There is no requirement for a nurse on site in ALCs. Seventy-five percent of ALCs provide social work services [1], with activities staff present more frequently in larger communities. Documentation and charting also varies, with state-specific regulations and scope of practice issues such as which AL staff, if any, are able to take verbal physician's or other healthcare professional's orders. State regulations and community-specific policies on which medical conditions may prohibit admission or give cause for discharge from an ALC vary. Ventilator dependency, stage IV decubiti, continuous intravenous fluids, and communicable airborne infections that require isolation may prohibit admission to AL. Most ALCs will admit residents with a moderate level of need for assistance, such as requiring help with or using wheelchairs (62–71 %). However, 44 % of ALCs will admit those who need assistance with transfers, and 53 % will *not* admit persons with moderate-to-severe dementia [3].

There is an increasing prevalence of dementia amongst AL residents. Zimmerman et al. [4] estimate that 71 % of AL residents have cognitive impairment (29 % mild, 23 % moderate, 19 % severe), and that 17 % of ALCs have *dementia special care units*, and 9 % *dementia-specific units*. A majority of residents with mild dementia go unrecognized by AL staff [4]. State regulations have begun focusing on dementia care especially related to resident safety, staff training, and provision of dementia-friendly activities. The Alzheimer's Association has developed AL-specific criteria and guidelines for dementia care [5]. Practitioners may notice a phenomenon in dementia-specific units that if a significant number of residents with dementia are admitted in a similar stage, at about the same time, that as these residents "age in place" and their disease progresses, many will be discharged from the AL community to a nursing community or hospice in a short period of time as they begin to require more complex medical and behavioral or end of life care. If antici-patory marketing has not been done, the community may experience a significant drop in occupancy rates that results in an impending financial crisis. AL residents may receive hospice care and continue to reside in the ALC depending on state regulation and each community's capabilities.

Resident Characteristics

Three-quarters of residents are either entirely (22 %) or partially (49 %) responsible for making the decision to move into an ALC, while for other residents, their adult children, children's spouse, or other family member commonly makes this decision. More than 70 % of residents move into an ALC from their own private home or apartment, and 60 % relocate within 10 miles of their previous permanent residence [6].

Similar to nursing communities, AL residents are typically female, white, with an average age of 87 years [6] and thus older than their nursing home counterparts [1]. The residents in AL do have increasing ADL needs [1] (Fig. 1) that generally correlate with declining overall health. This ADL dependency, though not as severe as those for nursing community residents, does exceed that seen in community-dwelling elderly. Data indicates that AL residents generally need assistance with two ADLs and have an average length of stay of 28 months.

AL residents often suffer from multiple medical problems. Half to three quarters have chronic conditions in three or more different general disease categories [7, 8]. As noted there is an increasing incidence and prevalence of dementia. Other common conditions include hypertension, heart disease, depression, arthritis, and osteoporosis [8].

Medication usage is an important issue in AL. Residents take an average of seven to eight prescriptions and two OTC medications daily, and 80 % require assistance with taking these medications [6]. Unlike skilled nursing communities, there is no federal mandate for a consultant pharmacist medication review, though many ALCs may provide this service. Use of over-the-counter medications, as well as alternative and herbal therapies are other potential concerns for the practitioner [9].

Overall, 60–90 % of residents are satisfied with their care in AL. The main two reasons residents leave the ALC are a change in health status or death. About 60 % move to a nursing community, 13 % move back home or to a child's or relative's home, 10 % transfer to another ALC, and 7 % go to a non-short-stay hospital [6].

Fig. 1 ADL Dependence

Assistance with	ALC	NH
Bathing	61%	96%
Eating	18%	56%
Dressing	45%	91%
Toileting	37%	87%

Understanding resident admission and discharge patterns is helpful to physicians when they discuss with residents and families the option of AL as it relates to the resident's care and illness trajectory.

Physicians and Other Providers

There is no federal mandate that requires an ALC to have a medical director, although some organizations have established this position. The ALW did not reach a majority consensus when considering a recommendation that ALCs have a medical director, but did reach a consensus that an "external professional consultant" should be used. One-quarter to one-third of ALCs have acquired a medical director [6]. There is increasing use of models where physicians either alone or in combination with nurse practitioners and/or physician assistants visit residents at the ALC on a regular basis. In general, most attending physicians continue to see residents in their private office. ALCs usually do not have a well-established "medical staff." Unlike nursing communities, where there are mandatory visits no less than every 60 days, *AL residents are required to be seen at a minimum of once yearly*. ALCs can contract with different services, including home health care and hospice agencies. Despite the lack of regulation in most states, a consultant pharmacist provides medication review and monitoring at 64 % of ALCs [6].

Financing

AL cost is significantly lower than that of a nursing community and is usually paid for privately with residents and families financing the majority of costs. Costs vary widely, depending on size of the AL residence, care requirements and geographic region (Fig. 2). The national median monthly rate in 2014 was $3500/month [10]. The national median yearly cost for a single ALC room was $42,000 (compared to a nursing home private room at $87,600) [10]. Fees usually include rent, meals and some level of basic services. Unlike the skilled nursing community, there are no Medicare payments to ALCs. But many states have developed Medicaid waiver programs under CMS to cover personal and skilled care services for qualified, low-income patients. Medicaid paid for at least some services for 19 % of all residents in 2010 [8]. Rendered services, *not* room and board charges, can be covered by Medicaid funds. These waivers are only available when a resident meets both the state's criteria for being "nursing home eligible" and the Medicaid financial eligibility requirement. Residents may experience a long delay before receiving such a

State	Low	High	Median
California	$987	$9000	$3750
Florida	$850	$7920	$3000
Illinois	$1048	$6500	$3805
Indiana	$1095	$8220	$3724
Iowa	$930	$8620	$3418
Maine	$3200	$8040	$4950
Massachusetts	$1263	$7613	$5247
New York	$1217	$10413	$3684
Oregon	$2196	$5463	$4000
Pennsylvania	$925	$7677	$3280
South Dakota	$1900	$6215	$3110
Texas	$825	$8605	$3523
Washington	$1000	$9000	$4250

Fig. 2 Variations in base rate costs for assisted living communities (one-bedroom single-occupancy monthly rate)

waiver and some ALC providers feel that they receive inadequate reimbursement under the waiver programs. Long-term care insurance is an occasional primary payment source. The lack of public funding for AL makes affordability a major concern for the future viability of the AL industry.

Another affordability concern is "a la carte" pricing policies at ALCs. ALC communities may charge extra when residents need additional help (i.e., a higher level of care/assistance) as illness progresses. Since many residents have limited funds, their families may be reluctant or even refuse to pay the increased fees and often subconsciously deny the existence of increasing frailty and medical risk.

Surprisingly, despite all these concerns about affordability, residents move out of an ALC due to financial reasons only 6 % of the time [6]. If a resident has to move out of the ALC for lack of funding, it is a difficult time for families. Not infrequently the resident is transferred to a hospital, which then assumes the responsibility of placing the resident at another healthcare community.

Physician Billing

Readers are referred to Part IV Special Issues in Long Term Care, Chap. "Documentation and Coding". Of note, the *custodial care codes* should be used (99324-99326 and 99334-99337) for ALC visits and *not* the home visit codes. AL coding uses *Place of Service Code 13*. Also note that reimbursement for AL medical services is generally higher than equivalent codes for other sites of service, such as the office and nursing home settings, which can be a financial incentive for physicians to make resident visits at the ALC.

Assisted Living Care

Direct Care Services

AL residents frequently require initial assessment by a physician prior to move-in, with this specific assessment varying by state. Unlike a formal mandatory plan of care in a nursing community, the ALC may develop a "service plan," which is similar in nature, and customized to the needs and preferences of the resident. Some service plans, however, may not incorporate a health care plan. Residents cannot be forced to move out of a community against their wishes, unless they meet discharge criteria exemplified by not being able to be cared for appropriately and safely. As previously mentioned, home care and hospice care may come into the community if the resident qualifies for these services.

Medication Management

Medication management is a significant issue in AL. As in other settings, medication management entails evidence-based prescribing, administration of medications, and e-prescribing. Healthcare providers should be knowledgeable about the basic tenets of geriatric prescribing (see Chap."Medication Management in Long Term Care"for a more detailed review). This includes the five "Rs"—the **R**ight medication at the **R**ight time, the **R**ight dose, and the **R**ight route of administration for the **R**ight patient. The Beers Criteria of "potentially inappropriate" medications for the elderly is a useful guide [11]. Many communities have a contract with a consultant pharmacist that can assist the community with medication management. Medication over- and undertreatment [12] is a problem in AL that consultant pharmacists can address with practitioners. The pharmacist may be especially helpful if they have advanced qualifications in geriatric pharmacy patient care.

Administration of medicines in the AL can be a problem because frequently non-licensed staff members give or assist with the dispensing of medications without adequate nurse supervision. Requirements for level of staff training and oversight of medication administration vary among states. Staff may lack assessment skills, so adverse medication side effects may be unrecognized. Unlike the nursing community, healthcare providers may not be notified when a resident has refused to take medications.

If the AL residents self-administer medications, over time this can become unsafe. When a resident with dementia has increasing memory loss and decreasing executive function, they struggle to self-administer medications. Even the definition of "self-administer" may be unclear—in some ALCs, this could simply mean that staff takes a medication from the med cart and places it into the resident's hand to self-administer.

Record keeping varies in ALCs, though some have more traditional patient charts. Medication delivery and storage in ALCs may be suboptimal. Order changes, inadequate medication monitoring, and multiple providers prescribing, all challenge safe medication management. Practitioners may have no influence on a particular ALC's structure, staff competency, ongoing quality improvement processes, or accountability in regard to medication administration and management, but could (and should) offer their expertise as a resource.

When applying the basic principles of medication management in the elderly, careful consideration must be given to the fact that the resident resides in AL. Any medication can cause almost any side effect in an elderly patient. Since the AL staff may not have formal training, common geriatric syndromes caused by medications (such as falls, urinary incontinence, change in appetite, and new or worsened confusion) may not be recognized. Without a formal chart or well-established notification channels, the attending physician (NP/PA) may be unaware that a new medication was prescribed or dose changed by another practitioner.

As in nursing communities, medications may be prescribed *without* a face-to-face visit by the practitioner. As such AL residents may receive unnecessary medications if the AL staff lacks assessment skills, or if underlying disease states go undiagnosed or untreated. The resident's quality of life needs to be carefully and continuously evaluated. As in all settings where the elderly receive care, a new or worsening condition may not need treatment if the treatment's potential side effects or risks outweigh the potential benefits.

Since the government categorizes an AL resident the same as a community-dwelling persons in regards to Medicare Part D, residents and their families may be presented with the problem of higher pharmacy costs when reaching the "donut hole" at which time residents are expected to pay for medications that were previously covered by pharmacy benefits. The residents may then end up paying more out-of-pocket cost for medication, which when combined with other AL fees can entail significant financial hardship for the resident and family.

Resident Rights

A common concern of residents and families is that they are often unaware of ALC services and costs. Ideally, marketing information should be consistent and residents should receive open disclosure of all ALC fees and services prior to signing the admission contract. The ALC need to inform residents and families on transfer and discharge policies to include the appeals process. The ALW recommendation regarding resident rights and provider responsibilities are listed in Tables 2 and 3 (where the ALC is also referred to as an assisted living residence or ALR).

Staff Training

Advocates stress that sufficient and experienced 24-h staffing should be available in the ALC. Not only should staff be aware of the changes seen with normal aging, but also be trained in the basics of medication management; and the recognition and

Table 2 Resident rights

Within the boundaries set by law, residents have the right to
• Be shown consideration and respect
• Be treated with dignity
• Exercise autonomy
• Exercise civil and religious rights and liberties
• Be free from chemical and physical restraints
• Be free from physical, mental, fiduciary, sexual and verbal abuse, and neglect
• Have free reciprocal communication with and access to the long-term care ombudsmen program
• Voice concerns and complaints to the ALR orally and in writing without reprisal
• Review and obtain copies of their own records that the ALR maintains
• Receive and send mail promptly and unopened
• Private unrestricted communication with other
• Privacy for phone calls and right to access a phone
• Privacy for couples and for visitors
• Privacy in treatment and caring for personal needs
• Manage their own financial affairs
• Confidentiality concerning financial, medical and personal affairs
• Guide the development and implementation of their service plans
• Participate in and appeal the discharge (move-out) planning process
• Involve family members in making decisions about services
• Arrange for third party services at their own expense*
• Accept or refuse services
• Choose their own physicians, dentists, pharmacists, and other health professionals
• Choose to execute advance directives
• Exercise choice about end-of-life care
• Participate or refuse to participate in social, spiritual, or community activities
• Arise and retire at times of their own choosing
• Form and participate in resident councils
• Furnish their own rooms and use and retain personal clothing and possessions
• Right to exercise choice and lifestyle as long as it does not interfere with other residents' rights
• Unrestricted contact with visitors and others as long as that does not infringe on other residents' rights
• Come and go rights that one would enjoy in their own home
• In addition, residents' family members have the right to form and participate in family councils

*An ALR may require that providers of third party services ensure that they and their employees have passed criminal background checks, are free from communicable diseases and are qualified to perform the duties they are hired to perform

general handling of common problems seen in the elderly resident. AL staff also needs to be able to determine when to contact the practitioner when a significant change of condition occurs in a resident [13]. In general, state regulations are moving towards more rigorous staff and administrative training in AL.

Table 3 Provider responsibilities

In the context of resident rights, providers have a responsibility to
• Promote an environment of civility, good manners and mutual consideration by requiring staff, and encouraging residents, to speak to one another in a respectful manner
• Provide all services for the resident or the resident's family that have been contracted for by the resident and the provider as well as those services that are required by law
• Obtain accurate information from residents that is sufficient to make an informed decision regarding admission and the services to be provided
• Maintain an environment free of illegal weapons and illegal drugs
• Obtain notification from residents of any third-party services they are receiving and to establish reasonable policies and procedures related to third-party services
• Report information regarding resident welfare to state agencies or other authorities as required by law
• Establish reasonable house rules in coordination with the resident council
• Involve staff and other providers in the development of resident service plans
• Maintain an environment that is free from physical, mental, fiduciary, sexual and verbal abuse, and neglect

Community Operations

State regulations generally address various areas affecting ALCs and their residents. These include resident activities, food preparation, transportation, environmental management, fire safety, disaster and emergency planning, life safety, and building codes [2].

Barriers to Care

Studies have shown that the most common resident/family complaints and survey deficiencies cited in AL are related to medication administration (48 %), staffing and staff qualifications (41 %), and sufficiency of services to meet resident needs (36 %) [14].

Problems arise when ALC staffs lack education in basic geriatrics principles. For example, some AL residents have dementia that remains undiagnosed because untrained staff do not identify and report observations that would lead to earlier recognition and treatment. As noted, most physicians see AL residents as outpatients, probably due to time constraints. *One study showed 50 % of physicians visited an AL setting once a year or less*, while only 20 % visited weekly or more [15]. Many attending physicians caring for an AL resident are neither a geriatrician nor specialty trained in geriatrics. Untrained physicians may bring an age bias to their practice or not recognize the special challenges and needs of the aging AL patient; such as being cognizant of the dangers inherent to hospitalization of these residents (e.g., delirium, inappropriate prescribing and nosocomial infections). Physician confidence in AL staff has been shown to be increased with smaller ALC size, nursing presence, and the physician being the medical director [15]. In addition to the higher reimbursement that the custodial care codes entail, there are a myriad of other benefits for *physicians who travel to see residents at the ALC* (Table 4).

Effective communication is a goal in all medical settings, not just AL. Communication problems in the AL occur at multiple levels. ALC Staff may not have a formalized "sign out" between shifts, sufficient assessment skills or know when to contact providers. Healthcare practitioners may not get accurate information from staff (especially after hours). Nor may practitioners be aware of the ALC's capabilities. Many physicians who only practice in the hospital and/or the community are unaware of the differences in the provision of care and services between ALCs and nursing communities. This is problematic either if a resident is sent back (from the ER or hospital) to an ALC that lacks the ability to provide adequate monitoring and/or treatment, or if a resident is kept at the ALC when the AL is no longer able to adequately care for the resident.

Because of the impending tsunami of the elderly population and the ever increasing number of persons who will reside in AL, some warn that the federal and state governments will eventually need to address the concerns regarding the AL industry [16].

Optimal Medical Care

Physician Practice

The physician's role in AL has been largely undefined, due in part to the industry's history of distinguishing between the "medical" vs. "social" models of care [17]. At this time, there is scant data in the literature, but Schumacher advocates for proactive

Table 4 Benefits of physicians seeing AL residents in a community

• Physician learns about AL capabilities
• Sees resident in their own environment
• Improved communication with AL staff
• Increased reimbursement from CMS for domiciliary codes
• No need for community transportation/ escort costs
• No need for family transport time/costs
• More efficient use of physician and staff time
• Increased resident/family/community satisfaction
• Potential for more patients for the physician
• Potential for improved resident care
• Potential for reduced medical errors
• Better marketing/public relations for community

development of relationships between ALCs and residents' medical providers [18]. He notes that "some ALCs appear to mistakenly interpret a "social model" of care as one that discourages the ALC's involvement with any medical providers due to (community) concerns about medicalization, staff time constraints, and cost issues." He recommends clear and timely communication with medical providers regarding medication management, that information be accurate, and residents' health status be documented longitudinally. He also recommends the development of a medical provider education packet describing the relevant services of each ALC.

AMDA — The Society for Post-Acute and Long Term Care Medicine convened a consensus conference to address the needs and issues related to AL residents with multiple chronic conditions. The main areas of concern were medication management, communication with practitioners, AL clinical practice guidelines, clinical direction and the physician's role in the AL. Recommendations were made to develop standard assessment tools and clinical protocols in order to improve the clinical care that residents receive in the AL setting [19].

Several of the issues and concerns mentioned in this chapter, including recommendations for both physicians and communities, were elaborated upon in the AMDA The Society for Post-Acute and Long Term Care Medicine policy statement on "Physicians Role in Assisted Living" (March 2009) with a commitment to expand efforts to promote quality of care in AL (March 2015).

Transitions of Care

Lapses in care commonly occur when patients are either newly admitted to an ALC or readmitted from the hospital. Renewed attention is focused on such scenarios. The National Transitions of Care Coalition Website includes information and tools for both consumers and healthcare professionals. ALCs should facilitate resident transitions to other settings. When a resident is hospitalized, the physician can inform hospital staff about the capabilities of the ALC. Physicians and hospital discharge planners can help assure that residents are being transferred back to an ALC only when it is safe (being knowledgeable as to what care the ALC can provide). Similar to when there is a discharge from hospital to home, extra services provided by home care agencies, in addition to private pay geriatric care or companion services may be necessary to help the resident safely remain in the ALC. On occasion, staff from the ALC may be able to evaluate the resident *prior* to their return from the hospital or skilled nursing community in order to ensure a safe, appropriate, and timely transition of care.

Hospice Services

Statistics show that hospice services are actually utilized more frequently in AL (90 % of communities) than in nursing homes (about 80 %) [1]. This is understandable, as the addition of hospice care may allow an AL resident to stay in the ALC during their final days. The federal government is beginning to scrutinize hospice payments in this setting as these Medicare payments in AL have more than doubled between 2007 and 2012. The U.S. Department of Health and Human Services Office of Inspector General (OIG) released a report in January 2015 titled "Medicare Hospices Have Financial Incentives to Provide Care in Assisted Living Communities" as part of a mandate for reform of the hospice payment system as stipulated in the Patient Protection and Affordable Care Act. The median length of stay on hospice per beneficiary is 98 days in ALCs, as compared to 50 days in nursing homes, 30 days in skilled nursing communities and 45 days in the home. The OIG concluded that hospices are incentivized to target ALCs because they offer the greatest financial gain to the hospice agency. Targeted reviews, adoption of claims-based measures of care, and making hospice data available to beneficiaries are among the recommendations being considered by the Centers for Medicare and Medicaid Services (CMS). The entire report is available at www.oig.hhs.gov.

Quality Assurance/Performance Improvement

The AL industry will probably be following some nursing home trends as resident acuity increases. One of these is the use of the Quality Assurance/Performance Improvement (QAPI) process to analyze data and improve care. AHCA/NCAL has established *The Quality Initiative for AL*, which is concentrating on four core areas with measurable goals: safely reducing hospital readmissions, reducing the off-label use of antipsychotics, increasing staff stability, and increasing customer satisfaction. Measurement summaries and business cases can be downloaded from the NCAL website. ALCs can start to track and measure data related to each goal. Physician leadership can greatly assist with these types of initiatives.

INTERACT-AL

INTERACT (Interventions to Reduce Acute Care Transfers) is a quality improvement program that focuses on the management of acute change in resident condition. It includes clinical and educational tools and strategies for use in every day practice in long-term care communities. INTERACT was originally designed for skilled nursing centers to use for improvement of the early identification, management, documentation and communication of acute changes in condition of residents; thereby *preventing avoidable hospitalizations*. The program has now expanded to include tools specifically for AL providers. After years of INTERACT use in skilled nursing communities, the program began testing its tools in ALCs through the support of a CMS Innovation Grant. Pilot communities assessed and provided feedback on the four categories of INTERACT tools (quality improvement, communication, decision support, and advance care planning) to help finalize the Assisted Living Version 1.0 tools that are now publicly available. The Version 1.0 tools can be accessed via the INTERACT website at http://interact2.net.

The Future of Assisted Living

A roundtable was convened by the CEAL in October 2014 entitled "The Future of Assisted Living: Consumer Preferences and the Era of Healthcare Reform." *Three main factors are driving change in AL*: steadily increasing resident healthcare acuity levels, the provision of healthcare being pushed out of traditional settings into the community, and the increased expectations of baby boomers. The provision of healthcare is being pushed out of traditional settings into the community through the creation of Accountable Care Organizations and other models of care. Baby boomers, because of a higher level of education, more work experience and increased technology savvy, have higher healthcare expectations. These societal changes are having a cascading effect upon numerous operational aspects of AL by influencing state regulatory limitations, accelerating the need for coordinated healthcare systems with processes for seamless information transfer, as well as advocating for shared healthcare outcomes with penalties for poor outcomes (e.g., high rate of hospital readmissions). The CEAL identified 14 major themes (Table 5), with Personnel, Data, State Regulations, and Affordability identified as key areas of focus. As of 2015 both a white paper and a report to determine the most feasible ways that CEAL can help providers facilitate AL transitions are in process.

Technology

While most ALCs lag behind hospitals and nursing communities in the use of technology, advances are expected in the future. Operational technology such as the electronic health record could impact care in AL and assist seamless transitions. High-tech sensor devices and other innovations are already being used in a few ALCs to better monitor residents. Smart home technology is being increasingly utilized, such as

Table 5 Emerging themes in AL (*Key)

• Aging in place
• Diverse models
• Future market
• Assisted living without walls
• Value proposition
• State regulations*
• Data*
• Technology in AL
• Personnel*
• Keeping the "home" in AL
• Risks and choice
• Affordability*
• Consumer education
• Flexibility

the TabSafe In-Home Medication Dispensing System that enables older adults to remain independent as it assists them with medication management, and allows providers to make medication adjustments and monitor as-needed medications. Smart shirts, smart toilets and bladder scanners are already available for monitoring residents in some ALCs. Extensive savings can occur when Robot "companions" enable AL corporations to virtually visit communities or telemedicine enables clinicians to promptly assess residents in remote areas. Future residents will be increasingly familiar with the use of the Internet and communication technology that will enable them to speak with and see distant family members. Computerized game systems are already being used to supplement resident activities and assist with therapy.

Suggestions on Improving Care

The following lists suggestions for healthcare providers aimed at *optimizing one's practice in AL*. Some of the suggestions will be easier to address if a medical director position has been established.

- *Adapt already established and evidence-based policies and procedures to AL.*
  Many health care practitioners familiar with the workings of nursing communities also take care of AL residents. **Residents** of nursing communities are required to be seen at a minimum of every 60 days—with the increasing acuity and frailty of ALC residents approaching that in nursing communities, it behooves physicians to establish a routine of seeing AL residents at least quarterly or more often if medically necessary. Pertinent guideline areas can be adopted for use in ALCs, such as fall prevention, notification protocols, and reduction of antipsychotic medication. Use of a consultant pharmacist for monthly or quarterly medication reviews is encouraged. Suggestions for efficient time management in LTC are still applicable to physician care in AL as well (Table 6) [20].
- *Meet regularly with the community administrator.*
  Getting buy-in from the administrator is an important strategy that helps improve resident care. The physician may bring up topics for discussion, or ask the administrator how physician involvement can help with state survey compliance and marketing of the community's image in the community. Improvement in physician communication and documentation is generally an area of mutual concern. Scheduled meetings can vary, from monthly to less often. Minutes from previous meetings should be kept, and it is recommended that the focus on an identified area of concern be continued until the problem is resolved, prior to addressing another area. If the administrator is unable to make meetings, physicians should at least keep in regular contact with head of the nursing staff. A physician could also have an opportunity to participate as a member of an "advisory committee" for a rehabilitation, hospice and/or home care agency that is delivering services to a large percentage of the ALC's residents.
- *Provide in-services to staff/residents.*

Table 6 Time management guidelines

• Limit practice to only 1–2 ALCs you know well
• Use a midlevel practitioner for management of routine problems
• Have a regular day for seeing residents at a particular community
• See the sickest patients first
• Develop protocols for common problems such as constipation, weight loss, falls, behavioral problems, and fever
• Train staff to limit after-hour telephone calls to urgent problems and provide mechanisms for staff to address non-urgent problems (such as daily telephone calls, regularly checked message lines or e-mails, or regular rounds by the healthcare practitioner)
• Speak with residents and families about advance directives shortly after admission and with major status changes. Document these discussions clearly
• Anticipate future events and discuss expectations with the family in advance to aid in decision-making and the adjustment process
• Learn as much as possible about family dynamics to eliminate any surprises when health care decisions need to be made. Communicate your expectations through discussions with staff, standing orders and in-service programs
• Educate yourself about assisted living regulations, especially those affecting provision of medical and nursing services
• Work as a partner with the staff and care providers

It is widely accepted that a well-educated staff is a critical component of providing good care. Accordingly, the physician or the physician's NP/PA can present educational sessions for front-line staff on such topics as geriatric principles, medication administration and adverse drug effects, best practices in communication, the *Choosing Wisely* campaign(s), and common illnesses in the elderly (dementia, hypertension, diabetes, stroke, mental health disorders, etc.). There is a series of AL-specific articles in nursing journals that may be beneficial for staff. Residents and families are often eager to learn more about common geriatric conditions, advance directives and medication issues. Some ALCs have "family nights" where physician-led "Q and A" or "Ask the Doc" sessions can be invaluable. Many communities have resident and/or family councils. Physician attendance at these can be of great value, whether to improve education and communication, or to help to identify other issues within the community.

• *Ensure effective communication.*
Physicians can help communities establish a process for timely attending physician notification when there is a change in patient status, medication error, or any treatment ordered by a consultant. The community should timely convey accurate and standard information whenever a resident leaves the community for any medical reason such as to see a different physician (Table 7), and even more importantly, any critical resident information during urgent or emergency transfers. Vitally important is to include the current medication regimen and copies of any advance directives. As such, physicians can help ALCs develop a packet of information that could be available in an emergency and also include copies of items such as insurance information, family contact numbers, activity, diet, and treatment orders as well as past medical history, pertinent consultant reports, and lab work.

Table 7 Standard information recommended for AL transfer/ communication forms

Patient name	Community phone number
Patient date of birth	Medication list
Attending physician	Reason for transfer/consultation
Community name	Relevant H&P/progress notes/labs/X-rays

Developing relationships and communicating with local emergency department providers and emergency medical services can be helpful. Inappropriate use of these resources can lead to unnecessary transfers, hospitalizations, patient/family stress, and excess costs [21]. Many of these problems can be either alleviated or resolved with use of the INTERACT-AL tools. Transferred residents should have clear identification that they reside in an ALC.

As mentioned, an ALC may not have a resident medical chart. If so, a physician can bring an office chart with them to the ALC. Use of a communication book in the ALC can be a useful practice to leave messages for practitioners from the AL nurse/staff. If there is a chart, a physician should request a separate section for physicians' progress notes. Copying or faxing the ALC note to the medical office can keep office records updated. Providers must also assume responsibility for returning calls promptly and professionally. One of the major problems identified by the AL industry is the poor response time from primary care providers. Primary care providers should establish a protocol where the ALC knows *how to contact their office for non-urgent and emergent calls.* Having a system to contact the ALC can be useful, as well as identification of a point person to contact, and calling regularly at specific time of day. Returning a call during the same shift can help decrease miscommunication between shifts.

Communicating with families can prevent many problems and increase resident, family and staff satisfaction. Calls received from the family should be returned as promptly as possible and with respect. Family should be contacted when there is a change in status and when a resident is transferred out of the ALC. Discussing family expectations upon resident admission can help identify unrealistic expectations. Medication issues and medication costs are a frequent concern and should be discussed with the family at appropriate intervals.

- *Focus on high-risk medications and medical problems.*

Certain common geriatric disease states lend themselves well to risk reduction strategies. As in nursing communities, special attention should be given to the prevention of falls and decubitus ulcers, diabetic management (especially hypoglycemia), and resident elopement. Some medication errors have more potential for significant harm than others, such as anti-coagulants (e.g., warfarin) diabetic drugs (both oral and injectable), opioids and antipsychotic medications. Many of the materials related to the *CMS National Partnership to Improve Dementia Care* and the reduction of antipsychotic use are applicable to AL (and is referred to in the title of the January 2015 GAO report "Antipsychotic Drug Use: HHS Initiatives to Reduce Use in Older Adults in Nursing Homes, but Should Expand

Efforts to Other Settings"). The AMDA-The Society for Post-Acute and Long Term Care *Medicine Quality Prescribing Campaign*, (based on an IOM report to prevent medication errors and promote safe prescribing) will also help improve care for AL residents.

- *Initiate discussions on advanced directives for healthcare*
  While a recent report notes that advance care planning is 5–10 % higher in residential care/AL than in nursing communities [22], many ALC residents either have no advance healthcare directive or have one that will not be applicable in an emergency situation. A physician encouraging their use, as well as resident and staff education, can be instrumental in clarifying residents' preferences for care. For example, use of the POLST (Physician Orders for Life Sustaining Treatment). This is another area where use of the INTERACT-AL tools can be of assistance.

- *Encourage preventive medicine and person-centered care.*
  The importance of health promotion, disease prevention and wellness services for AL residents has been well recognized. ALCs represent exceptional opportunities for treatment and management of chronic conditions, with the potential for enormous benefit to residents [21]. Examples include screening for Alzheimer's disease, hypercholesterolemia, and osteoporosis, as well as using immunization protocols and promoting exercise programs.
  Person-centered care has been recognized as an important component of quality of life for AL residents, yet no measures had existed until recently to describe, quantify, and ultimately improve it [23]. The Person-Centered Practices in AL (PC-PAL) questionnaires were developed to improve person-centeredness by measuring care from the perspectives of residents and staff, and is supported by multiple national organizations [23]. Medical leadership can help bring this to the attention of ALC administration and encourage its use.

- *Urge hiring of a medical director.*
  The ALC administration or corporation may be unaware of the advantages of a contracting with a medical director and/or are concerned about the financial burden of paying the physician. Appropriate medical direction can improve patient care, communication and marketing, as well as potentially lower liability risk.
  As a significant number of ALCs neither have written policies and procedures for quality improvement regarding medication management, nor policies regarding drug regimen review and monitoring for adverse drug events [24], improving medication management for example would be an ideal opportunity for medical director leadership. AMDA The Society for Post-Acute and Long Term Care Medicine's *Position Statement on Assisted Living* lists some potential roles and responsibilities of an AL medical director (the ALC is referred to as an ALR– Table 8). The challenge to the physician is convincing the ALC of the significant benefits this may provide. There is evidence that having a full-time physician at the ALC by itself can improve care. One study showed statistically significant decreases in hospitalizations and hospital days, and a suggestion of a decrease in falls [25]. ALCs might consider the concept of having a medical director on retainer, not as a dedicated position, but as an administrative position who is available as needed. Many ALCs often have a physician who sees a majority of their

Table 8 Potential roles and responsibilities of AL medical director

Practitioner services
• Assist the ALR in ensuring that residents have appropriate physician coverage and ensure the provision of physician and healthcare practitioner services
• Assist the ALR in developing a process for reviewing physician and healthcare practitioners' credentials
• Provide specific guidance for physician and healthcare practitioner performance expectations
• Assist the ALR in ensuring that a system is in place for monitoring the performance of healthcare practitioners
• Facilitate feedback to physicians and other healthcare practitioners on performance and practices
• Assist ALR with resident assessment and development of the clinical component of the service plan, when necessary
Clinical care
• Participate in administrative decision making and the development of policies and procedures related to resident care and medication management
• Participate in administrative decision making on staffing levels, coverage, licensing, and training requirements for resident-care staff
• Assist in developing, approving, and implementing specific clinical practices for the ALR to incorporate into its care-related policies and procedures, including areas required by laws and regulations
• Review, respond, to and participate in federal, state, local, and other external inspections
• Assist in reviewing policies and procedures regarding the adequate protection of residents' rights, advance care planning, and other ethical issues
Quality of care
• Assist the ALR in establishing systems and methods for reviewing the quality and appropriateness of clinical care, medication management, and other health-related services and provide appropriate feedback
• Participate in the ALR's quality improvement process
• Advise on infection control issues and approve specific infection control policies to be incorporated into ALR policies and procedures
• Assist the community in providing a safe and caring environment with optimal levels of family and community involvement
• Assist in the promotion of employee health and safety
• Assist in the development and implementation of employee health policies and programs
Education, information, and communication
• Promote a learning culture within the community by educating, informing, and communicating
• Assist the ALR in developing medical information and communication systems with staff, residents, families, and others
• Assist in establishing appropriate relationships with other healthcare professionals

residents, becoming a sort of "de facto" medical director. This position will not have any coverage for administrative liability. However, the physicians may find themselves empowered to suggest or enact changes beneficial for resident care.

• *Guide families and colleagues to available resources.*
  Physicians often play a role when patients are no longer able to be cared for at home. Several organizations offer information about the ALCs in the community

Table 9 Factors influencing AL growth and structure

• Shifting population demographics
• Evolving patient mix and acuity levels
• Health status and life-span of target populations
• Cost structure (e.g., liability insurance and higher costs to serve patients with more demanding service needs)
• Regulatory landscape
• Medical and technological advances
• Adequacy of public financing
• Availability of small ALCs

and guides to choosing an ALC (National Center for Assisted Living, AARP, Assisted Living Federation of America, etc.). Hospital social workers may not be aware of some of these resources or of the existence of the CEAL or AL-specific consumer groups. Some areas of the country have literature available to families that list housing options including AL (such as the SourceBook: Guide to Retirement Living for several eastern states).

• *Champion state "mini-ALWs".*

One of the recommendations from the national ALW was to have state-level public meetings to review their recommendations. Virginia has already convened such a meeting. This can be challenging, as many different factors influence the growth and structure of the AL industry (Table 9) [26]. Wisconsin has developed an innovative collaborative called the Wisconsin Coalition for Collaborative Excellence in Assisted Living (WCCEAL) which includes regulatory and public funding agencies, the state ombudsman's program, as well as the state AL and residential care provider associations. The Collaborative has developed performance measures and satisfaction surveys that can be voluntarily used by Wisconsin AL providers as QAPI tools. A physician interested and involved in AL may be able to spearhead a "mini-ALW" or similar collaborative in their state.

Summary

Physicians as well as nurse practitioners and physician assistants play an essential role in the treatment of patients in ALCs. The trend of increasing resident medical acuity and recognition of the importance of healthcare providers in AL makes this an exciting time to practice in this setting. Understanding the capabilities of the ALC where residents live is essential. The potential for clinician collaboration in ALCs in establishing seamless community-based care, promotion of preventive care and wellness, early identification of patient sentinel events, and contribution to quality-of-life outcomes shows great promise [27]. Ideally, the physician can be a "middle man," advocating for resident care and helping to establish a safety net for patient care [19] while understanding ALC concerns and trying to maintain affordability for residents.

Pearls for the Practitioner

- Assisted living communities (ALCs) are regulated by the states and currently there are no mandatory federal regulations. This leads to significant state-to-state variability in rules, requirements, and terminology.
- ALCs themselves vary significantly in size, patient characteristics, philosophy, staff, and patient care capabilities.
- Staff number, availability, training, and capabilities also vary greatly by state and location, leading to potential problems with communication, medication management, and overall patient care.
- Seeing patients in the ALC has many benefits for all concerned.
- Many of the barriers to care in AL can be addressed and overcome by increased physician attention and involvement.

Acknowledgements The author is grateful to the editors of this book, as well as to Dave Kyllo, Lindsay Schwartz, Dave Smith, and Sheryl Zimmerman for their assistance.

References

1. National study of long-term care providers. 2013.
2. The Assisted Living Workgroup. Assuring quality in assisted living: guidelines for federal and state policy, state regulation and operations. A report to the US Senate Special Committee on Aging. April 2003.
3. Hawes C, Phillips CD, Rose M, et al. A national survey of assisted living communities. Gerontologist. 2003;436(6):875–82.
4. Zimmerman S et al. Dementia prevalence and care in assisted living. Health Aff. 2014;33(4): 658–66.
5. Alzheimer's Association Campaign for Quality Residential Care. Dementia care practice: recommendations for assisted living residences and nursing homes
6. Overview of assisted living. A collaborative research project of AAHSA, ASHA, ALFA, NCAL & NIC. 2009
7. McNabney M et al. The spectrum of medical illness and medication use among residents of assisted living communities in central Maryland. J Am Med Dir Assoc. 2008;9(8):558–64.
8. Caffrey C. Residents living in residential care communities: United States, 2010. NCHS data brief no 91. Hyattsville, MD: National Center for Health Statistics; 2012.
9. Carder P. Beyond the radar screen: access to and use of OTC and as-needed medication by AL residents. AMDA annual symposium presentation. 2009.
10. Genworth. Cost of care survey. 2014.
11. AGS 2012 Beers Criteria Update Expert Panel. AGS updated beers criteria for potentially inappropriate medication use in older adults. J Am Geriatr Soc. 2012;60:616–31.
12. Sloane PD et al. Medication undertreatment in assisted living settings. Arch Intern Med. 2004;164:2031–7.
13. Stefanacci R, Podrazik P. Assisted living communities: optimizing outcomes. J Am Geriatr Soc. 2005;53:538–40.
14. U.S. Department of Health and Human Services. State residential care and assisted living policy: 2004. April 2005.
15. Sloane P et al. Physician perspectives on medical care delivery in assisted living. J Am Geriatr Soc. 2011;59:2326–31.

16. Levenson S. Assisted living: shall we learn from history or repeat it? J Am Med Dir Assoc. 2008;07(003):539–41.
17. Utz R. Assisted living: the philosophical challenges of everyday practice. J Appl Gerontol. 2003;22:379–404.
18. Schumacher J. Assisted living communities and medical care providers: establishing proactive relationships. Seniors Hous Care J. 2005;13(1):35–48.
19. Vance J. Proceedings of the AMDA assisted living consensus conference, Washington, DC October 24, 2006. J Am Med Dir Assoc. 2008;9(6):378–82.
20. Anderson EG. Nursing home practice: 10 tips to simplify patient care. Geriatrics. 1993; 48:61–3.
21. Schumacher J. Examining the physician's role with assisted living residents. J Am Med Dir Assoc. 2006;7(6):377–82.
22. Daaleman T et al. Advance care planning in nursing homes and assisted living communities. J Am Med Dir Assoc. 2009;10(4):243–51.
23. Zimmerman S et al. A measure of person-centered practices in assisted living: The PC-PAL. J Am Med Dir Assoc. 2015;16:132–7.
24. Mitty E. Medication management in assisted living: a national survey of policies and practices. J Am Med Dir Assoc. 2009;10(2):107–14.
25. Pruchnicki A. Full time primary care in an assisted living community. AMDA poster submission, annual symposium. 2005.
26. Novartis. The senior care source facts figures and forecasts. 2008;5:34–44.
27. Schumacher J. Physicians and their assisted living residents: adventures in falls (mis) communication. AMDA annual symposium presentation, March 2009.

Resources

28. American Medical Directors Association (AMDA). The Society for Post-Acute and Long Term Care Medicine Policy statement physicians role in assisted living March 2009 and promoting the quality of care provided in assisted living communities. March 2015.
29. American Geriatrics Society (AGS). Assisted living communities position statement. May 2004.
30. ASCP pharmacy policy and procedure manual for assisted living. 2008.
31. Namazi K, Chafetz Paul editors. Assisted living: current issues in community management and resident care. 2001.
32. NCAL assisted living state regulatory review (yearly).
33. Zimmerman Sheryl. Assisted living, needs, practices and policies in residential care for the elderly. 2001.
34. AARP. www.aarp.org.
35. Assisted Living Federation of America (ALFA). www.alfa.org.
36. Alzheimer's Association. www.alz.org.
37. American Medical Directors Association (AMDA). www.amda.com.
38. Center for Excellence in Assisted Living (CEAL). www.theceal.org.
39. National Center for Assisted Living (NCAL). www.ncal.org.
40. National Transitions of Care Coalition. www.ntocc.org.
41. POLST. website www.polst.org.
42. National study of long-term care providers (biennial report). 2013. http://www.cdc.gov/nchs/nsltcp.htm.
43. Daniel Haimowitz, Richard Stefanacci. Geriatric nursing series on assisted living. 2012. www.gnjournal.com/.

PACE

Laura Trice

Introduction

Effective and value-based healthcare for older people is becoming increasingly important as the number of older adults who require high-quality long-term care for chronic illness continues to increase. How can healthcare providers best serve the needs of those who are both frail and elderly? Models of care must incorporate cost containment without compromising participants' quality of care or quality of life. Though frail elders say they want to remain at home in their community, frequently, complex medical conditions and lack of financial and community resources may make nursing home placement the only option [1].

PACE is a unique health care delivery system that strives to successfully integrate a full spectrum of services for frail persons 55 years of age and older. PACE organizations deliver a combination of primary, specialist, acute, long-term and home-based care as well as palliative care to its enrollees. Use of interdisciplinary team care, managed care services, and care coordination result in improved health outcomes and reduced expense over time.

The average PACE enrollee is 80 years old, has an average of eight acute and chronic medical conditions and three limitations in activities of daily living (ADLs). Over 90 % of PACE participants continue to live in the community [2]. Comparing this to the data for older adults living in assisted living facilities, who require assistance with two or more ADLs and average three chronic medical conditions, the PACE member population is more frail.

L. Trice, MD (✉)
Physician Hospital Organization, TriHealth,
4750 Wesley Avenue, Cincinnati, OH 45206, USA
e-mail: laura_trice@trihealth.com

© Springer International Publishing Switzerland 2016   37
P.A. Fenstemacher, P. Winn (eds.), *Post-Acute and Long-Term Medicine*,
Current Clinical Practice, DOI 10.1007/978-3-319-16979-8_3

PACE History

PACE originated in 1971 in San Francisco's Chinatown, with a $2,000 federal grant to the Chinatown-North Beach Health Care Planning and Development Corporation (later renamed On Lok Senior Health Services). Marie-Louise Ansak, a Swiss social worker, developed a long-term care model for an elderly Chinese population that considered nursing home placement culturally unacceptable. Ansak developed the concept for the original PACE site out of the British Day Hospital's model which offered therapeutic and minor medical services, with patients returning home at the end of the day. The American version, "On Lok" (Cantonese for peaceful abode) expanded these provisions, thereby creating a global approach to managing patient cases, which included offering housing, a full range of medical and social services, and therapies.

On Lok continued to succeed and grow in the 1970s, and by the 1980s On Loc had received waivers from Medicare and Medicaid to pilot a new financing system that allowed the PACE programs to provide full medical services for a fixed monthly payment for each enrollee in the program [3]. In 1986, federal legislation allowed for other PACE sites and in 1997, PACE received permanent Medicare and Medicaid provider status under the Balanced Budget Act. Alexian Brothers Community Services in St. Louis became the first PACE site to become a permanently recognized part of the Medicare and Medicaid programs. When the Federal Interim Regulation for PACE was published in 1999 there were 30 programs in 19 states. PACE organizations became subject to both Federal and State regulation and surveys in a manner similar to those of long-term care facilities.

PACE expansion to rural markets was initiated by a 2005 Deficit Reduction Act with $7.5 million in funding. There are currently over 100 PACE programs in 31 states with more than 31,500 enrollees.

The National PACE Association (NPA) was founded in 1994 to support PACE programs. NPA provides education resources, communication forums, and collects *benchmarking data* to compare participant characteristics and service delivery across sites. NPA works closely with members of Congress, senior administration officials, and state policy makers to educate and to promote a reimbursement and regulatory environment that enables PACE programs to provide high-quality, individualized, and innovative care. The NPA Primary Care Committee develops resources to assist PACE clinicians, serves as a clinical resource to the NPA Board of Directors and promotes PACE to the wider medical community.

Financing

PACE offers an innovative financing model that integrates capitated Medicare and Medicaid dollars per enrollee. Once enrolled, PACE becomes the participant's sole source of Medicare- and Medicaid-covered services, including coverage of medications. Most PACE participants are dually eligible, i.e., have both Medicare and

Medicaid, but do have the option to pay privately if they do not. Medicare rates are calculated for each participant using a risk-adjusted payment methodology similar to Medicare Advantage plans. Medicaid rates are negotiated between each PACE organization and the state agency administering the Medicaid program. PACE organizations assume all financial risk for delivering all healthcare services that would normally be covered under Medicare Parts A, B, D and Medicaid. PACE programs are considered Medicare Advantage Programs, and are funded under Medicare Part C. PACE is in a unique position as both payor and provider of services that allows for payment flexibility, creativity, and innovation.

Outcomes

Although there are limited outcome studies on PACE, the results are generally positive: PACE has been shown to improve functional status and quality of life, and decrease mortality [4–6]. Findings also suggest that the very old (80–90 years), those living alone, using ambulation aids, cognitively impaired, and requiring assistance to perform instrumental activities of daily living (IADLs) benefit the most from a non-institutional long-term care approach such as PACE [7].

Rates of hospitalization, readmission and potentially avoidable hospitalization (PAH) are lower for PACE enrollees than for comparable Medicaid nursing home residents [6, 8–11]. The variation in study results across PACE sites reflects their heterogeneity in case mix, longevity and experience of the interdisciplinary team (IDT). The programs availability of transitional housing, contracts and agreements with local hospitals and skilled nursing facilities, as well as the local medical culture also caused the programs results to vary [6, 11].

A Day at the PACE Day Health Center (DHC)

The IDT

- Primary care physician
- Registered nurse
- Master's-level social worker
- Physical therapist
- Occupational therapist
- Recreational therapist or activities coordinator
- Dietician
- PACE site manager
- Home care coordinator
- Personal care attendant or his or her representative
- Driver or his or her representative

Case Scenario

Like other PACE enrollees, Anna enjoys attending the DHC an average of three times a week. Her home health aide (HHA) arrives at Anna's home early to prepare Anna for the day. Anna's daughter welcomes the aide into their small apartment. Anna depends on PACE HHAs for her daily personal care since a stroke left her wheelchair bound. Bathed and dressed, Anna waits in the living room for the PACE driver to pick her up for the trip to the DHC. Meanwhile in the kitchen, her daughter shares a list of concerns with the aide, which include financial and medical, as well as equipment and supply issues for her mother. The aide assures her daughter that everything will be addressed at the IDT meeting later in the morning. Her driver arrives to transport Anna to the DHC. A PACE driver for many years, he is very familiar with all the people on his route and Anna greets him like an old friend.

When Anna enters the DHC, staff greets her, while giving her a nametag. Her arrival time is entered into the electronic medical record, alerting clinical staff that plans to see her during the day. The DHC serves as the main medical center as well as the social services base for PACE participants. There is a full schedule of recreational activities that Anna may attend but she first heads for the therapy department. She had completed skilled therapy after a stroke 2 years ago, but like many PACE participants, benefits from an ongoing restorative therapy program.

Meanwhile, Anna's IDT is meeting in a conference room nearby. The IDT is responsible for the initial assessment, periodic reassessment, plan of care, and coordination of 24-h care delivery as written in the Code of Federal Regulation (42 CFR:460.104). Medical care is coordinated by the PACE IDT assigned to each participant. The IDT's members include physicians, nurse practitioners, behavioral health specialists, nurses, social workers, therapists, van drivers, aides, and other staff. This group meets regularly as the status of a PACE participant evolves.

The HHA has reported Anna's daughter's concerns to the home care coordinator, to be discussed at the IDT meeting. Problems with increased knee pain, questions about a new medication, issues with a defective wheelchair, and difficulties paying the rent are all discussed. Agreeing to a plan, IDT members will address these issues and concerns in the next few days.

Anna then arrives at the PACE clinic for an acute visit with her PACE primary care physician (PCP) who routinely sees Mary every 3 months alternating between reassessment and wellness visits. Because the clinic is physically part of the DHC, acute visits are flexible and frequent. Front-line staff, HHAs, and drivers are often the "eyes and ears" of a PACE program, often identifying changes in condition well ahead of clinic staff. The PCP was informed about Anna's new onset of left knee pain during the IDT meeting, that her daughter has noticed a decrease in her mobility and that the therapy staff also noticed decreased range of motion during the morning restorative exercises. After ordering conservative treatment measures, the physician reassures Anna she'll see her again on a subsequent DHC visit.

Working at a PACE is a "dream job" for the PCP. With a small patient panel, typically 100 or less, there is the opportunity to manage complex social and medical conditions of each enrollee and to see positive outcomes.

Anna's nurse, telephones to update her daughter, reassures her that her mother's vital signs and weight are stable, answers questions about any new medication and explains the plan of care for her mother's knee condition. Her occupational therapist has ordered a new part to fix her wheelchair and the social worker will schedule a meeting with her landlord.

During the next month at the DHC, Anna has the opportunity to see several PACE in-house specialist's from podiatry, optometry, dentistry, and behavioral health. PACE also schedules and provides transportation for any other specialist appointments approved by the IDT. Several times a year PACE admits Anna to a contracted nursing home for respite allowing her daughter to visit family in another state. Should Anna ever need a hospital or skilled nursing facility (SNF) stay, PACE clinical staff will continue to follow her at the SNF with the IDT authorizing and overseeing all care.

In the late afternoon, Anna leaves the DHC for her trip home. The driver will deliver all her medications, frozen meals, and incontinence products when he drops her off. Sarah knows there is a PACE nurse and physician on call 24/7 should any issues arise at home during the night or on the weekends.

Tired but happy, Anna is already looking forward to her next DHC visit!

PACE Model Practice

Beginning in 2006, the NPA Primary Care Committee began developing *Model Practices* as guides for key chronic conditions often seen in PACE participants. These model practices direct care along one of *three pathways* according to the directives and priorities of each participant: *achieving longevity*, *maintaining function*, or *receiving palliative care* [12]. Current Model Practices include the following:

- Diabetes mellitus (2009)
- Dementia (2013)
- Chronic heart failure (2011)
- Chronic kidney disease (2011)
- Chronic obstructive pulmonary disease (2012)
- Preventive care guideline (2010)

NPA encourages the use of these model practices. NPA members may obtain the documents at Members Only/Primary Care Resources/Model Practices. Non-member clinicians or organizations may not use, reproduce, or modify the model practices without the expressed written consent of the National PACE Association. To obtain permission, inquire at e-mail info@npaonline.org.

Role of the Medical Director in PACE

My inspiration and continued passion for geriatric healthcare are a direct result of a most challenging but rewarding position I held as a PACE Medical Director.
   42CFR:460.60 *The organization must employ a medical director who is responsible for the delivery of participant care, for clinical outcomes, and for the implementation, as well as oversight, of the quality assessment and performance program.*

A PACE Medical Director operates as both a director of diverse clinical services and an administrator of a health plan. The need to move from a provider to a payor role during the work day can be very challenging that includes reviewing and enrollees' charts and financial reports. Medical Directors who come to PACE with a long-term care background usually have a good understanding of federal and state regulatory compliance while those with a primary care practice background often better understand staffing and balance sheet issues.

Medical Directors must assure that participants receive quality geriatric care in every setting including the PACE clinic, hospital, SNF and home. Since PACE providers often provide all these direct services, the Medical Director has the opportunity to closely supervise all the clinical care the participants receive while monitoring the quality of contracted provider services. While clinical responsibilities are key, the Medical Director must also work closely with the Site manager and other administrative staff to manage the financial risk of the program and plan for expansion of the program.

Although PACE sites endeavor to recruit geriatricians for both the Medical Director and Primary Care Physician (PCP) roles, there is not always a supply to meet the need. Finding practitioners that have a passion for elderly care is always the priority. The typical PACE program is small, with an average of 300 participants; so many Medical Directors also function as the PCP in addition to their administrative duties. Recruiting, training and retaining PCPs are key responsibilities. Currently PACE regulation requires the PCP be a PACE employee which means the PACE participant must change from their current community PCP at the time of enrollment. The PACE PCP must be able to care for medically complex elderly using sound geriatric medicine principles. Working collaboratively as an IDT member is often a new experience for a PACE PCP and usually requires six months to become proficient in the role. Many PACE sites also successfully use non-physician providers such as nurse practitioners and physician assistants though existing PACE regulation stipulates that a physician must be a member of the IDT.

The Medical Director must also recruit and contract with a provider networks that include specialists, hospitals, SNFs, pharmacy and all ancillary services such as home care and durable medical equipment suppliers. While the program director will oversee and maintain contracts with each network member, the Medical Director must ensure that the network is educated about PACE and provides quality care.

Oversight of the Quality Assessment and Performance Improvement (QAPI) plan includes making sure that utilization of services, caregiver and participant satisfaction, and safety and clinical outcome measures are addressed. Similar to the functions of a nursing home quality committee, wound care, infections, and falls are routinely reviewed. Additional QAPI responsibilities include oversight of staff competency and tracking participant grievances.

There is great opportunity for the Medical Director to educate, mentor and participate in research. PACE sites often become centers of geriatric excellence for sponsoring health care organization, with fellows, residents, medical students, and nursing students routinely rotating with PACE clinical staff.

The Primary Care Committee of the National PACE Association (NPA) provides excellent training resources for all Medical Directors regardless of experience level or background. Education sessions are offered during the summer and fall NPA conferences and online resources are available for NPA member Medical Directors on the NPA website.

PACE in the Nursing Home

Although the goal of PACE is to care for nursing home eligible people in the community, about 10 % of PACE participants require skilled or custodial nursing care. Like all other contracted services, PACE sites must ensure that contracted nursing facilities are educated about PACE and provide quality care. Ideally, PACE sites contract with an adequate number of nursing homes to be able to offer enough geographic choice to meet participant and family preferences. PACE and nursing facility administrative and clinical teams need to collaborate to ensure that documentation and care plans are integrated. It is helpful to attend the Quality Assurance meetings at all contracted nursing facilities, as well as communicating frequently with the facility administrator, medical director, and director of nursing. CMS requires a comprehensive medical record at the PACE site even if the participant resides in a nursing facility.

The Future of PACE

Operational challenges have limited growth for PACE despite its attractive features [13]. Significant human and financial resources are required to run what is essentially a small health plan. Substantial "back-office" overhead costs to process Part A and B claims as well as Part D data requirements and federal and state reporting requirements mean less dollars for patient care [14]. Hiring qualified staff especially primary care physicians and geriatricians can be challenging.

Expanding PACE organizations is often limited by federal regulation that has not kept up with modern innovations [15]. NPA is working with Congress to support more operational flexibility, growth, and innovation. Issues to explore and address include expansion of service areas, engagement of community physicians, and utilization of alternative care settings.

Pearls for the Practitioner

- Nursing home-eligible participants that are aged 55 or older can continue living in their homes with comprehensive services through PACE.
- PACE is a unique model that delivers a full continuum of care.
- With capitated Medicare and Medicaid payments, PACE serves as a model for value-based care and payment innovation.

Websites

- National PACE Association www.npaonline.org
- Medicare.gov http://www.medicare.gov/your-medicare-costs/help-paying-costs/pace/pace.html
- Medicaid.gov   http://www.medicaid.gov/Medicaid-CHIP-Program-Information/By-Topics/Long-Term-Services-and-Supports/Integrating-Care/Program-of-All-Inclusive-Care-for-the-Elderly-PACE/Program-of-All-Inclusive-Care-for-the-Elderly-PACE.html

References

1. Trice L. PACE: a model for providing comprehensive healthcare for frail elders. Generations. Fall 2006;90–92.
2. National PACE Association. www.npaonline.org.
3. Eng C, Pedulla J, Eleazer GP, McCann R, Fox N. Program of All-inclusive care for the elderly (PACE): an innovative model of integrated geriatric care and financing. J Am Geriatr Soc. 1997;45:223–32.
4. White AJ, Abel Y, Kidder D. Evaluation of the program of all-inclusive care for the elderly (PACE) demonstration. A comparison of the PACE capitation rates to projected costs in the first year of enrollment. Baltimore, MA: Abt Associates Inc.; 2000.
5. Mancuso D, Yamashiro G, Filver B. PACE an evaluation. Olympia, WA: Department of Social and health Services, Research and Data Analysis Division; 2005.
6. Weiland D, Boland R, Baskins J, Kinosian B. Five year survival in PACE compared with alternative institutional and home and community based care. J Gerontol A Biol Sci Med Sci. 2010;65(7):721–6.
7. Branch LG, Coulam RF, Zimmerman YA. The PACE evaluation: Initial findings. Gerontologist. 1995;35:349–59.
8. Chatterji P, Burstein NR, Kidder D, White AJ. Evaluations of the Program of All-Inclusive Care for the Elderly (PACE)-demonstration the impact of PACE on participant outcomes. Boston: Abt. Associates; 2003.
9. Meret-Hanke LA. Effects of the Program of All-Inclusive Care of the Elderly on hospital use. Gerontologist. 2011;51:774–85.
10. Beauchamp J, Cheh V, Schmitz R, Kemper R, Hall J. The effects of the program of all-inclusive care for the elderly (PACE) on quality. Princeton NJ: Mathematica Policy Research Inc.; 2008.

11. Segelman M, Szydlowski J, Kinosian B, Mcnabney M, et al. Hospitalization in the program of all-inclusive care for the elderly. J Am Geriatr Soc. 2014;62:320–4.
12. Schamp RO. A day in the life of a PACE medical director. Caring for the Ages. 2011;June 20.
13. Boult C, Wieland DG. Comprehensive primary care for older patients with multiple chronic conditions "nobody rushes you through". J Am Med Assoc. 2010;304:1936–43.
14. Hirth V, Baskins J, Dever-Bumba M. Program of All-Inclusive Care (PACE): past, present, and future. J Am Med Dir Assoc. 2009;10:155–60.
15. Bloom S. PACE has shown path to improved elder care. Modern Healthcare. 2014;Mar 26.

Department of Veteran Affairs Options for LTC

Deborah Way

Introduction

The Department of Veterans Affairs (VA) has developed many options for long-term care that include traditional institutional care as well as innovative programs for community-based long-term and post-acute care. Not unlike The Center for Medicare and Medicaid Services, the VA is also focused on the provision of cost-effective care through community based services aimed at reducing hospitalizations and preventing long-term institutionalization. Services that the VA offers to community dwelling veterans include: *Hospital in Home*, *Home Based Primary Care*, *Telehealth,* and *Aide and Attendance*. End-of-life care is also available to veterans with eligibility based on clinical need. Veterans can receive nursing facility (NF) care, either at a community NF or at a community living center (CLC) if they meet service-connected status, level of disability, and income requirements.

Community-Based Care

Hospital in Home

The VA was one of the original participants in the Hospital at Home demonstration, pioneering the innovation of discharging patients from inpatient units and completing their treatment at home [1]. This model was called Program at Home. Hospital in Home is the VA's version of Hospital at Home and is currently operational at five

D. Way (✉)
Department of Palliative Care, Corporal Michael J. Crescenz VA Medical Center,
3900 Woodland Avenue, Philadelphia, PA 19104, USA
e-mail: Deborah.Way@va.gov

© Springer International Publishing Switzerland 2016
P.A. Fenstemacher, P. Winn (eds.), *Post-Acute and Long-Term Medicine*,
Current Clinical Practice, DOI 10.1007/978-3-319-16979-8_4

VA Medical Centers. With Hospital in Home, veterans can receive hospital-level services including parenteral infusion therapy and occasionally external ventilation. While on service they receive daily visits from a medical provider and skilled nursing. Other services can include physical therapy and aides. In this program patients can be transferred directly from the Emergency Department to home instead of being admitted to the hospital.

Most programs are staffed by VA employees. The VA provides the medical care and DME such as oxygen, while a partner home health agency/infusion pharmacy provides the skilled nursing and infusion services. The most common conditions treated by Hospital in Home are CHF, COPD, cellulitis, and pneumonia. In most programs over half of patients have CHF. Evaluations of the program have shown improved outcomes as well as a cost savings of 30–60 % for a comparative index hospitalization. Hospital in Home has lower readmission rates, and substantially lower hospital-associated adverse events such as falls, delirium, and catheter-related infections when compared to a traditional inpatient hospital stay.

Home Based Primary Care

Home-based primary care (HBPC)was established in 1972. The program was initially called hospital based home care, but in 1995 the name was changed to reflect the primary care focus of the program. HBPC is a comprehensive home care program that provides long-term care that specifically targets individuals with complex, chronic, and disabling illness, with the goal of maximizing independence and reducing preventable emergency room visits, hospitalizations, and long-term institutionalization.

The VA uses an interdisciplinary team including a physician, nurse, social worker, rehabilitation therapist, dietitian, psychologist, and pharmacist to care for the veterans. Other disciplines such as nurse practitioners, physician assistants, chaplains, and recreational therapists may also be included in the team. HBPC provides primary care in the homes of veterans for whom routine clinic-based care has not been effective [2]. In addition, the care provided in the veteran's home may include palliative care, disease management, and coordination of care. The frequency of visits and intensity of care in HBPC varies according to the needs of each veteran. If enrolled in Medicare, the veteran may also receive skilled services under Part B. It is possible for the VA to contract with community-based agencies to provide care if a veteran lives outside the coverage area of the team (generally 30–70 miles from a VA medical center or a community-based outpatient clinic) or HBPC doesn't provide the care needed [2].

The census of HBPC programs ranges from 70 to 900, although programs that focus on primary care rarely have more than 600 patients. Half of patients have dependency in two or more ADLs. The annual mortality rate averages 25 %. Patients have high multi-morbidity with an average of 19 diagnoses and 15 medications [3]. Almost 90 % of patients have hypertension and more than 60 % have coronary artery disease. Other conditions such as diabetes, depression, and dementia are also prevalent [4]. Patients receive on average 2–3 contacts every month from the various team disciplines, with a primary care visit usually every 4–6 weeks.

The success of the HBPC program is attributable to the *team-based care planning* with attention to both the medical and psychosocial factors that affect each veteran [5]. When the cost of the program was evaluated, a reduction in both VA and Medicare costs was seen for those veterans who were dually enrolled with overall cost reductions in excess of 10 % [5]. Enrollment in HPBC has been associated with decreased hospital bed days, decreased nursing home bed days, and decreased hospital readmission rates [2]. The VA's National Patient Satisfaction Survey showed that 83 % of patients rated HBPC care as very good or excellent [5].

Telehealth

Home Telehealth can connect a veteran to a VA hospital from their home using regular telephone lines. The VA provides training on how to use Telehealth so that clinicians and patients can use video technology and a messaging device. Usually a nurse or social worker is the point of contact. Telehealth can provide medical and mental health services.

Aide and Attendance

Through the Aide and Attendance program at the VA, homemakers and home health aides can provide personal services, case management, and assistance with basic activities of daily living and/or instrumental activities of daily living. These services can be combined with other VA services to help avoid or delay admission to a nursing facility. The VA contracts with outside agencies to provide this care.

Nursing Facility Care

Community Nursing Facilities and Community Living Center

The VA contracts with community NFs to provide care to eligible veterans. VA payment for care at the NF is based on service-connected status, level of disability, and income. If these requirements are not met, then care is paid from the veteran's own financial resources or Medicaid. The CLC or *Community LivingCenter* is a nursing facility owned and operated by the VA. The services provided at the CLC are similar to those provided in community nursing facilities. Eligibility for the CLC is also based on service-connected status, level of disability, and income.

End of Life Care

Hospice and Palliative Care

Veterans Health Administration (VHA) policyrequires the presence of an *interdisciplinary palliative care consult* team at each VA facility. Hospice and palliative care are part of the VA Standard Medical Benefits Package. All enrolled veterans are eligible if they meet the clinical need for these services.

There is no policy at this time that prevents veterans from receiving the Medicare hospice benefit along with other VA care, but this is subject to interpretation by each VA facility. There are *some VA facilities that will authorize hospice and pay for treatments that are palliative in nature*, for example palliative brain irradiation or palliative chemotherapy.

Pearls for the Practitioner

- Remember to ask patients if they are a veteran, if so, they may be entitled to additional care funded thought the VA.
- The VA offers community veterans a variety of LTC services: *Hospital in Home, Home-Based Primary care, Telehealth,* and *Aide and Attendance.*
- VA payment for care at NFs is based on service-connected status, level of disability, and income.
- Hospice and palliative care are part of the VHA Standard Medical Benefits Package.
- To contact your local VA, access the website www.va.gov/geriatrics/.

References and Websites

1. Leff B, Weston C, Garriguea S, Patel K, Ritchie C. Home based primary care practices in the United States: current state and quality improvement approaches. J Am Geriatr Soc. 2015;63:963–9.
2. Leftwich Beales J, Edes T. Veteran's Affairs home based primary care. Clin Geriatr Med. 2009;25:149–54.
3. HBPC Master Files FY 2014 – an internal VA database.
4. VA Decision Support System Report, FY2014, Primary Care, HBPC Cohort – an internal VA database.
5. Edes T, Kinosian B, Vuckovic N, Nichols L, Becker M, Hossain M. Better access, quality, and cost for clinically complex veterans with home-based primary care. J Am Geriatr Soc. 2014;62:1954–61.
6. www.va.gov/geriatrics/.

Behind the Scenes at Nursing Facilities

Richard G. Stefanacci, George Brown, and Shelley Reich

Introduction

While the delivery of long-term care (LTC) continues to become more community-based, the traditional model of LTC remains the skilled nursing facility (SNF) with over 16,000 Medicare and Medicaid certified nursing facilities in the USA and almost 1.5 million residents. State Medicaid programs pay for the majority of the frail elderly care. Typically, residents of SNFs require skilled nursing care for the management of multiple chronic conditions, taking on average 8–10 medications per day. The care in nursing facilities is highly regulated through both state and federal regulations developed to ensure appropriate resident care. This care is provided through an interdisciplinary team that strives to have each resident attain the highest practicable level of well-being.

A transition of care often occurs when an older person, living at home, has an acute change in condition that requires that they be admitted to a hospital and then discharged to a nursing facility. During their stay at the nursing facility, it is not uncommon that another acute event occurs that then requires readmission to the

R.G. Stefanacci, DO, MGH, MBA, AGSF, CMD (✉)
Thomas Jefferson University, College of Population Health, MercyLIFE,
Philadelphia, PA, USA

Chief Medical Office, The Access Group, 400 Connell Drive FL2, Berkeley Heights,
NJ 07922, USA
e-mail: RStefanacci@theaccessgp.com

G. Brown, PhD
Director of Clinical Services, The Access Group, 400 Connell Drive FL2, Berkeley Heights,
NJ 07922 USA
e-mail: GBrown@theaccessgp.com

S. Reich
The Access Group, 400 Connell Drive FL2, Berkeley Heights, NJ 07922, USA
e-mail: SReich@theaccessgp.com

© Springer International Publishing Switzerland 2016
P.A. Fenstemacher, P. Winn (eds.), *Post-Acute and Long-Term Medicine*,
Current Clinical Practice, DOI 10.1007/978-3-319-16979-8_5

hospital and subsequently back to the nursing facility. Such transitions in care require careful coordination to protect against adverse outcomes to maximize outcomes and ensure quality, Medicare is now requiring improvements in transitions of care by holding acute care hospitals accountable for avoidable readmissions occurring within a 30-day time frame. This focus on quality care especially with regard to hospitalizations and quality of life for the SNF resident will continue to be a growing focus on SNFs [1].

The Interdisciplinary Team

An interdisciplinary team of health care professionals who provide both a comprehensive and coordinated assessment and management of each resident's medical, psychological, social, and functional needs is essential for resident well-being in LTC (Table 1). This in fact is mandated in nursing facilities but is also a practical approach to provide care for the elderly in the assisted living facility and home as well.

Regulations: OBRA 87

Prior to 1987 nursing facility care was characterized by the prevalent use of physical restraints, inappropriate use of psychotropic medication, overuse of urinary catheters, and a high occurrence of urinary incontinence, pressure ulcers, weight loss, and behavioral problems. Because of widespread poor quality of care in nursing facilities, Congress requested that the Institute of Medicine (IOM) study how to improve the quality of care in the nation's Medicaid and Medicare certified nursing facilities. In its 1986 report, *Improving the Quality of Care in Nursing Homes*, the IOM expert panel recommended:

- A stronger Federal role in improving quality.
- Revisions in performance standards and the inspection, i.e., survey process.
- Better training of staff.
- Improved assessment of resident needs.
- And a dynamic and improved regulatory process [3].

The Omnibus Reconciliation Act of 1987 (OBRA) contained the Nursing Home Reform Act, which was written by federal legislators in response to these recommendations proposed by the IOM. The "Campaign for Quality Care" was organized by the National Citizens' Coalition for Nursing Home Reform in order to both implement the IOM recommendations and to support these Federal reforms. National organizations representing consumers, nursing facilities (both for profit and nonprofit) and health care professionals including AMDA-The Society for Post-Acute and Long-Term Care Medicine, as well as the American Geriatrics Society, have worked and continue to work together to create consensus positions on major nursing facility issues.

Table 1 The interdisciplinary care team in nursing facilities

Title	Scope of practice	Education	Annual mean salary [2]
Certified nurses aids	Work under the supervision of a nurse and provide assistance to patients with daily living tasks	In addition to a high school diploma or GED, completion of a 6–12-week CNA certificate program at a community college or medical facility	$26,020
Licensed practical nurse	Provide the patient care on a very personal level. They usually report directly to physicians and RNs, and are usually responsible for taking vitals and monitoring in-and-out volumes, treating common conditions like pressure sores, and preparing or performing several procedures such as dressing wounds, bathing and dressing, and giving enemas. In some, but not all, states LPNs and LVNs may administer prescribed medicines or start IV fluids	Required to pass a licensing examination, known as the NCLEX-PN, after completing a State-approved practical nursing program. A high school diploma or its equivalent usually is required for entry	$42,910
Registered nurse	Work directly with patients and their families. They are the primary point of contact between the patient and the world of health care, both at the bedside and in outpatient settings. RNs perform frequent patient evaluations, including monitoring and tracking vital signs, performing procedures such as IV placement, phlebotomy, and administering medications. Because the RN has much more regular contact with patients than physicians, the RN is usually first to notice problems or raise concerns about patient progress	The three major educational paths to registered nursing are a bachelor's degree, an associate degree, and a diploma from an approved nursing program. Nurses most commonly enter the occupation by completing an associate degree or bachelor's degree program. Individuals then must complete a national licensing examination in order to obtain a nursing license	$62,010
Registered Nurse Assessment Coordinator (RNAC)	The Registered Nurse Assessment Coordinator (RNAC) will assist the Director of Nursing (DON) with ensuring that documentation in the center meets Federal State and Certification guidelines. The RNAC will coordinate RAI process assuring the accuracy timeliness and completeness of the MDS RAPS and Interdisciplinary Care Plan. The Registered Nurse Assessment Coordinator (RNAC) conducts the nursing process—Assessment Planning Implementation and Evaluation—under the state's Nurse Practice Act for Registered Nurse Licensure		$80,190
Director of Nursing (DON)	The Director of Nursing has the responsibility of overseeing the standards of nursing practices for the organization's nursing services. The DON participates with other members of Nursing Services and Administration in the development of patient care programs, policies and procedures to meet all requirements including ethical and legal concerns		$107,200

(continued)

Table 1 (continued)

Title	Scope of practice	Education	Annual mean salary [2]
Social worker	Assist people by helping them cope with issues in their everyday lives, deal with their relationships, and solve personal and family problems	All States and the District of Columbia have licensing, certification, or registration requirements regarding social work practice and the use of professional titles. Although standards for licensing vary by State, a growing number of States are placing greater emphasis on communications skills, professional ethics, and sensitivity to cultural diversity issues. Most States require 2 years (3,000 h) of supervised clinical experience for licensure of clinical social workers	$52,520
Dietitian	Plan food and nutrition programs, supervise meal preparation, and oversee the serving of meals. They prevent and treat illnesses by promoting healthy eating habits and recommending dietary modifications. They perform nutrition screenings for their clients and offer advice on diet-related concerns such as weight loss and cholesterol reduction	At least a bachelor's degree. Licensure, certification, or registration requirements vary by State	$56,300
Physical therapist	Physical therapists provide a variety of medical services to help individuals who have been injured or physically affected by illness to recover or improve function. A physical therapist must be able to evaluate a patient's condition and devise a customized physical rehabilitation and treatment plan to enhance strength, flexibility, range of motion, motor control, and reduce any pain, discomfort and swelling the patient is experiencing	Graduate from a physical therapist educational program with a master's or doctoral degree	$87,250
Occupational therapist	Occupational therapists help patients improve their ability to perform tasks in living and working environments. They work with individuals who suffer from a mentally, physically, developmentally, or emotionally disabling condition. Occupational therapists use treatments to develop, recover, or maintain the daily living and work skills of their patients. The therapist helps clients not only to improve their basic motor functions and reasoning abilities, but also to compensate for permanent loss of function. The goal is to help clients have independent, productive, and satisfying lives	A master's degree or higher in occupational therapy is the minimum requirement for entry into the field	$77,890

Recreational therapist	Recreational therapists devise programs in art, music, dance, sports, games, and crafts for individuals with disabilities or illnesses. These activities help to prevent or to alleviate physical, mental, and social problems	Bachelor's degree with some additional training is usually required for this field	$45,520
Attending primary care physician	Responsibility for initial patient care and support discharges and transfers. Also make periodic, pertinent on-site visits to patients and insure adequate ongoing coverage (see Chap. "The Role of Practitioners and the Medical Director")	In addition to 4 years of medical school most nursing home attending physicians complete a primary residency, which is typically 1–3 years. Some go on to complete a geriatric fellowship as well.	$188,440
Medical director	Roles and responsibilities of the medical director in the nursing home can be divided into four areas: physician leadership, patient care–clinical leadership, quality of care, and education. Nursing facilities are required to have a medical director as outlined in OBRA 87 (see Chap. "The Role of Practitioners and the Medical Director")	Currently Maryland is the only State that requires Medical Directors to be a Certified Medical Director (CMD) in Long Term Care or have similar training. CMD was established by the American Medical Directors Association to professionalize the field of medical direction	$90.60 per hour[a]
Nurse practitioner	Advanced practice nurses who provide high-quality health care services similar to those of a doctor. NPs diagnose and treat a wide range of health problems. They have a unique approach and stress both care and cure. Besides clinical care, NPs focus on health promotion, disease prevention, health education and counseling (see Chap. Nurse Practitioners, Clinical Nurse Specialists and Physician Assistants)	The entry-level training for NPs is a graduate degree. At this time, NPs complete a master's or doctoral degree program. This means that NPs earn a bachelor's degree in nursing (4 years of education), then their graduate NP degree (2–4 years of education)	$95,070
Consultant pharmacists	Focuses on reviewing and managing the medication regimens of patients, particularly those in institutional settings such as nursing homes. Consultant pharmacists ensure their patients' medications are appropriate, effective, as safe as possible and used correctly; and identify, resolve, and prevent medication-related problems that may interfere with the goals of therapy	The Doctorate of Pharmacy (Pharm.D.) is the only professional Pharmacy degree, and the 5-year Bachelors of Science in Pharmacy is being phased out as a professional degree. Since this program traditionally follows 2 years of pre-pharmacy education, students typically take 6 years of post-secondary education to obtain their Pharm.D	$107,220
Nursing home administers	Responsibility as the managing officer of the facility to plan, organize, direct, and control the day-to-day functions of a facility and to maintain the facility's compliance with applicable laws, rules, and regulations The administrator shall be vested with adequate authority to comply with the laws, rules, and regulations relating to the management of the facility	Typically requirement of a certificate program of about 120 h is required before sitting for a licensing examination. Most are required to have completed a bachelor degree program as well as preceptor training as a NHA	$97,870

[a]Part-time position
Bureau of labor Statistics, May 2013. http://www.bls.gov/oes/current/oes291141.htm

Under OBRA 1987, surveyors of nursing facilities have shifted focus from the nursing facility to *resident outcomes*. The *quality of life* and the *quality of care* of each resident now became the two basic areas for review. Under quality of life, the concept of the living environment maintaining or improving the residents' "well-being" was now *the* major focus. In addition to physical and mental health, well-being includes the resident's functional status, dignity, self-esteem, relationships, physical appearance as well as their social and spiritual needs.

The changes that OBRA incorporated into the care of residents are noteworthy with the most important provisions being:

- Emphasis on resident *quality of life* as well as the *quality of care.*
- A resident assessment process leading to development of an *individualized care plan.*
- New *expectations that each resident's ability* to walk, bathe, and perform other activities of daily living *will be maintained or improved* unless an underlying medical condition precludes it.
- The right to be *free* of unnecessary and inappropriate *physical and chemical restraints.*
- The right to *choose a personal physician* and to *access their medical records.*
- The right to organize and participate in a *resident or family council.*
- The right to *return* to the nursing facility after a hospital stay or have an overnight visit with family and friends.
- The right to safely *maintain personal funds* with the nursing facility.
- The *right to remain* in the nursing facility *unless* non-payment, dangerous resident behavior, or a significant change in the resident's medical condition.
- Prohibitions on asking family members to pay for Medicare and Medicaid services.
- *Uniform certification standards* for Medicare and Medicaid homes.
- 75-h of training for paraprofessional staff.
- New opportunities for residents with mental retardation or mental illness to access services *inside* and *outside* the nursing facility.
- New *penalties* for certified nursing facilities that fail to meet minimum federal standards.

Under OBRA, state surveyors no longer spend their time exclusively with staff or with review of facility records. Conversations with residents and families are now an important part of the survey process. Observations of resident dining and medication administration are other focal points of the survey. Since OBRA has been implemented, it has indeed changed the care and lives of residents of nursing facilities across the USA. Significant improvements have occurred in the comprehensiveness of care planning, antipsychotic drug use has declined by 28–36 %, and physical restraints reduced by 40 %.

Nursing Facility Regulations

The Resident Assessment Instrument (RAI) provides a comprehensive assessment of each resident's functional capabilities and helps the nursing facility staff identify each resident's health problems. Care Area Assessments (CAAs), previously called Resident Assessment Protocols (RAPs) are a major part of this process and provide the foundation upon which a resident's individual care plan is developed by the interdisciplinary team. Use of the Minimum Data Set (MDS) is part of the federally mandated tool for clinical assessment of each resident and usually "triggers" several CAAs. MDS assessments are required to be completed on admission to the nursing facility and updated quarterly and annually, as well as when there is a significant change in condition (worsened or improved). These assessments focus on many areas including: tasks of daily living (basic ADLs), mobility, cognition, continence, mood, behaviors, nutritional status, vision and communication, recreational activities, psychosocial well-being, pain, falls, and injuries.

Once the MDS information is entered into a computer database by the MDS coordinator, it is then transmitted from the nursing facility to the state database. From the state database, it is then sent to the national database at the Centers for Medicare and Medicaid Services (CMS). The information in the MDS determines the resident's Resource Utilization Group (RUG) that in term *determines the per diem rate paid to the facility* for the resident's stay under Medicare Part A, i.e., skilled care. The MDS data also determines each facility's quality measures (QM) report, several of which are publicly reported and routinely used by surveyors during the pre-survey and survey process (Table 2).

MDS 3.0 version and the Quality Indicator Survey (QIS) process are gradually being introduced to many states (Table 3). Specifics of the MDS 3.0 can be obtained at the Centers for Medicare and Medicaid Services website at: http://www.cms.hhs.gov/NursingHomeQualityInits/25_NHQIMDS30.asp

CMS Reference

http://www.cms.hhs.gov/NursingHomeQualityInits/25_NHQIMDS30.asp

Table 2 Uses of MDS data

• Payment Resource Utilization Groups (RUGs) Facility Prospective Payment System (PPS)
• Care planning Resident assessment protocols (Resident assessment instrument)
• Quality measures Quality improvement activities Available to state surveyors Available for posting at the Medicare "nursing home compare" website

Table 3 MDS 3.0: goals, changes and anticipated results

Goal of MDS 3.0	MDS 3.0 changes	Anticipated results
Improving the: Reliability Accuracy Usefulness Length Staff satisfaction and perception of clinical utility	Introduce advances in assessment measures: Increase the clinical relevance of items Improve accuracy and validity Increase the resident's voice by introducing more resident interview items Briefer assessment periods for clinical items	Improve identification of resident needs Enhance resident-focused care planning Enhance communication among providers

Regulations: State Operations Manual (SOM)

The State Operations Manual (SOM) sets out survey investigative protocols and interpretive guidelines to provide guidance to state surveyors. These serve to clarify and explain the intent of the Federal regulations. Furthermore, these protocols and guidelines direct the surveyor's attention when preparing for the survey, conducting the survey, and evaluating the survey findings. The survey is conducted to determine whether a citation of non-compliance is appropriate. Deficiencies are based on a violation of the state and/or federal regulations, as supported by surveyor observations of the nursing facilities' staff performance and care practices. Chart review, interview of staff, residents, family, and possibly practitioners and the facility medical director are also the basis for surveyor evaluations. The Interpretive Guidelines include three parts: survey tag number; wording of the regulation; and guidance to surveyors, including additional survey procedures and probes if warranted.

The regulations emphasize the need for continuous, rather than annual cyclical compliance. The enforcement process mandates that policies and procedures are established to remedy deficient practices and to ensure that correction is lasting. Facilities must take the initiative and responsibility for continuously monitoring their own performance to sustain compliance. Measures to meet the requirements for an acceptable *plan of correction* in response to survey deficiencies emphasize the need to achieve and maintain compliance. A second requirement is that all survey deficiencies will be addressed promptly. A third requirement is that all residents will receive the care and services they need to attain their highest practicable level of functioning.

Quality Initiative: Medicare Five Star Program

With three million older Americans admitted to nursing facilities each year of which, 1.5 million stay long enough to consider the nursing facility their main residence, it should come as no surprise that nursing facilities are strictly surveyed in order to assure appropriate care. Despite this, one in five nursing facilities nationwide was cited for deficiencies that caused actual harm or immediate jeopardy to their residents [4].

Some major concerns of quality that were identified by facility medical directors include the following: telephone conversations, transitional care, falls and hip fractures, warfarin usage, pressure ulcers, inappropriate medications, pain control, urinary incontinence, weight loss and exercise of residents [5]. The CMS "Nursing Home Compare" website publically reviews the survey deficiencies received by nursing facilities but does not reflect the entire inspection report (form HCFA-2567). The complete survey inspection report and the nursing facility's subsequent *plan of correction* to address the deficiencies are available either from the State survey agency or from the nursing facility itself that can be accessed by the resident and family member.

The Department of Health and Human Services (DHHS) has a national Nursing Home Quality Initiative for improving nursing facility care. A critical part of this initiative is CMS's public posting of the quality measures for every nursing facility, also known as "report cards" [4]. These report cards can be used by consumers to make better-informed decisions and motivate providers to improve care; but there is concern that these nursing home report cards fail to adjust for risk differences in resident populations of various long-term care facilities [5]. The CMS quality initiative continues to redirect focus on the care needs of frail elders who reside in nursing facilities. Under CMS, the Nursing Home Quality Initiative has also expanded and refined its measures in order to improve resident outcomes and care effectiveness, e.g., reducing the occurrence of pressure ulcers and avoiding potentially preventable hospital admissions. The CMS quality measures are divided between those focused on the short-term (SNF) and long stay residents. These quality measures include the following [6]:

Short-Stay Facility Quality Measures

- Percent of residents who self-report moderate to severe pain.
- Percent of residents with pressure ulcers that are new or worsened.
- Percent of residents who were assessed and appropriately given the seasonal influenza vaccine.
- Percent of residents assessed and appropriately given the pneumococcal vaccine.
- Percent of short-stay residents who newly received an antipsychotic medication.

Long Stay Facility Quality Measures

- Percent of residents experiencing one or more falls with major injury.
- Percent of residents who self-report moderate to severe pain.
- Percent of high-risk residents with pressure ulcers.
- Percent of residents assessed and appropriately given the seasonal influenza vaccine.
- Percent of residents assessed and appropriately given the pneumococcal vaccine.
- Percent of residents with a urinary tract infection.

- Percent of low-risk residents who lose control of their bowels or bladder.
- Percent of residents who have/had a catheter inserted and left in their bladder.
- Percent of residents who were physically restrained.
- Percent of residents whose need for help with activities of daily living has increased.
- Percent of residents who lose too much weight.
- Percent of residents who have depressive symptoms.
- Percent of long-stay residents who received an antipsychotic medication.

Beginning in 2015, CMS will implement the following improvements to the Nursing Home Five Star Quality Rating System [7]:

- *Nationwide Focused Survey Inspections*: Effective January 2015, CMS and states will implement focused survey inspections nationwide for a sample of nursing homes to enable better verification of both the staffing and quality measure information that is part of the Five-Star Quality Rating System. In fiscal year 2014, CMS piloted special surveys of nursing homes that focused on investigating the coding of the Minimum Data Set (MDS) that are specifically based on resident assessment and used in the determination of the quality measures.
- *Payroll-Based Staffing Reporting*: CMS will implement a quarterly electronic reporting system that is auditable back to payroll to verify staffing information. This new system will increase accuracy and timeliness of data and allow for the calculation of quality measures for staff turnover, retention, types of staffing, and levels of different types of staffing. Implementation will be improved by funding provided in the recently enacted, bipartisan Improving Medicare Post-Acute Care Transformation Act (IMPACT) of 2014.
- *Additional Quality Measures*: CMS will increase both the number and type of quality measures used in the Five-Star Quality Rating System. The first additional measure, starting January 2015, will be the extent to which antipsychotic medications are in use. Future additional measures will include claims-based data on rehospitalization and community discharge rates.
- *Timely and Complete Inspection Data*: CMS will also strengthen requirements to ensure that States maintain a user-friendly website and complete inspections of nursing facilities in a timely and accurate manner for inclusion in the rating system.
- *Improved Scoring Methodology*: In 2015, CMS will revise the scoring methodology by which we calculate each facility's quality measure rating, which is used to calculate the overall Five Star rating. We also note that sources (independent of self-reporting by nursing facilities) already are weighted higher than self-reported components in the scoring methodology.

Financing

The complexity of nursing facility care is further complicated by a fragmented payment system [8]. All of Medicare Parts A, B, C, and D, as well as Medicaid are involved in some aspect of funding services for SNF and NF residents (Table 4).

Table 4 Medicare benefit coverage

Medicare part	Title	Coverage
A	Hospital insurance	Hospital, subacute care, hospice
B	Medical insurance	Physician and NP/PA services
		Certain vaccines
C	Medicare advantage	Managed care
D	Prescription drug coverage	Prescription drugs

Table 5 Skilled versus non-skilled nursing facility care

	Eligibility	Room and board	Physician services	Medication
Skilled	For Medicare beneficiaries requiring skilled nursing care following a 3-day acute hospitalization	Part A	Part B	Part A
General nursing care (nonskilled)	ADL/IADL needs	Medicaid	Part B	Part D
		LTC insurance		
		Private payment	Part C	

Within most nursing facilities, residents are typically receiving either skilled or non-skilled nursing care (Table 5). *Skilled care* occurs when a resident requires more intensive nursing and rehabilitation services. Skilled care is available to Medicare beneficiaries following a hospitalization under Medicare part A. *Non-skilled general nursing facility care* is typically paid for by state Medicaid programs or privately.

Currently, more than 60 % of LTC funding comes from Medicaid, and this funding is expected to increase with the expansion of Medicaid under the Patient Protection and Affordable Care Act [9].

The dollar value of family caregiving exceeds that of all spending on long-term services and supports (LTSS). Family caregiving had an estimated economic value of $450 billion in 2009 as compared with $220 billion spent on LTSS in 2012 [10]. In addition, the cost to US businesses due to lost productivity from full-time family caregiver employees (e.g., reduced hours, replacement of employees, absenteeism, distractions) was estimated at approximately $34 billion in 2004 [11].

Private LTC insurance has been sold in the USA for more than 30 years, but only 10 % of the potential market of Americans older than 50 years is insured [9]. Therefore, any hope of it serving a large percentage of the population has not been realized. In fact, the rate of issuing new policies has declined, and a significant number of insurers have left the private LTC insurance market and closed blocks of policies for several reasons, including low interest rates that have affected the products' financial performance and unexpectedly low forfeiture rates. The policies that remain have recently been forced to substantially increase their premiums.

Today, there is no comprehensive approach to care coordination for many individuals and caregivers, although there are models, such as the Program for All-Inclusive Care (see chapter "PACE") in which nursing home–eligible community dwelling older adults who are cared for by an interdisciplinary team focused on care coordination and supportive services. Outside of PACE, the fragmentation and lack of coordination of the LTSS delivery system is due in part to the misalignment of benefit structures, conflicting rules, separate funding streams of Medicare, Medicaid, and other public and private programs.

Medicare Part A

Medicare beneficiaries who need short-term skilled care (nursing or rehabilitation services) following a hospital stay require at least 3 days of hospitalization (i.e., admissions days). Hospital observation days do not qualify for covered services in a SNF. The Medicare SNF benefit pays facilities a predetermined daily rate for each day of care up to 100 days (Table 6). The prospective payment system (PPS) rates are determined through Resource Utilization Groups (RUGs). Residents are assigned to one of 53 RUGs based on resident characteristics and expected service use: skilled nursing and rehabilitation. After the first 21 days of a skilled facility stay Medicare Part A no longer covers 100 % of the cost, but only 80 % with a 20 % daily copayment.

Medicare Part B

Medicare Part B covers practitioner (physician, physicians' assistant and nurse practitioner) and rehabilitation services (OT, PT, or ST) for *non-skilled residents*. Medicare Part B also covers vaccines like the influenza and pneumococcal.

Medicare Part C

Medicare is expanding programs that care for beneficiaries who reside in and outside of traditional nursing facilities. Under Medicare Part C (also called Medicare Advantage), managed care organizations are responsible for providing all the benefits available under Medicare Part A, B, and D. United Healthcare launched the Evercare program in 1987. Evercare utilizes nurse practitioner (NPs) within nursing facilities to provide timely care and thereby reduce emergency room evaluations and hospital admissions and to increase preventive care. The Evercare program is also able to provide a skilled level of services at nursing facilities without Medicare's requirement for three admission days of hospitalization.

Table 6 Medicare daily base rates for fiscal year 2014 (MedPAC) [12]

Rate component	Nursing	Therapy	Room and board	Total
Urban	$169.28	$127.51	$86.39	$383.18
Rural	$161.72	$147.02	$87.99	$396.73

More recently, the Medicare Modernization Act allowed for the continuing development of these types of programs as well as a broader range of options under Medicare Advantage (MA) and Special Needs Plans (SNP). SNPs are authorized to focus on one of three distinct patients groups: residents of nursing homes, dually eligible seniors (those who are entitled to Medicare Part A and/or Part B *and* are eligible for some form of Medicaid benefit), or those suffering from multiple chronic illnesses. The SNFs under such programs receive financial incentives to provide care that improves resident outcomes and prevents hospitalizations.

Medicare Part D

Part D is the prescription drug benefit that started in 2006 for Medicare beneficiaries. For the dually-eligible residents (who have both Medicare and Medicaid) their drug coverage previously under Medicaid is now covered under Medicare Part D without any copayments or premiums.

Medicaid

All state Medicaid programs have two eligibility requirements that regulate which persons may obtain Medicaid financial support for their nursing facility stay(s). The first is financial eligibility, and the second, medical eligibility. With respect to medical eligibility, CMS has allowed states to adopt their own procedures and set of criteria. While Medicaid no longer pays for Part D covered medications for the dually eligible, Medicaid does cover non-Part D medications such as benzodiazepines that were excluded from Part D coverage. Medicaid also covers the daily cost of nursing facility room and board for non-skilled stays for those finically indigent.

Transitions of Care

Quality of care can be affected (for better or worse) during the transition of care from one setting to another. When residents transition from the long term care facility to other settings they are at high risk for the adverse effects of prescribing or transcription errors. Just admitting a patient into an unfamiliar environment like an emergency department can result in severe patient decompensation, and lead to medical errors [13]. Overlooked appointments, diagnoses, or laboratory tests as well as a missed or duplication of medication are just a few of the potential errors that can occur. Seamless transitions from the hospital to home, skilled nursing care, and home health care can all reduce these errors [14]. Quality Improvement Organizations (QIOs) under contract with CMS are trying to improve care coordination; promote seamless transitions; and reduce rehospitalizations [1]. Medicare is striving to improve these transitions by encouraging provider investments in health information technology as well as anticipating a "bundled" payment system that would financially tie hospitals and nursing facilities together for an episode of resident care. Medicare is also encouraging the development of systems that will hold hospitals financially accountable for poor outcomes during transitions of care. The system that Medicare is encouraging will have interdisciplinary teams working on assuring improved transitions. The CMS Hospital Readmissions Reduction Program is currently focused on readmissions that occur in Medicare beneficiaries with a diagnosis of pneumonia, MI, CHF, and eventually COPD and diabetes [1].

As each patient is unique in the needs and specifics of his/her illness, so is each care transition. The transition plan must consider caregiver availability for the patient, as well as patient abilities and responsibilities. Financial and insurance issues are important factors and must be taken into account when deciding the appropriate level of care for each patient. When the patient transitions to a skilled nurse facility/nursing facility (SNF/NF) from the acute care hospital (ACH), clinical information must be sent to ensure a seamless plan of care, and hospital clinicians must remain available to answer questions about transfer orders and to oversee patient care until SNF/NF clinicians have assumed clinical responsibility. As many patients are often elderly and vulnerable physically and mentally, transitioning from the ACH setting to the SNF/NF is often traumatic to the patient and family. Planning for the patient's discharge and transition as early as possible during the hospital stay may lessen patient and family stress and anxiety.

Transitions from ACH to SNF/NF

Communication is the key to a successful transfer of care, ideally from physician-to-physician [13]. This is typified in medical home models and PACE (Program for All-inclusive Care for the Elderly) programs where a patient has a physician (medical point of contact) who ideally is the attending in the ACH, who at discharge continues as the attending in the SNF/NF, and who upon return of the patient to the community continues to serve as the patients physician. Frequently, however, this degree of continuity is not possible. The patient may not have a community practitioner nor participate in a medical home. Having a different practitioner at each subsequent setting of patient care raises important issues on information transfer between facilities, medication reconciliation, and patient/caregiver education [14].

The best time for information transfer is before the patient discharges to the SNF/NF. Inter-facility transfer forms are common method for transferring information; however, these forms are not standardized and can lead to miscommunication or non-communication of information. The ACH may not be able to provide patient information on baseline cognitive and functional status prior to hospitalization. Additionally, transfer forms may have incorrect information, be incomplete, or have errors. Despite the best efforts of ACH case managers/social workers/discharge planners and SNF/NF admission coordinators; patient transition is still an area of with significant problems. A recent survey of directors of nursing in SNF/NFs revealed that patient hospital discharge information was shared with the SNF/NF medical director only 3.3 % of the time. Furthermore, more than half of attending physicians (57.6 %) in the SNF/NF "rarely" or "never" discussed patients with the transferring physicians [15].

The hospitalist section of the Society of Hospital Medicine and the American College of Physicians has published standards for essential components of a discharge summary. This is to include

- Reason for SNF/NF referral and whether a return to the community is the intent;
- Recommendations of specialty consultants;
- Pending laboratory or other diagnostic study results;
- Recommended follow-up and management plans.

A greater the degree of transfer standardization coupled with increased hospital staff education are critical elements in information transfer to the SNF/NF that will help to decrease medical errors [16].

Central to information transfer is medication reconciliation. It has several components:

- Assembling a currently, complete list of all prescription and OTC drugs, vitamins, and supplements;
- Recording their dose and frequency at each site of care; and
- Reconciling the medication list to ensure there is clear indication for use of a drug and the reason as to why it is not to be discontinued.

Oversight, review, and discussion of the medication regimen before and after a transition can include the consultant pharmacist, the attending physician, nurse practitioner, physician assistant, hospital nurse, community PCP or pharmacist, SNF/NF nurse, and other health care team members as deemed appropriate.

Transitions of care can cause great anxiety for patients and caregivers. It is common for patients and their families to have unrealistic expectations of what the care and services the SNF/NF will provide. Such information should be provided to families in all settings and not just ACH discharge. SNF/NFs should develop information packages and discuss the differences between SNF/NF care role and that of ACHs. Patients and families should be educated and empowered as much as possible to be active participants in their own care.

https://www.nhqualitycampaign.org/files/Transition_of_Care_Reference.pdf

Future Changes

Long-term care (LTC) is undergoing major changes that will impact all LTC providers. These changes are occurring as a result of a focus to decrease LTC costs, which are expected to occur through reductions in both LTC utilization as well as reimbursement. These cuts are occurring not directly through Medicare and Medicaid but through private payers, such as managed care organizations and other groups newly responsible for provision of LTC services. Skilled nursing facilities and other LTC facilities succeeding in the face of these regulatory and practice shifts will be those that understand these changes and have developed processes to efficiently and effectively deliver care. Reducing the use of emergency and hospital services for SNF residents will be especially important. This will require SNFs to deliver outcomes for which they are held financially accountable. In addition, SNFs will need an enhanced focus on medication management. The following section briefly reviews bundled payment changes, Accountable Care Organizations (ACOs), managed Medicaid, pay-for-performance requirements, and the increased complexity of medication management [17].

Bundled Payments

The plan to decrease LTC costs is a focus of the Bundled Payments for Care Improvement (BPCI) initiative that was announced in January 2013[1]. BPCI participant organizations enter into payment arrangements that entails financial and performance accountability for a patient's episode of care. There are four models of care. According to CMS, these models are anticipated to lead to "higher quality, more coordinated care at a lower cost to Medicare." [18]. The model that is most relevant to long-term care is the third model—Retrospective Post-Acute Care Only—which occurs when an episode of care is triggered by an acute care hospital stay and begun upon starting of post-acute care services with a participating SNF, inpatient rehabilitation facility, LTC hospital, or home health agency. The post-acute care services included in the episode must begin within 30 days of discharge from the inpatient hospital stay and will end either after a minimum of 30, 60, or 90 days. Participants in this model can select up to 48 different clinical condition-related episodes of care, which are listed at http://innovation.cms.gov/initiatives/bundled-payments.

If the CMS Innovation Center finds this initiative to be successful, they will introduce this program on a national basis such that all Medicare funds for post-acute services would be channeled through the hospital. This would require SNFs to contract with their local hospitals. SNFs operating in the most efficient and effective manner with regard to *length of stay* and *reduction in avoidable hospital readmissions* will benefit, as these will be to whom hospitals will preferentially refer.

Currently Medicare makes separate payments to each provider for the services they furnish to beneficiaries for a given illness or course of treatment. This has led to fragmented care with poor coordination across providers and health-care settings [18]. This approach bases payment on the extent of services (i.e., how much a provider does), rather than on the outcome of that care. Research has shown that bundled payments can better align incentives for providers—hospitals, post-acute care providers, physicians, and other practitioners—to partner closely across all specialties and settings in order to improve the patient's experience of care not only during a hospital stay for acute care, but also during their post-discharge recovery [19, 20].

In the third model, the bundle will include physicians' services, care by other post-acute providers, related hospital readmissions, and other Medicare Part B services included in the "episode" of care definition. These would include clinical laboratory services, costs for durable medical equipment, prosthetics, orthotics, and supplies, and Part B drugs [21]. This means that physicians caring for post-acute patients will be tied to the SNF for payment just as SNFs will be tied to health systems/hospitals for their payment. This will likely increase the use of the so-called *SNFist*, a physician who specializes in the care of patients in skilled nursing settings. Accordingly many hospitalists will likely become attending physicians at the SNF with which the hospital has partnered.

Under this third model, a target price is set based on historical fee-for-service payments for that type of episode of care, less a discount, after which the aggregate Medicare payment for the episode is reconciled against the bundled payment target price. Any reduction in expenditures below the discount reflected in the target price would then be paid to the participant organization and be shared among their provider partners. Any expenditure that was reimbursed above the target price would be repaid to Medicare by the health care system/hospital [18].

Accountable Care Organizations

An ACO is a provider network typically run by hospitals, physicians, or, sometimes, nursing facilities that share the responsibility of managing and coordinating care of the Medicare fee-for-service beneficiaries assigned to them. The ACO is held accountable for the quality, cost, and overall care of these individuals. Under the Affordable Care Act, an ACO is responsible for at least 5,000 Medicare beneficiaries for at least 3 years [22]. Medicare continues to pay the providers in an ACO for services provided on a fee-for-service basis. However, if the ACO is able to provide better care at significant cost savings to Medicare, then the ACO providers ultimately share in those savings. The benefit of an ACO to the patient is that it reduces the incentive for providers to treat, test, and perform more procedures for fiduciary gain, which also results in health care savings.

The importance of LTC settings in ACO partnerships has been increasingly recognized since 2011, when CMS issued a final regulation allowing nursing facilities as ACO participants. With the goal of providing high quality LTC and reducing hospital readmissions, nursing facilities are in the position to lower costs to the ACO. However, nursing facilities that are trying to align themselves with an ACO will need to stand out in a competitive marketplace. For instance, an ACO may not want to partner with a nursing facility that has a low quality rating or does not have an electronic health records (EHRs) system in place. As a recent commentary stated, "In the ACO [world], one physician, one nursing home, or one hospital participant in the ACO that performs poorly could affect the bottom line by reducing the amount of the shared savings from the government" [23]. The hope is that the benefits of inclusion in an ACO partnership will motivate nursing facility administrators to further improve quality assessment and performance improvement (QAPI).

Medicaid Managed Care and SNF Room and Board Reimbursement

Increasingly, states are moving to mandatory managed care for all Medicaid beneficiaries. According to 2011 data collected by CMS, 74.2 % of the more than 57 million Medicaid beneficiaries in the USA were in a managed Medicaid program [24]. Historically, Medicaid beneficiaries who reside in SNFs had been exempt from the requirement for managed Medicaid, but that is rapidly changing. As a result, we are seeing programs emerge such as New York State's Fully Integrated Dual Advantage. New York is one of 15 states to receive a federal grant to develop a demonstration program to coordinate care for "dual eligibles" (i.e., individuals with both Medicare and Medicaid). The initial enrollment for the New York program was scheduled for July 2014 but was moved forward to January 2015. The program is being funded through the Federal Coordinated Health Care Office, which is housed in the CMS Innovation Center [25]. These programs are responsible for all LTC services, including the payment of the SNF room and board component and other Medicaid benefits. These programs will require SNFs to contract with each of their states' Medicaid LTC managed care plans for reimbursement.

Nursing Home Value-Based Purchasing

While there are many model programs being piloted, this does not assure that they will be introduced as national programs. One demonstration project that recently concluded with limited success is the Nursing Home Value-Based Purchasing (NHVBP) Demonstration [26]. The NHVBP was launched in 2009 as a 3-year CMS demonstration in three states: Arizona, New York, and Wisconsin. *Value-based purchasing* is a payment methodology that rewards quality of care rather than volume of services through payment incentives and transparency.

In its final evaluation, it was concluded that the NHVBP demonstration neither lowered Medicare spending nor improved quality for nursing home residents [27]. The summary report noted that the results may have revealed more about specific flaws in the design of the demonstration rather than actual problems with pay-for-performance. The report offered six potential changes aimed at optimizing payment incentive responses and improving the quality of any Medicare programs moving forward with pay-for-performance models in nursing homes. As such, modifications to the design of any future NHVBP program might include:

- Simplified payment and reward rules.
- Increased payout pools.
- Relaxation/elimination of budget neutrality restrictions such that the likelihood of payout to a facility does not hinge on the efforts of other participating facilities.
- Offering more immediate payouts.
- Real-time feedback on performance and quality activity results.
- Providing increased education and guidance on best practices to providers, such that the program could become more prescriptive by mandating that participating providers undertake specific training or utilize best practices in order to qualify for a reward payment [5].

Despite the findings of the NHVBP, the direction of CMS and states is clear: motivate SNFs to deliver care in a more efficient and effective manner especially with regard to length of stay, hospital readmission rates, and overall facility-based LTC services.

Meaningful and Useful?

The CMS incentives to increase the use of EHRs will turn into penalties in 2015. A 1 % Medicare pay cut will be applied to qualified providers who do not demonstrate meaningful use of a certified EHR by October 2014 unless they have applied for a hardship exemption [28]. *Qualified* providers are those who are considered ambulatory providers, meaning that more than 10 % of one's patient encounters are outside of a hospital [29]. Post-acute care and LTC settings are counted as ambulatory.

The hardship exemption can be applied if more than half of a physician's encounters are in the SNF and those settings do not provide or support EHR technology that meets meaningful use criteria. In these situations, a physician cannot utilize their own EHR. The bottom line for SNF providers is that the SNF's record system must be utilized whether an EHR or paper. If the SNF uses a paper-based record system, the physician would be exempt. For assisted living communities, as they are not required to maintain records, the physician would be required to use his or her own records system and, as such, could not be exempt simply because the assisted living facility does not have its own EHR.

There are also penalties for failing to participate in the Physician Quality Reporting System (PQRS). PQRS is a reporting program that uses a combination of incentive payments and payment adjustments to promote reporting of quality information by eligible professionals [6]. CMS describes the program as providing incentive payment to practices that satisfactorily report data on quality measures. Eligible professionals who do not satisfactorily report data on quality measures for covered professional services are subject to a payment adjustment under PQRS beginning in

2015. Specifically, those penalties will result in a payment adjustment in 2015 of 1.5 % of those providers' total Medicare payments. For 2016 and subsequent years, the payment adjustment is 2.0 % [30]. These two penalties mean that an LTC provider who fails to deliver on their PQRS and EHR requirements would see a 2.5 % reduction in their total 2015 Medicare payments; increasing to 3.0 % in 2016 [31].

For example, an LTC provider with $225,000 in Medicare payments would see a reduction of $5,625 in 2015 and $6,750 in 2016. It is important to note that while this number is deducted from total Medicare payments, it ultimately comes out of the physician's salary. In this example, an LTC provider previously collecting $225,000 in Medicare payments who has expenses of $50,000 for malpractice, billing, and other operating expenses, will take home less than $170,000 compared with $175,000. Avoiding these penalties will require LTC providers to submit the required documentation to CMS in a timely and accurate manner [7].

Summary

As a result of concern over escalating costs and care issues in the nation's SNF, the focus of regulation and payment has shifted to the attainment of better quality outcomes at less cost.

Changes in payment are occurring in every aspect of the Medicare system: Medicare A that covers the initial skilled stay within a nursing facility, physician services under Medicare Part B, Medicare managed care under Part C and the Medicare prescription drug program under Part D. Not only is payment reform occurring, but also improved reporting of data both to Medicare and to the public. Through the establishment of the Medicare Five Star Program hospital discharge planners, patients and their families can know better identify nursing facilities that deliver higher quality care and services.

Pearls for the Practitioner

- The Omnibus Reconciliation Act of 1987 (OBRA '87) was the beginning of focusing on quality outcomes in SNFs and NFs. Today, that is being continued and refocused through innovative delivery models of care promoted through the CMS Innovation Center.
- Changes in reporting quality data are occurring through the MDS and Medicare's Five Star Program.
- Care in nursing facilities is best delivered through an Interdisciplinary Team working in a coordinated manner within the local health care system.
- Knowledge of the benefits under Medicare's Parts A, B, C, and D is crucial to improve the development of relationships and processes between health care providers.
- Practitioners and nursing facilities need a positive attitude and work ethic toward future change in order to ensure their future success.

References

1. Payment/AcuteInpatientPPS/Readmissions-Reduction-Program.html. https://www.nhquality-campaign.org/files/Transition_of_Care_Reference.pdf.
2. Bureau of Labor Statistics. May, 2013. http://www.bls.gov/oes/current/oes291141.htm.
3. http://www.iom.edu/Reports/1986/Improving-the-Quality-of-Care-in-Nursing-Homes.aspx.
4. Nursing home reform: continued attention is needed to improve quality of care in small but significant share of facilities. Testimony before the Special Committee on Aging, US Senate. Washington, DC: General Accounting Office, 2007.
5. Morley JD. Rapid cycles, an essential part of the medical director's role. J Am Med Dir Assoc. 2008;8(1):535–8.
6. http://www.cms.gov/medicare/quality-initiatives-patient-assessment-instruments/nursing-homequalityinits/nhqiqualitymeasures.html.
7. http://www.cms.gov/Medicare/Provider-Enrollment-and-Certification/CertificationandComplianc/FSQRS.html.
8. Stefanacci RG. Determining the future of long-term care. Ann LTC. 2014;22:5.
9. Commission on Long-Term Care. Report to Congress. www.gpo.gov/fdsys/pkg/GPO-LTCCOMMISSION/pdf/GPO-LTCCOMMISSION.pdf. Published September 30, 2013. Accessed 28 Apr 2014.
10. Feinberg L, Reinhard SC, Houser A, Choula R. Valuing the invaluable: 2011 update the growing contributions and costs of family caregiving. http://assets.aarp.org/rgcenter/ppi/ltc/i51-caregiving.pdf. Accessed 16 Apr 2014.
11. O'Shaughnessy CV, National Health Policy Forum. National Spending for Long-Term Services and Supports (LTSS), 2012. www.nhpf.org/library/the-basics/ Basics_LTSS_03-27-14.pdf. Accessed 1 Feb 2013.
12. Skilled nursing facility services paymentbasics payment system. Revised, October, 2014. www.MEDPAC.gov.
13. Kripalani S, LeFevre F, Phillips CO, et al. Deficits in communication and information transfer between hospital-based and primary care physicians: implications for patient safety and continuity of care. JAMA. 2007;297(8):831–41. https://www.nhqualitycampaign.org/files/Transition_of_Care_Reference.pdf.
14. Lester P, Stefanacci RG, Chen DG. Nursing home procedures on transitions of care. J Am Med Dir Assoc. 2009;10(9):634–8.
15. Louden K. Creating a better discharge summary: is standardization the answer? ACP Hospitalist. 2009. http://www.acphospitalist.org/archives/2009/03/discharge.htm. Accessed 23 Feb 2010.
16. Snow V, Beck D, Budnitz T, et al. Transitions of care consensus policy statement: American College of Physicians, Society of General Internal Medicine, Society of Hospital Medicine, American Geriatrics Society, American College of Emergency Physicians, and Society for Academic Emergency Medicine. J Hosp Med. 2009;4:364–70.
17. Stefanacci RG. Long-term care regulatory and practice changes: impact on care, quality, and access. Ann LTC. 2014;22:11.
18. Bundled payments for care improvement initiative: general information. Centers for Medicare and Medicaid Services website. http://innovation.cms.gov/initiatives/bundled-payments. Accessed 8 Oct 2014.
19. Changes in ACO participants and ACO providers/suppliers during the agreement period. Centers for Medicare & Medicaid website. www.cms.gov/Medicare/Medicare-Fee-for-Service-Payment/sharedsavingsprogr. Updated 27 Aug 2014. Accessed 8 Oct 8 2014.
20. Delisle DR. Big things come in bundled packages: implications of bundled payment systems in health care reimbursement reform. Am J Med Qual. 2013;28(4):339–44.
21. O'Byrne TJ, Shah ND, Wood D, et al. Episode-based payment: evaluating the impact on chronic conditions. Medicare Medicaid Res Rev. 2013;3(3).

22. Chandra A, Dalton MA, Holmes J. Large increases in spending on postacute care in Medicare point to the potential for cost savings in these settings. Health Aff (Millwood). 2013;32(5): 864–72.
23. Bilimoria NM. ACOs and long-term care: it's all about readmissions. Readmissions News. 2013;2(2):1,5,6. www.setma.com/In-The-News/pdfs/Readmissions-News-Feb-2013. pdf. Accessed 8 Oct 2014.
24. Centers for Medicare & Medicaid Services. Medicaid managed care enrollment report: summary statistics as of July 1, 2011. www.medicaid.gov/Medicaid-CHIP-Program-Information/ By-Topics/Data-and-Systems/Medicaid-Managed-Care/Medicaid-Managed-Care-Enrollment-Report.html. Accessed 15 Oct 2014. See more at: http://www.annalsoflongtermcare.com/article/ long-term-care-regulatory-and-practice-changes-impact-care-quality-and-access#sthash. E7AAhu72.dpuf.
25. Federal coordinated health care office. Centers for Medicare & Medicaid website. www.cms. gov/About-CMS/Agency-Information/CMSLeadership/Office_FCHCO.html. Updated 1 Aug 2014. Accessed 15 Oct 2014.
26. Nursing home value-based purchasing demonstration. Centers for Medicare & Medicaid Services website. www.cms.gov/Medicare/demonstration-Projects/demoProjectsEvalRpts/ downdload. Accessed 15 Oct 2014.
27. Evaluation of the nursing home value-based purchasing demonstration: Year 3 and final evaluation report. Washington, DC: L&M Policy Research LLC, 2013. http://innovation.cms.gov/ Files/reports/NursingHomeVBP_EvalReport.pdf. Accessed October 15, 2014. - See more at: http://www.annalsoflongtermcare.com/article/long-term-care-regulatory-and-practice-changes-impact-care-quality-and-access#sthash.E7AAhu72.dpuf.
28. Are there penalties to providers who don't switch to electronic health records? HealthIT.gov. www.healthit.gov/providers-professionals/faqs/are-there-penalties-providers-who-don%E2%80%99t-switch-electronic-health-record. Updated 15 Jan 2013. Accessed 15 Oct 2014. See more at: http://www.annalsoflongtermcare.com/article/long-term-care-regulatory-and-practice-changes-impact-care-quality-and-access#sthash.E7AAhu72.dpuf.
29. Eligibility. Centers for Medicare & Medicaid website. www.cms.gov/Regulations-and-Guidance/Legislation/EHRIncentivePrograms/el.Updated May 2012. Accessed 15 Oct 2014.
30. Physician quality reporting system. Centers for Medicare & Medicaid Services website. www. cms.gov/Medicare/Quality-Initiatives-Patient-Assessment-Instruments/PQRS/index.html. Updated Jun 2014. Accessed 15 Oct 2014. See more at: http://www.annalsoflongtermcare. com/article/long-term-care-regulatory-and-practice-changes-impact-care-quality-and-access#sthash.E7AAhu72.dpuf.
31. Payment adjustment information. Centers for Medicare & Medicaid Services website. www. cms.gov/Medicare/Quality-Initiatives-Patient-Assessment-Instruments/PQRS/Payment-Adjustment-Information.html. Updated Sept 2014. Accessed 15 Oct 2014. See more at: http:// www.annalsoflongtermcare.com/article/long-term-care-regulatory-and-practice-changes-impact-care-quality-and-access#sthash.E7AAhu72.dpuf.

The Role of Practitioners and the Medical Director

Steven A. Levenson

Introduction

The role of nursing facilities in the USA has changed along with the health care system. Traditionally, nursing facilities had provided personal and nursing care in a residence primarily for cognitively and functionally impaired elderly. Today, while nursing facilities still provide this residential care, they now admit much more medically complex people from acute or specialty hospitals. These long-term care residents and post-acute care patients are often unstable and typically have multi-morbidities as well as risk factors for geriatric syndromes such as pressure ulcers, anorexia, and falling. Managing these patients requires the application of proficient clinical reasoning and problem solving skills. Accordingly, nursing facilities require more physician and practitioner involvement in assessing and managing their patients [1].

Long-term residents often need acute and chronic medical care and *short-stay patients* may have an extended stay or become long-term residents after completing their post-acute treatment. Persons who live in nursing facilities are commonly referred to as residents; those who come to nursing facilities primarily to receive short-term medical and skilled care after an acute care stay at the hospital are often referred to as patients. Physicians serve a vital role in providing nursing facility care, whether as a medical director, attending physician, or consultant. All are crucial to facilitate effective collaboration amongst the interdisciplinary team members because of their primary responsibility to the patient's medical care [2].

S.A. Levenson, MD, CMD (✉)
Genesis Healthcare, Baltimore, MD, USA
e-mail: salanlev@cs.com

© Springer International Publishing Switzerland 2016
P.A. Fenstemacher, P. Winn (eds.), *Post-Acute and Long-Term Medicine*, Current Clinical Practice, DOI 10.1007/978-3-319-16979-8_6

73

While many medical directors also serve as attending physicians, the roles and functions of a medical director are separate from those of an attending physician. The attending physician provides direct resident care; the medical director oversees and coordinates the facility's medical care and helps the facility oversee and improve its overall care and services.

As of 2015, Maryland has implemented substantial state regulations regarding expectation for the medical director and physicians [3]. Several other states have developed or in the process of developing requirements for increased oversight. Although concern related to physician performance and practice is enduring and widespread, opinions about the desirability and impact of such requirements are still mixed [4].

The Role of the Practitioner

Many community-based physicians have had a history of poor involvement in long-term care. While many physicians provide high quality care and clinical leadership, others have shown little interest in the care of the chronically ill and an unwillingness to take care of nursing facility residents [5]. Other physicians may lack pertinent knowledge about the care of the complex frail elderly patient or the clinical approaches required for post-acute and long-term medical care.

According to the regulatory requirements of the Omnibus Reconciliation Act of 1987, every nursing facility resident or patient must have an attending physician to supervise his or her medical care [6]. "Supervising the care" means participating in the assessment and management of patients, monitoring changes in their medical status, and providing consultation or treatment when needed. It also includes prescribing new treatment as indicated and conducting required routine visits or delegating and supervising nurse practitioners or physician assistant visits. In addition, it involves reviewing the pertinence and effectiveness of care provided by other physicians and licensed health care professionals and practitioners who provide care to their patients. Table 1 describes the basic physician functions and tasks based on federal OBRA '87 requirements.

Increasingly, physicians have a more intensive involvement with long-term and post-acute care facilities. Traditionally the practitioner who occasionally visited his or her patients and did the minimum *has changed* to one of active involvement to assess and provide in-depth management of patients, to avoid hospitalization wherever possible, and to address the many issues (for example, adequate diagnosis, delirium, medication-related complications) that arise before and after admission to a long-term and post-acute care facility. Currently, AMDA—The Society for Post-Acute and Long-Term Care Medicine is developing a curriculum and certification program for attending physicians covering diverse areas of physician competency and to promote a more uniform standard of practitioner knowledge and skill.

Table 1 Attending physician functions and tasks in the nursing facility based on Federal OBRA'87 regulations

Roles	Related functions and tasks
Supervise individual resident care	• Approve a resident's admission to the facility, e.g., this may be done by giving and approving orders upon admission • Be familiar with, and contribute to, a patient's assessment and care planning; e.g., by helping staff identify and manage underlying causes of impaired function and significant condition changes • Ensure that there is backup medical coverage if the attending physician is unavailable; e.g., by providing the facility with information about on-call coverage and addressing any issues with that coverage

Make resident visits	• Take an active role in supervising their patients' care
	• At the time of each visit:
	  – Review the total program of care, including medications and treatments rendered by other disciplines
	  – Write, sign, and date a progress note
	  – Sign and date all orders except immunization orders that may be periodic without a new order
	  – Evaluate the resident's condition and continued appropriateness of the current medical regimen

Make timely visits	• See a patient at least once every 30 days for the first 90 days after admission, and at least once every 60 thereafter (the next scheduled visit date should be determined by this interval, not by the actual date that the last visit occurred; a visit is timely if it occurs not later than 10 days after the date it was required) • Make all required physician visits personally (required visits after the initial visit may alternate between visits by the attending physician and visits by a physician assistant, nurse practitioner, or clinical nurse specialist under the physician's supervision)
Arrange for provision of emergency services	• Designate backup coverage; e.g., individual physician, physician group, or advance practice nurse • Ensure that backup coverage is available as needed • Address issues related to backup coverage, as needed by the facility
Delegate tasks appropriately	• Delegate tasks to physician assistants, nurse practitioners, or clinical nurse specialists consistent with OBRA'87 requirements and state requirements related to licensure and scope of practice

As the health care system changes, hospitals are partnering more with long-term and post-acute care facilities to develop integrated care models (see chapters "Behind the Scenes at Nursing Facilities" and "Preventing Hospital Admissions and Readmissions" for further discussion). In the process, more hospitalists are becoming involved in providing care in these non-hospital settings.

Table 2 identifies key practitioner responsibilities in long-term care that are integral to quality resident care [7]. The practitioner must work with the facility's leadership, usually its administrator and nursing staff as conflicts or problems arise.

Table 2 Practitioner's roles and related functions and tasks

Practitioner's role	Related functions and tasks
Accept responsibility for resident care	• Assess new admissions in a timely fashion
	• Seek, provide, and analyze information regarding a patient's current status, recent history, medications, and treatments
	• Provide information and documentation that helps staff determine appropriate level of care for a new admission
	• Authorize admission orders in a manner that enables the facility to provide safe, appropriate, and timely care
	• If pending transfer, continue to provide all necessary medical care and services, until another physician takes over the care
Support discharges and transfers	• Follow up, as needed, when an acutely ill or unstable patient is transferred from the facility
	• Provide necessary documentation and other information needed at the time of transfer to enable care continuity
	• Provide a pertinent discharge summary within 30 days of patient discharge or transfer from the nursing facility
Make periodic, pertinent resident visits	• Visit patients in a timely fashion, based on their needs and on regulatory requirements, including an alternate visit schedule as appropriate
	• Maintain progress notes that cover pertinent aspects of a patient's condition, current status, and goals
	• Review and approve a patient's treatment and care program
	• Determine a patient's medical condition and address active issues at visits
	• Respond to issues requiring a physician's expertise, such as diagnosis of causes of a recent condition changes and review of current medications and treatments for continued relevance and safety
	• Provide legible progress notes in a timely manner
Provide adequate ongoing coverage	• Designate alternate coverage
	• Update the facility about communicating with his/her practice and designated alternate coverage
	• Help ensure that alternate coverage provides adequate and timely support
	• Notify the facility of any extended absence and related coverage arrangements

Provide appropriate resident care	• Perform accurate, timely, and relevant medical assessments • Define and describe resident symptoms and problems, clarify and verify diagnoses, and help establish prognosis and realistic care goals • Help determine appropriate services and programs for the patient • Verify the medical necessity and appropriateness of treatments and services, including rehabilitation services, in accordance with relevant practice standards and regulatory requirements • Respond in an appropriate time frame to emergency and routine notification by staff • Analyze and address laboratory and other diagnostic test results • Assess and promptly manage significant acute changes in a patient's condition when notified • Guide ethics-related decisions (for example, options for life-sustaining treatments) • Order appropriate comfort and supportive measures as needed • Periodically review continued relevance of all prescribed medications for patients and identify and address possible medication-related adverse consequences
Provide appropriate and timely medical orders	• Provide timely and legible medical orders • Sign and verify the accuracy of verbal orders
Provide appropriate, timely, and pertinent documentation	• Document pertinent explanations of medical decisions, helping the facility comply with its legal and regulatory requirements • Complete all physician information required on death certificates in a timely manner
Perform and act appropriately	• Abide by pertinent facility and medical policies and procedures, and collaborate with the medical director/facility leadership to help the facility provide high-quality care • Contact the medical director/facility leadership about issues and concerns • Keep the well-being of patients in mind in all situations • Be alert to any observed or suspected violations of resident rights, including abuse or neglect • Interact in a courteous, professional manner with facility staff, patients/residents, family/significant others, facility employees, and management • Inform the medical director/facility leadership of disputes or problems or problems with other parties (e.g., staff, patients, or other practitioners) that the physician cannot readily resolve

Clinical Reasoning and Diagnostic Quality

Medical practitioners play a crucial role in a facility's care quality by their individual performance and practice as well as by influencing facility processes related to clinical decision making and cause identification.

Diverse disciplines (e.g., therapists, nurses, and dieticians) in long-term and post-acute care facilities must work collaboratively to solve clinical problems and to make clinical decisions. However, many clinical decisions are often made in other settings before patients are admitted to a long-term or post-acute care facility. Staff, patients, and families need to query whether the right decisions were made. Thus all disciplines have a great responsibility to think critically and act prudently. *The care delivery process is key to providing safe, effective, efficient, patient-centered, equitable, and timely evidence-based care.* Using the care delivery process of recognition, cause identification/diagnosis, management, monitoring and continual reassessment of response to treatment interventions is critical. The medical practitioner's role is to paint an accurate picture of the patient over time and to determine what is causing and contributing to illness and impairment. Patients often have symptoms that require a detailed and thoughtful differential diagnosis. Improving function and reducing or preventing further impairments is essential to the provision of *patient-centered care*.

Key steps in developing and implementing a patient-centered medical plan include:

1. Clarifying relevant medical issues (including physical and psychiatric conditions as well as patient prognosis).
2. Determining decision-making capacity.
3. Identifying the primary or proxy decision maker.
4. Identifying the "big picture."
5. Reviewing an individual's values, goals, wishes.
6. Reconciling patient goals and medical goals.
7. Ordering appropriate interventions.
8. Monitoring and when needed, adjusting those interventions.

All staff, practitioners and the medical director must support a culture of consistent care, competent clinical reasoning, and problem solving that actively supports the QAPI process. *Diagnostic quality* includes efforts to minimize and recognize diagnostic errors that contribute to adverse events. Facilities and medical practitioners should be able to recognize and distinguish between a proper and "misguided" care process where skipped critical steps lead to diagnostic errors and inappropriate or harmful treatment.

The Role of the Medical Director

Medical directors serve in various other settings, including hospitals, insurance companies, specialty programs or services (e.g., dialysis, hospice, wound care, PACE), and assisted living facilities (only some of which have a medical director).

However, medical directors are predominantly in nursing facilities as a result of federal regulation where the role of the medical director is defined as "a physician who oversees the medical care and other designated care and services in a health care organization or facility" [8].

Medical Director Characteristics

The background, characteristics, and performance of medical directors have been researched over the years [9, 10] and also investigated by AMDA: The Society for Post-Acute and Long-Term Care Medicine (formerly known as the American Medical Directors Association). In nursing homes, most medical directors have an internal medicine or family medicine background, and approximately 23 % are also geriatricians [11]. A medical director may cover one or several facilities. Although most medical directors also serve as attending physicians in their facilities, a significant number act solely as a medical director with no individual patient care responsibilities.

Origins of the Medical Director Role

The need for a nursing facility medical director concept evolved out of government investigations stemming from a 1970 salmonella outbreak in a Maryland nursing facility [12, 13]. In the 1970s, the American Medical Association's Committee on Aging attempted to define the roles and functions of a medical director and promoted educating physicians about these basic roles and responsibilities [14]. By 1974, every skilled nursing facility (those certified to provide skilled nursing services to Medicare beneficiaries) was required to retain a full- or part-time medical director [15].

The 1987 Omnibus Budget Reconciliation Act (OBRA) and its related regulations expanded the medical director requirements to include residential as well as skilled portions of nursing facilities. For regulatory purposes, both skilled and residential facilities were referred to as "nursing facilities." Subsequently, surveyor guidance (as written in 42 CFR 483.75(i) Medical Director [F501]) has clarified expectations. Beginning in the late 1980s and early 1990s, physicians serving as medical directors [16, 17] and their representative organization (AMDA) [18] have reviewed and summarized information and perspectives on medical direction. In 2001, the Institute of Medicine recommended that nursing facility medical directors be given greater authority and that structures and processes be developed not only to enable but also to require a more focused and dedicated physician participation [19].

Key Medical Director Responsibilities

Based on these initiatives, there are now regulatory and professional organizations that have developed the *medical director's roles and responsibilities*. Collaboration among physician organizations and regulatory agencies has helped to make those requirements more consistent throughout the USA. In contrast, requirements for medical direction in assisted living facilities vary among states. As of 2015, most states did not require a medical director in assisted living facilities.

Regulatory Foundation

Federal regulations require everynursing facilityin the USA to retain a physician to serve as its medical director. The primary source of medical director regulations is OBRA '87 and the State Operations Manual on surveyor guidance; but there may also be some individual state regulations regarding medical director's responsibilities [20]. Federal nursing facility regulations divide requirements into discrete segments called "F-Tags," related to one or more specific regulatory requirements and used for state and Federal survey purposes.

A specific section of federal regulations (F-Tag 501) cover the roles and responsibilities of the medical director. The actual regulations regarding medical direction are brief, requiring that the *medical director is responsible for implementation of resident care policies and coordination of medical care in the facility.* Surveyor guidance provides additional information and instructions on how to survey a facility for compliance with federal regulations, including that of the medical director (F-Tag 501) (Table 3) [21]. A nursing facility can be cited for a deficiency if it does not have a medical director who is fulfilling these requirements. F-Tag 501 cannot be cited alone, but would be attached to another F-Tag deficiency if the latter was found to be at least *partially attributable to noninvolvement of the medical director.* Table 3 summarizes the guidance for surveyors to interpret whether facilities meet the requirements of F-Tag 501.

F-Tag 501 surveyor guidance emphasizes the medical director's role in helping facilities identify *whether their care is consistent with current standards of practice.* The guidance defines "current standards of practice" as "approaches to care, procedures, techniques, treatments, etc., that are based on research and/or expert consensus and that are contained in current manuals, textbooks, or publications, or that are accepted, adopted or promulgated by recognized professional organizations or national accrediting bodies" [21]. *The facility is expected to obtain the medical director's input into all clinical policies, including services provided by other disciplines.*

Table 3 Medical director responsibilities based on F-Tag 501

Roles	Related functions and tasks

Coordination of medical care	• Help the facility obtain and maintain timely and appropriate medical care that:
	  – Supports the health care needs of the residents
	  – Is consistent with current standards of practice
	  – Helps the facility meet its regulatory requirements.
	• Help the facility identify, evaluate, and address/resolve medical and clinical concerns and issues that:
	  – Affect resident care, medical care, or quality of life
	  – Are related to the provision of services by physicians and other licensed health care practitioners
	• Help the facility develop a process to review basic physician and health care practitioner credentials (e.g., licensure and pertinent background)
	• Help the facility develop systems to ensure that other licensed practitioners (e.g., nurse practitioners) who may perform physician-delegated tasks act within the regulatory requirements and within the scope of practice as defined by State law
	• Help the facility ensure that residents have primary attending and backup physician coverage

Implementation of resident care policies	• Collaborate with facility leadership, staff, and other practitioners and consultants to help develop, implement, and evaluate resident care policies and procedures that reflect current standards of practice • Review and help revise existing policies • Provide clinical leadership regarding application of current standards of practice for resident care and new or proposed treatments, practices, and approaches to care • Advise on availability, qualifications, and clinical functions of staff necessary to meet resident care needs
Support for improving quality of care	• Help coordinate and evaluate the medical care within the facility • Review and evaluate aspects of practitioner care and services • Help the facility identify, evaluate, and address health care issues related to the quality of care and quality of life of residents • Promote attainment of optimal resident outcomes • Guide facility staff regarding when to contact a practitioner, including information that should be gathered prior to contacting the practitioner for a clinical issue/question or change in condition
Survey-related support	• Provide input to surveyors on physician issues, individual residents' clinical issues, and the facility's clinical practices • Clarify for surveyors clinical questions or information about the care of specific residents • Attend exit conference or otherwise demonstrate interest and help the facility analyze the nature and scope of its deficiencies • Help the facility identify corrective actions for survey citations

Professional Foundations of the Medical Director Role

Medical director responsibilities have also originated from the recommendations of professional associations. AMDA is a national organization that represents long-term care medical directors and other practitioners and has produced consensus statements on many topics including medical director roles and related functions and tasks (Table 4) [22]. AMDA recommendations go beyond those delineated in the federal regulations to include aspects of medical direction that this organization has identified as vital for high quality medical direction in LTC.

Table 4 Medical director responsibilities as identified by AMDA

Role	Related functions and tasks
Physician leadership	• Help ensure appropriate physician coverage and provision of physician and health care practitioner services • Help develop a process for reviewing practitioner credentials • Give the practitioners performance expectations • Help develop and implement a system to monitor practitioner performance and give the practitioners feedback
Patient care/clinical leadership	• Help develop policies and procedures related to resident care • Help identify specific clinical practices for the facility to incorporate into its care-related policies • Help guide staff about contacting practitioners and the medical director • Review and consider consultant recommendations that affect the facility's care-related policies and procedures or individual resident care • Help protect resident rights, including advance care planning and other ethical issues
Quality of care	• Review and be available for external surveys and inspections • Help develop effective ways to review the quality and appropriateness of clinical care and services • Participate in quality improvement processes • Advise on infection control issues and approve specific infection control policies • Help the facility provide a safe and caring environment • Help promote employee health and safety • Help develop and implement employee health policies and programs
Education, information, and communication	• Promote a learning culture within the facility • Provide information to help the facility provide care consistent with current standards of practice • Help develop medical information and communication systems • Represent the facility to the professional and lay community on medical and resident care issues • Maintain knowledge of social, regulatory, political, and economic factors that affect medical and health services of long term care residents • Help establish appropriate relationships with other health care organizations

Medical Director Relationships with Practitioners

The medical director is responsible for the coordination of medical care in the facility. As identified in the federal surveyor guidance for F-Tag 501, the medical director "helps the facility obtain and maintain timely and appropriate medical care that supports the healthcare needs of the residents, is consistent with current standards of practice, and helps the facility meet its regulatory requirements" [21].

The medical director is expected to help the facility:

- Ensure that residents have primary attending and backup physician coverage
- Obtain physician and other health care practitioner services to help residents attain and maintain their highest practicable level of functioning, consistent with regulatory requirements
- Develop a process to review basic physician and health care practitioner credentials (e.g., licensure and pertinent background)
- Address and resolve concerns and issues between the physicians, health care practitioners, and facility staff
- Help the facility address issues related to continuity of care and transfer of medical information and patients between the facility and other care settings.

The medical director needs to define the lines of accountability between the administration, governing body or owner, and the physicians. According to the OBRA'87 surveyor guidance, *practitioners are responsible to the medical director for their performance and practice.* As with the medical director, physicians may also be accountable to others for their performance as attending physicians; for example, a program director in academia or a supervisor of a group practice. In order to oversee physician practice and care, the medical director must clarify practitioner responsibilities and performance expectations. Therefore, the medical director must understand and convey federal and state requirements (e.g., requirements for frequency of patient visits), facility policies, and related standards of practice to the physicians and other practitioners who provide care in the facility.

Practitioner Responsibilities

The medical director clarifies practitioner responsibilities by:

- Promulgating expectations
- Explaining how to fulfill those expectations
- Establishing criteria for satisfactory performance
- Determining whether those expectations are being met
- Giving practitioners feedback on their performance and practice.

Practitioner responsibilities in nursing facilities relate to the needs of the population and to the specific requirements of the practice setting. Medical practice in long-term care is a hybrid of ambulatory, office-based, and hospital-based practice. Nursing facility residents and SNF patients are often medically complex. Their care often involves those of other disciplines in assessment and monitoring, identifying problems, and conveying concerns to the physician.

Assisted living residents may be less functionally impaired and medically complex. Assisted living facilities typically have fewer direct care staff than do nursing homes.

The medical director provides clinical leadership by educating practitioners about providing care in the proper context. Medical care must take into account the expectation that facilities are to identify and to address various risk factors (e.g., impaired nutrition, fall risk) and to explain the basis for clinical decisions that impact outcomes (e.g., decisions not to hospitalize, choice of medications and treatments). Clinicians who recognize these factors can be more supportive and provide more effective medical care compared to those who are not.

The medical director helps the facility educate and inform the staff and practitioners about medical conditions and current geriatrics practices. Appropriate clinical practices for the long-term care population have been identified and discussed in the literature for several decades [23]. Practitioners should try to minimize complications (secondary and tertiary prevention), including those related to iatrogenic illness. In conjunction with the staff, the medical director identifies clinical conditions and risks pertinent to the facility's population such as adverse drug events (ADEs), common causes of acute changes in condition, fall risks, exacerbation of heart failure, altered mental status, and decline in function. The medical director's clinical knowledge and understanding of a *facility's case mix* can help the facility develop relevant policies and procedures. The medical director and attending physicians also have an essential role in promoting diagnostic quality in the facility and in effectively diagnosing causes of symptoms in individual patients.

The Medical Director's Relationship with the Facility

*The administrator, director of nursing, and medical director are the key management leadership in the nursing facility.*The management leadership is ultimately responsible for the facility's care processes and practices. Unlike a medical staff president or chief of staff, who primarily represents the physicians to a facility or organization, a medical director in LTC plays a meaningful role for the facility as well the practitioners.

Through its administrator, a facility should guide their physician leader on how to perform the job of medical director. The facility leadership must know what is needed from their medical director (and vice versa) by understanding regulatory requirements and professional recommendations that affect the medical director's responsibilities. Across the country, medical director performance varies considerably. Many facilities are still challenged to find qualified and competent attending physicians and medical directors. In other settings, physicians may find themselves stymied in trying to assert themselves to improve practices and hold practitioners accountable.

The OBRA '87 surveyor guidance does not specify how a nursing facility must arrange for medical director services. It simply requires that each nursing facility designate a medical director who must be currently licensed as a physician in the state where the facility is located. The facility may employ or contract directly with the medical director, or may contract with a company or academic program that employs the physician. In multi-facility organizations, arrangements for such services may be made by corporate or regional offices, and policies may be developed at a corporate level. In these instances, it is still expected that medical director will be involved in their facility to ensure that clinical policies are applied appropriately.

It is desirable for the medical director to develop a job description in conjunction with the administrator. This job description should describe specific functions and tasks of the medical director and should be developed after reviewing the facility's needs, as well as required and desired medical director responsibilities. A medical director should review the job description and consider whether it is realistic, pertinent, and clearly delineates expectations. The facility should give the medical director adequate support and compensation. Facilities may have diverse criteria for choosing a medical director and may vary in their expectations of the medical director. For example, some facilities are primarily interested in physicians who will fulfill medical director roles regardless of whether they also provide primary patient care, while many facilities want the medical director to be the attending physician for a number of residents and a referral source for their facility.

Medical directors need facility support to fulfill their job responsibilities. As pointed out in the OBRA '87 surveyor guidance on medical direction, the medical director may not have control over some things that influence outcomes; e.g., the performance of nursing and other disciplines. A facility can also assist the medical director by creating an environment conducive to practicing competent medicine. For example, before contacting a practitioner, the staff should be expected to:

• Perform proper assessments and coordinate phone calls.
• Provide accurate information to describe a situation in detail.
• Be prepared to answer the physician's questions about the patient.
• Know what questions to ask the physician.
• Know when to notify the medical director about physician issues and clinical concerns.

The Medical Director's Role in Facility Quality

Increasing attention is being paid to measuring quality in all health care settings. This is being done for several reasons, including trying to improve overall results, improve patient satisfaction and safety, and identify and focus on care that makes a difference and reduce wasted resources. Medical directors are a key part of a facility's management, in that they oversee and coordinate medical care. They should also be considered part of a facility's leadership, in that they help clarify and support the goals and objectives of care, help the organization articulate and strive to meet its goals, show the staff and practitioners how to achieve desired performance, help solve and prevent problems, and help improve employee and patient health, safety, and welfare. There is some evidence of the medical director's potential impact on facility quality. For example, facilities with a certified medical director (a medical director who has met the AMDA's certification requirements) have been shown to have greater improvements in their quality results as compared to nursing facilities that do not have a certified medical director [24].

Surveyor guidance related to F-tag 501 acknowledges that various factors influence optimal outcomes, such as resident characteristics and preferences, individual attending physician actions, and facility support. The medical director should help the facility identify and address potentially remediable issues such as the impact of physician performance and practices. The medical director should guide the facility in determining whether clinical policies and protocols are consistent with applicable standards of medical and geriatric practice.

The medical director can learn much about regulatory expectations for facilities as well as details about his or her role as medical director by reviewing in some detail CMS' State Operations Manual (SOM) for surveyors, which guides state survey agencies about how to assess every nursing home for regulatory compliance. Doing this review can help the medical director understand the basis for facility and staff approaches to care and identify whether the care a facility provides has a clinically sound foundation or may be based on misinterpretation of regulations.

The medical director can also refer to various resources to better understand the efforts to improve quality and to compare performance of his or her facility to benchmarks and the performance of other facilities in areas such as staffing and rehospitalization. One example is CMS' "Nursing Home Compare" website (https://www.medicare.gov/nursinghomecompare) that reports quality measures data based on the Minimum Data Set (MDS), as well as staffing and compliance (i.e., survey deficiencies).

In addition, the medical director should engage in case reviews along with other disciplines, looking for care quality and safety issues that not identified by aggregate quality measures. The medical director should provide guidance on risk management concerns such as adverse drug events, medication errors, and falls; review accidents and incidents; and advise on infection control issues by providing input on specific infection control policies and practices.

The medical director can help the facility identify *internal quality measures* such as rates of unplanned hospital transfers and the incidence of adverse drug events. The medical director should be able to help staff review and discuss quality data and educate them on clinical topics such as pressure ulcers, pain management, and unplanned weight loss as part of the quality assurance process and at quality assurance meetings. The medical director can also help a facility develop and implement a program to evaluate the care and performance of physicians and other licensed health care practitioners whom the medical director oversees.

The medical director helps the facility ensure that all the patients receive adequate and appropriate medical care. When needed, the medical director may intervene directly in the care of other physicians' patients by examining a patient or giving orders. For example, medical director intervention may be needed if another practitioner does not respond in a timely manner to notification of a significant acute change of condition, or if a physician is acting in a manner that impedes facility compliance with legal and regulatory requirements.

Pearls for the Practitioner

- Physicians play an important role in long-term care, both in providing direct care and in providing oversight as medical directors.
- Expectations for performance and practice for both practitioners and medical directors come from both regulatory and professional sources, and have increasingly become more uniform and widely known.
- Collectively, the physicians and medical director play a vital role in supporting care quality, including clinical reasoning, problem solving, and diagnostic quality.
- A facility's approach to its practitioners greatly influences the success of practitioner participation and, in turn, many aspects of the facility's results. This includes—but is not limited to—support for the medical director and holding practitioners accountable for resident care.
- Practitioners should view their roles in the proper context, related to both the system in which they operate and to medical decision making about individual residents.
- Clinician performance and participation have varied substantially over the years, ranging from excellent to highly problematic, but expectations are now increasing.
- Changes in the health care system and the increasing provision of post-acute care as well as the initiatives to reduce hospitalizations from nursing homes has required increased and more dedicated physician involvement
- The medical director can have a major impact on a facility's care, by influencing both the facility's practices and the practitioners' performance.
- The medical director is accountable to the facility administrator while licensed health care practitioners and attending physicians should be accountable to the medical director.

- The medical director informs and educates practitioners on expectations and reviews and gives feedback on performance.
- Effective medical direction and attending physician care can go far towards improving and sustaining high quality care.

References

1. Levenson SA. Subacute care. In: Capezuti E, Siegler G, Mezey MD, editors. The encyclopedia of elder care. 2nd ed. New York: Springer; 2007.
2. Dimant J. Roles and responsibilities of attending physicians in skilled nursing facilities. J Am Med Dir Assoc. 2003;4:231.
3. Boyce BF, Bob H, Levenson SA. The preliminary impact of Maryland's medical director and attending physician regulations. J Am Med Dir Assoc. 2003;4:157.
4. Levenson SA. The impact of laws and regulations in improving physician performance and care processes in long-term care. J Am Med Dir Assoc. 2004;5:268.
5. Mitchell JB, Hewes HT. Why won't physicians make nursing facility visits? The Gerontologist. 1986;26:650.
6. Centers for Medicare and Medicaid Services (CMS). State operations manual: Appendix PP - guidance to surveyors for long term care facilities, Revision 52. Physician Services (F483.40). http://www.cms.hhs.gov/manuals/downloads/som107ap_pp_guidelines_ltcf.pdf.
7. Levenson SA. Medical Director and Attending Physicians Policy and Procedure Manual for Long-term Care. Dayton, OH: Med-Pass; 2013.
8. http://www.cms.hhs.gov/manuals/downloads/som107ap_pp_guidelines_ltcf.pdf
9. Zimmer JG, Watson NM, Levenson SA. Nursing facility medical directors: ideals and realities. J Am Geriatr Soc. 1993;41:127.
10. Department of Health and Human Services, Office of Inspector General. Nursing facility medical directors survey. http://oig.hhs.gov/oei/reports/oei-06-99-00300.pdf
11. Resnick HE, Manard B, Stone RI, Castle NG. Tenure, certification, and education of nursing facility administrators, medical directors, and directors of nursing in for-profit and not-for-profit nursing facilities: United States 2004. J Am Med Dir Assoc. 2009;10:423.
12. Gladue JR. Evolution of the Medical Director concept. J Am Geriatr Soc. 1974;22:43.
13. Reichel W. Role of the medical director in the skilled nursing facility: historical perspectives. In: Reichel W, editor. Clinical aspects of aging, vol. 570. 2nd ed. Baltimore: Williams and Wilkins; 1983.
14. Gruber HW. The medical director in the nursing facility - a catalyst for quality care. J Am Geriatr Soc. 1977;25:497.
15. HEW guidelines and survey procedures--medical director. J Am Health Care Assoc. 1975;1:29.
16. Levenson SA. Medical direction in long-term care. a guidebook for the future. 2nd ed. Durham, NC: Carolina Academic Press; 1993.
17. Pattee JJ, Otteson O. Medical direction in the nursing facility. Minneapolis: Northridge Press; 1991.
18. Pattee JJ, Altemeier TM. Results of a consensus conference on the role of the nursing facility medical director. Annu Med Direct. 1991;1(1):5.
19. Institute of Medicine. Improving the quality of long-term care. Washington, DC: National Academy Press; 2001.
20. Levenson SA. The Maryland regulations: rethinking physician and medical director accountability in nursing facilities. J Am Med Dir Assoc. 2002;3:79.

21. Centers for Medicare and Medicaid Services (CMS). State operations manual: Appendix PP - guidance to surveyors for long term care facilities, Revision 52. F501- Medical Director (F483.75(I). http://www.cms.hhs.gov/manuals/downloads/som107ap_pp_guidelines_ltcf.pdf

22. American Medical Directors Association. Roles and responsibilities of the medical director in the nursing facility: position statement A03. J Am Med Dir Assoc. 2005;6:411.

23. Ouslander JG. Medical care in the nursing facility. JAMA. 1989;262:2582.

24. Rowland FN, Cowles M, Dickstein C, Katz PR. Impact of medical director certification on nursing facility quality of care. J Am Med Dir Assoc. 2009;10:431.

Nurse Practitioners, Clinical Nurse Specialists, and Physician Assistants

Pamela Z. Cacchione and Reshma Shah

Introduction

Nursing facility residents' care needs have become more complex [1]. In part, this may be due to more options for community-based care such as adult day service centers and Programs of All-inclusive Care for the Elderly (PACE). Residents in nursing facilities are often the most vulnerable elderly due to multi-morbidities, neurocognitive disorders, and psychosocial issues. The complexity of resident needs coupled with the increased burden on physicians providing care in long-term care has increased awareness on the need for physician, nurse practitioner and physician assistant collaboration to enhance medical care in nursing facilities [2].

Nurse practitioners are Registered Nurses (with a Baccalaureate degree in nursing and duly licensed as registered nurses) who have then obtained either a Master's degree of nursing (MSN) or a clinical doctoral degree as a Doctor of Nursing Practice (DNP). The DNP was developed in order to recognize professional parity with those pharmacists and physical therapists that have acquired a clinical doctorate. Nurse practitioners with a DNP have additional education and clinical training

P.Z. Cacchione, PhD, CRNP, BC, FGSA, FAAN (✉)
Department of Family and Community Health, University of Pennsylvania,
418 Curie Blvd., Philadelphia, PA 19194, USA
e-mail: pamelaca@nursing.upenn.edu

R. Shah, MBBS
Living Independently For Elders (LIFE), University of Pennsylvania,
4508 Chestnut Street, Philadelphia, PA 19139, USA
e-mail: drreshmashah@gmail.com

© Springer International Publishing Switzerland 2016
P.A. Fenstemacher, P. Winn (eds.), *Post-Acute and Long-Term Medicine*,
Current Clinical Practice, DOI 10.1007/978-3-319-16979-8_7

related to quality improvement, leadership, and health policy. Nurse practitioners who commonly practice in nursing facilities are usually a gerontological, adult, adult-gerontological, or family NP. Recently the psychiatric mental health Clinical Nurse Specialist education *has been switched to that of a* psychiatric mental health *nurse practitioner* education at both the MSN and DNP level. Nurse practitioners have greater than 6 years of academic and clinical training [3].

Advanced practice nurses, both nurse practitioners (NP) and clinical nurse specialists (CNS) are associated with improvements in several measures of health and behavior of residents in long-term care as well as improvements in family satisfaction [4]. The NP and CNS are autonomous and collaborative members of the interdisciplinary team who can enhance the accessibility and quality of primary care in nursing facilities, and serve as a resource to the nursing staff who are challenged by the increasingly complex needs of residents [5].

There are over 205,000 NPs licensed in the USA [3]. Of these only 2.8 % work in long-term care facilities. The majority work in primary care settings [6]. Nurse practitioners are trained to perform complete histories and physical exams, diagnose and treat acute illness, and manage chronic conditions. Nurse practitioners can order and interpret laboratory tests, diagnostic reports such as X-rays, Doppler studies, and cardiac studies. Nurse practitioners are skilled in primary, secondary, and tertiary prevention including immunizations. They can prescribe medication including controlled substances depending on state regulations. NP's also provide health teaching, anticipatory guidance, and supportive counseling to patients [6, 7]. As of 2015, there were 22 *full practice states* with practice and licensure law allowing NPs to evaluate patients, diagnose, order and interpret diagnostic tests, initiate and manage treatments, including prescribing medications (under the licensure authority of the state boards of nursing). This is the model that has been recommended by the Institute of Medicine and National Council of State Boards of Nursing [8]. Additionally there are 17 states with *reduced practice*, meaning the state practice and licensure law reduces the ability of NPs to engage independently in at least one element of NP practice. These States require a regulated *collaborative agreement* with another health discipline in order for the NP to provide patient care [8]. The remaining 12 states have *restricted practice* due to state practice and licensure laws those restrict the ability of a NP to engage in at least one element of NP practice. Some States require supervision, delegation or team-management by an outside health discipline in order for the NP to provide patient care [8]. The map showing which states fit into these different categories can be found at http://www.aanp.org/component/content/article/66-legislation-regulation/state-practice-environment/1380-state-practice-by-type

It is essential when collaborating with a NP or CNS to have a thorough understanding of their scope of practice. The Institute of Medicine report *The Future of Nursing*: *Leading change*, *Advancing Health* acknowledged that nurses should practice to the full extent of their education, training and scope of practice in order to best meet our nation's health care needs [7]. This report also emphasized that nurses should be full practice partners with physicians.

Partnering with a Nurse Practitioner or Physician Assistant

With NPs as members of the primary care team, nursing facility residents can better achieve health care goals without adding to the cost of care. Another study that looked at the impact of both NPs and physician assistants (PAs) in long term care demonstrated reduced hospital use and costs [9]. The Evercare program has shown that nursing facilities having an NP managing resident's care had half the number of hospitalizations of nursing facilities that did *not* have NP managing the resident's care [10]. NPs can recognize and improve quality and accessibility of primary health care services for an ever-increasing complex resident population by being approachable and respectful of patient, family, and staff [11]. Nursing staff trusts NPs and value their knowledge [11, 12]. Consistent with other studies in primary care [4], NPs in nursing facilities care for the majority of the day-to-day needs and concerns of residents and families. Recent meta-analysis studies and systematic reviews have demonstrated the following *positive results of NP practice in long-term care*:

- High patient satisfaction, decreased hospitalizations, and decreased all cause mortality compared to physician alone practices [13].
- Reduced hospitalizations and emergency department transfers [14].
- Lower rates of depression, urinary incontinence, pressure ulcers, use of restraint, and aggressive behaviors in the residents [4].
- Practice with a high degree of collaboration with the interprofessional team [5].
- Provide leadership activities within nursing facility including educating the interdisciplinary staff, quality improvement, facilitating evidence-based practice and implementing practice innovation [5].

Clinical Nurse Specialists

Clinical Nurse Specialists (CNS) are nurses with a Master's degree who have specialized in a particular area of clinical nursing and though most frequently employed in Magnet hospitals, they can have a significant positive impact when working in post-acute and long-term care. These advanced practice nurses are clinical nursing experts in the diagnosis and treatment of illness, health promotion and implementation of evidence based practice in a given population [15]. The presence of a CNS in a long term care facility has been shown to reduce urinary incontinence, pressure ulcers, aggressive behavior, use of restraints (both physical and pharmacological), decrease fall related injuries, and improved affect in cognitively impaired residents. The domains of the CNS role that contributed to these improved outcomes were education and consultation with the staff [4]. Adult and gerontological CNSs are expanding their practice in wound care, quality improvement, and education and leadership positions within long-term care settings. Psychiatric mental health CNS and NPs are trained in behavioral management in persons afflicted with dementia and can assist in the management of residents with serious mental illness.

Physician Assistants

There are over 100,000 Physician Assistants (PAs) working currently in the USA and this number is projected to increase by 38 % by the year 2022 [16]. In 2013, a national survey by the American Academy of Physician Assistants, reported that 0.9 % of PAs were employed by a nursing facility or other long-term care facility [17]. PA training programs are commonly located at medical schools, hospitals and other health care facilities. Teaching sessions and clinical rotations are often taken alongside medical students. This helps to cultivate a future close working relationship between these two groups of professionals.

The first year of the 26-month long PA program covers the basic medical sciences followed by clinical rotations in all major medical specialties. Having over 2000 h of clinical skill training, PAs are well suited to perform histories and physical exams, diagnose, order, interpret investigations and manage acute and chronic conditions, *in collaboration with physicians* [18]. To be able to practice as a PA, one must pass the Physician Assistant National Certifying Exam (PANCE) and pursue continuing education in order to recertify every 10 years [19].

Each PA's scope of practice is defined by four parameters: *education & experience, state law, facility policy and the needs of the patients.* Each must be met in order to promote effective patient-centered care [20]. PAs are expected to perform patient care tasks at a similar skill level and competency as a physician. However, state boards do not require the PA to be proficient in any specific tasks. Although PAs are ultimately responsible for their own practice, in cases of medical malpractice or professional misconduct, the collaborative physician and the long-term care facility could be held liable [21].

Collaboration does not necessarily require the constant presence of the physician. In fact in some rural areas the PA is the patient's primary care provider with the supervising physician "checking-in" once or twice a week [22]. The PA's scope of practice continues to grow, adapting to changes within the medical profession and states' legislatures. *It is imperative that the supervising physicians and the long-term care facility employer keep abreast of the changing regulations.*

Prescribing Privileges

A significant difference in prescribing privileges should be noted between NPs and PAs. Currently all states allow PAs to prescribe as long as a physician is either directly involved or available. Most commonly this association is through *delegation* (19 states) and *authorization* (18 states) with the rest (13 states) specifying a physician be involved directly in a *supervisory nature*. Only Arizona has *specified collaboration* [23]. *In contrast, 24 states allow NPs to have prescriptive authority* where states have regulations allowing NPs to diagnose and treat patients

Table 1 DEA classification of scheduled drugs [24]

Schedule	Medical use/effects	Abuse potential	Examples
I	• No medical use • Research use only	Highest	Heroin, Marihuana, LSD, MDMA
II/IIN	• Severe psychic or physical dependence liability • Narcotic, Stimulant, Depressant drugs	High	*Narcotic*: Opium, Codeine, Hydromorphone, Methadone, Hydrocodone *Non-narcotic*: Amphetamine, Methamphetamine, Nabilone
III/IIIN	• Moderate or Low psychical or physical dependency	High	Narcotic: Acetaminophen with Codeine, Buprenorphine Non-narcotic: Ketamine, Anabolic steroids
IV	• Limited psychological or physical dependency	Low	Chlordiazepoxide, Diazepam, Barbital, Phenobarbital, Clorazepate, Alprazolam
V	• Over the counter or prescription drugs with limited amounts of narcotics • Used for analgesic, antitussive, antidiarrheal	Lowest	Buprenorphine, Propylhexedrine

independently [23]. The remaining states require varying levels of collaboration, delegation, and supervision. Prescribing of scheduled drugs is regulated and enforced by individual states through the Drug Enforcement Agency (DEA) (Table 1).

Controlled (scheduled) drug prescribing is allowed for PAs in the majority of states through their collaborative practice with physicians. However, 15 states restrict this privilege to schedule III–V. Florida and Kentucky do not allow for any controlled substance to be prescribed by a PA. All states (except for Florida) allow NPs to prescribe controlled substances: the majority of states allow Schedule II through V; however, 8 states restrict this to Schedule III through V [8, 23].

*The registration procedure with the DEA is the same for all Advanced Practitioners who are designated as "**mid-level practitioners**" by this agency.* After successfully completing all requirements imposed by the state in which they will practice and successfully receiving a state license, mid-level practitioners are able to apply for a DEA registration via Form 224a. Subsequently they will receive a DEA number beginning with "M" [25].

There is a significant lack of PAs practicing in long-term care even though 20 % work in primary care. To date, it appears that PA schools have shown a propensity to fill gaps in orthopedics, urgent care, and in-patient care. Data has shown that PAs have a favorable attitude towards the elderly and would welcome incorporation of a rotation in long-term care during their training as a means to increase their knowledge in geriatrics [26].

Collaboration

How and when to develop *Collaborative Practice Agreements* is beyond the scope of this chapter; however, some general comments are important. *Interprofessional team care is becoming the gold standard in long-term care.* Within this concept, team members include physicians, Advanced Practice Nurses (NPs and CNS), and PAs. Currently NP and CNS can work independently (depending upon state regulations), whereas PAs at this time must work in collaboration with a physician. There are *six models of care* in collaborative NP/ physician practice at long-stay nursing facilities: collaborator, clinician, care coordinator/manager, coach/educator, counselor, and communicator/cheerleader [26, 27]. Combining these models of care can create synergy that rewards the physician, NP, residents, resident families, facilities, and staff. *There are at least seven different forms of collaboration* in practice which include (1) NP hired by the physician; (2) NP and physician both employed by the long-term care setting; (3) NP contracted (self-employed) or employed by an NP practice; (4) NP employed directly by the nursing facility; (5) NP employed by the payer (e.g., Optum); (6) NP in a specialty collaborative practice that includes consulting; and (7) NP in independent practice employs a physician [28].

It is encouraging to see the progress that has been made in acknowledging the crucial role that advanced practitioners play in the realm of long term care and geriatric practice. In 2014, AMDA—The Society for Post-Acute and Long-Term Care Medicine, House of Delegates, voted to permit full membership to NPs and PAs. This resolution allows NPs and PAs to stand for board positions and to contribute their expertise to improving patient care [29].

Resources for developing collaborative practice agreements can be found through professional organizations including AMDA—The Society of Post-Acute and Long Term Care Medicine (www.amda.com), the Gerontological Advanced Practice Nurses Association (www.gapna.org), the American Association of Nurse Practitioners (www.aanp.org), and American Academy of Physician Assistants (www.aapa.org).

Pearls for the Practitioner

- Nurse practitioners and clinical nurse specialists are autonomous collaborative members of the interprofessional team in both post-acute and long-term care settings.
- Nurse practitioners scope of practice ranges from state to state: full practice, reduced practice, and restricted practice.
- Physician assistant scope of practice is determined by education/training, experience, state law, and facility policy.
- Prescribing privileges differ between NPs and PAs and from state to state.
- The DEA designates NPs and PAs as "mid-level practitioners."
- Collaborative practice agreements are often necessary for NPs, CNSs, and PAs.

References

1. Bakerjian D. Care of nursing home residents by advanced practice nurses: a review of the literature. Res Gerontol Nurs. 2008;1(3):177–85. doi:10.3928/00220124-20091301-01.
2. Caprio TV. Physician practice in the nursing home: collaboration with nurse practitioners and physician assistants. Ann Long Term Care. 2006;14(3):17–24.
3. American Association of Nurse Practitioners. NP Fact Sheet. 2015. http://www.aanp.org/all-about-nps/np-fact-sheet. Accessed 11 Jun 2015.
4. Donald F, Martin-Misener R, Carter N, Donald EE, Kaasalaienen S, Wickson-Griffiths A, DiCenso A. A systematic review of the effectiveness of advanced practice nurses in long-term care. J Adv Nurs. 2013;69(10):2148–61. doi:10.1111/jan.12140.
5. Martin-Misener R, Donald F, Wickson-Griffiths A, Akhtar-Danesh N, Ploeg J, Brazil K, Taniguchi A. A mixed methods study of the work patterns of full-time nurse practitioners in nursing homes. J Clin Nurs. 2014;24:1327–37. doi:10.1111/jon.12741c.
6. American Association of Nurse Practitioners. 2013–2014 National Nurse Practitioner Practice Site Census. 2015. http://www.aanp.org/images/documents/research/2013-14nationalnpcensusreport.pdf. Accessed on 11 Jun 2015.
7. Institute of Medicine. The future of nursing: leading change, advancing health. Washington, DC: The National Academies Press; 2010. Accessed online @ http://nap.edu.
8. American Association of Nurse Practitioners. States categorized by type. 2015. http://www.aanp.org/component/content/article/66-legislation-regulation/state-practice-environment/1380-state-practice-by-type. Accessed 18 Jun 2015
9. Intrator O, Zinn J, Mor V. Nursing home characteristics and potentially preventable hospitalizations of long-stay residents. J Am Geriatr Soc. 2004;52:1730–6.
10. Kane RL, Keckhafer G, Robst J (2002) Evaluation of the Evercare Demonstration Program: final report. http://www.cms.gov/Medicare/Demonstration-Projects/DemoProjectsEval Rpts/Downloads/Evercare_Final_Report.pdf. Accessed 11 Jun 2015
11. Sangster-Gromley E, Carter N, Donald F, Misener RM, Ploeg J, Kaasalainen S, McAiney C, Wickson-Griffiths A. A value-added benefit of nurse practitioners in long-term care settings: increased nursing staff's ability to care for residents. Nurs Leadersh. 2013;26(3):24–37. doi:10.12927/cjnl.2013.23552.
12. Borbasi SE, Emmanuel B, Farrelly B, Ashcroft J. Report of an evaluation of a Nurse-led Dementia Outreach Service of People with the behavioral and psychological symptoms of dementia living in residential aged care facilities. Perspect Public Health. 2011;131(3):124–30.
13. Martinez-Gonzalez NA, Djalali S, Tandjung R, Huber-Geismann F, Wensing M, Rosemann T. Substitution of physicians by nurses in primary care: a systematic review and meta-analysis. BMC Health Serv Res. 2014;14(214):1–17.
14. Christian R, Baker K. Effectiveness of nurse practitioners in nursing homes: a systematic review. JBI Database Syst Rev Implement Rep. 2009;7:133–1352.
15. National Association of Clinical Nurse Specialists. Statement on clinical nurse specialist practice and education. Harrisburg, PA: National Association of Clinical Nurse Specialists; 2004. p. 1–102. http://www.nacns.org/docs/NACNS-Statement.pdf. Accessed 18 Jun 2015.
16. Bureau of Labor Statistics, U.S. Department of Labor. (2014–2015). Occupational outlook handbook physician assistants. NE Washington, DC. 2015. http://www.bls.gov/ooh/health-care/physician-assistants.htm. Accessed 17 Jun 2015.
17. American Academy of Physician Assistants. 2013 Annual survey report. Alexandria, VA: American Academy of Physician Assistants. 2013. p. 11. https://www.aapa.org/WorkArea/DownloadAsset.aspx?id=2902. Accessed 19 Jun 2015.
18. Cawley J, Hooker R. Physician assistants in American medicine: the half-century mark. Am J Manag Care. 2013;19(10):e333–41.
19. NCCPA. National Commission on Certification of Physician Assistants (NCCPA). Johns Creek, GA. 2015. www.nccpa.net. Retrieved 2015.

20. American Academy of Physician Assistants. Professional issues. Alexandria, VA: American Academy of Physician Assistants. March 2014. www.aapa.org/WorkArea/DownloadAsset. aspx?id=583. Retrieved 2015.
21. Department of Veterans Affairs. Utilization of Physician Assistants, VA Directive 1063. Washington, DC. 2013. http://www.va.gov/VHAPUBLICATIONS/ViewPublication.asp?pub_ ID=2958. Accessed 17 Jun 2015
22. Henry LR, Hooker RS. Retention of physician assistants in rural health clinics. J Rural Health. 2007;23:207–14. doi:10.1111/j.1748-0361.2007.00092.x.
23. Gadbois EA. Trends in state regulation of nurse practitioners and physician assistants, 2001 to 2010. Med Care Rev. 2015;72(2):200–19. doi:10.1177/1077558714563763.
24. Drug Enforcement Agency. Mid-level practitioners authorization by state. Springfield, VA. June 2015. http://www.deadiversion.usdoj.gov/drugreg/practioners/mlp_by_state.pdf. Retrieved 17 Jun 2015.
25. Drug Enforcement Agency. Office of Diversion Control, Registration. 2011. www.deadiversion.usdoj.gov/drugreg/index.html. Retrieved 17 Jun 2015.
26. Bell-Dzide D, Gokula M, Gaspar P. Effect of a long-term care geriatrics rotation on physician assistant student's knowledge and attitudes towards the elderly. J Physician Assist Educ. 2014;25(1):38–40.
27. Abdallah LM, Van Etten D, Lee AJ, Devereaux Meliello K, Remington R, Gautam R, Gore RJ. A Medicare current beneficiary survey-based investigation of alternative primary care models in nursing homes. Res Gerontol Nurs. 2015;8(2):85–93. doi:10.3928/19404921-20150121-01.
28. Bakerjian D, Caprio T, Crecelius C, Leible K, Rapp MP, Resnick B. The nuts and bolts of NP/ physician collaborative agreements in long term care. Accessed online on 18 Jun 2015.
29. Casey T. AMDA—dedicated to long term care medicine. Ann Long Term Care Clin Care Aging. 2014;22(3).

Additional References

American Academy of Physician Assistants. The six key elements of a Modern Physician Assistant Practice Act. State law issues. Alexandria, VA: American Academy of Physician Assistants. March 2011. Accessed 17 Jun 2015. https://www.aapa.org/WorkArea/DownloadAsset.aspx?id=628.
Buerhaus P, DesRoches CM, Dittus R, Donelan K. Practice characteristics of primary care nurse practitioners and physicians. Nurs Outlook. 2015;63:144–53. dx.doi.org/10.1016/j.outlook. 2014.08.008.
Ersek M, Sefcik JS, Lin F-C, Lee TJ, Gillam R, Hanson LC. Provider staffing effect on a decision aid intervention. Clin Nurs Res. 2014;23(1):36–53. doi:10.1177/1054773812470840.
Hurlock-Chorostecki C, van Soeren M, MacMillan K, Sidani S, Collins L, Harbman P, Donald F, Reeves S. A survey of interprofessional activity of acute and long-term care employed nurse practitioners. J Am Assoc Nurse Pract. 2015. doi:10.1002/2327-6924.12213.
Kaasalainen S, Papaioannou A, Burges J, Van der Horst ML. Exploring the nurse practitioner role in managing fractures in long-term care. Clin Nurs Res. 2015;1–22. Online ahead of print. doi:10.1177/1054773815577577.
Meuller CA, Tetzlaff B, Theile G, Fleishmann N, Cavazzini C, Geister C, Hummers-Pradier E. Interprofessional collaboration and communication in nursing homes: a qualitative exploration of problems in medical care for nursing home residents – study protocol. J Adv Nurs. 2015;71(2):451–7. doi:10.1111/jan.12545.
Sangster-Gormley E, Firsch N, Schreiber R. Articulating new outcomes of nurse practitioner practice. J Am Assoc Nurse Pract. 2013;25:653–8. doi:10.1002/2327-6924.12040.

Common Clinical Conditions in Long-Term Care

Naushira Pandya

Introduction

The management of medical conditions in the frail elderly who reside in post-acute (PA) and long-term care facilities (LTC) can be challenging. This chapter will review some of the common clinical conditions that are frequently encountered in patients in post-acute and residents in the LTC continuum. The treatment and treatment goals for these conditions often differ from those of patients in other settings, and thus require an approach that evaluates the risk/benefit of treatment guided by discussion with the resident or surrogate decision-maker. The conditions to be reviewed are:

- Hypertension
- Anemia
- Heart failure
- COPD
- Type 2 diabetes
- Hypothyroidism
- B_{12} deficiency
- Skin Disorders: scabies, herpes zoster
- *Clostridium difficile*
- Multidrug-resistant organisms

N. Pandya, MD, CMD, FACP (✉)
Department of Geriatrics, Nova Southeastern University College of Osteopathic Medicine,
3200 S. University Drive, Fort Lauderdale, FL 33328, USA
e-mail: pandya@nova.edu

© Springer International Publishing Switzerland 2016
P.A. Fenstemacher, P. Winn (eds.), *Post-Acute and Long-Term Medicine*,
Current Clinical Practice, DOI 10.1007/978-3-319-16979-8_8

Hypertension

Although (HTN) is not a normal part of aging, its prevalence increases steadily with age. Many physiologic changes of aging that contribute to elevated blood pressure include arterial stiffness, decreased baroreceptor sensitivity, increased activity of the sympathetic nervous system, decreased alpha and beta-adrenergic receptor responsiveness, decreased ability to excrete a sodium load, low plasma renin activity, obesity and insulin resistance. Systolic HTN is highly prevalent, more common than diastolic HTN and more closely related to cardiovascular risk than diastolic HTN. The National Health and Nutritional Examination Survey (NHANES) reported a 50–75 % prevalence of HTN among those aged 65 years or older, with an earlier onset and more prevalent in African–American women. In a nursing facility study of 202 individuals, HTN was present in 71 % (mean age 73 years) [1]. Older adults treated for HTN are less likely to be adequately controlled than younger adults, suggesting that clinicians may be reluctant to add a second or third antihypertensive drug for treatment.

Benefits of Treatment

In addition to the well-ascribed risk factors for stroke and cardiovascular disease, persons with HTN are also at risk for atrial fibrillation, congestive heart failure (CHF), peripheral arterial disease (PAD), chronic kidney disease (CKD), and cognitive impairment (each with an increased relative risk between two and fourfold). Cardiovascular morbidity and mortality have been shown to progressively increase as the systolic and diastolic blood pressures increase. The benefits of treating HTN in the elderly have been firmly established. The Cochrane Review of essential HTN treatment in elderly patients (15 trials with 24,055 subjects ≥60 years) reported a reduction in total mortality, (RR 0.90) and a reduction in total cardiovascular morbidity and mortality, (RR 0.72) with hypertension treatment. *In very elderly patients ≥80 years, the reduction in total cardiovascular mortality and morbidity* was similar (RR 0.75). However, there was no reduction in total mortality, (RR 1.01) [2]. Residents with more cardiovascular risk factors (e.g., diabetes, family history of heart disease, left ventricular hypertrophy) will have more cardiovascular events prevented with antihypertensive therapy than those at lower risk. The benefit of antihypertensive treatment in patients age 80 years and older has been demonstrated by the HYVET study in which 3845 healthy community individuals over age 80 years with a sustained SBP of ≥160 mmHg were randomized to indapamide or placebo with the addition of perindopril or placebo to achieve a target BP of 150/80. The benefits of treatment were apparent at 1 year, and further increased at 2 years, with a 30 % reduction in the incidence of fatal or nonfatal stroke, a 39 % reduction in fatal stroke, and a 21 % reduction in all cause mortality [3]. Other randomized trials of HTN treatment in the elderly (SHEP: Systolic Hypertension in the Elderly Program; STOP: Swedish Trial in Old Patients; Sys-Eur: European Systolic Hypertension in the Elderly; Syst-China: Chinese Trial on Isolated Systolic Hypertension in Elderly) have shown a 32–47 % reduction in stroke, 13–30 % reduction in coronary disease, and 29–58 % reduction in heart failure. A meta-analysis of the PROGRESS, Syst-Eur, and the Rotterdam studies has shown that antihypertensive therapy also reduced vascular dementia and cognitive impairment.

Evaluation

The diagnosis of hypertension should be made carefully. In addition to using an appropriate cuff size and measuring blood pressure in a seated position at rest, it is important that hypertension be diagnosed on the basis of the average of two readings that are obtained on at least three occasions. This is especially important in older adults due to blood pressure variability. In the long-term care setting, BP may be highest in the morning and low after meals. Stage I hypertension is defined by the Joint National Committee on the Prevention, Detection, Evaluation and Treatment of High Blood Pressure (JNC 8) as a SBP of 140–159 mmHg, or DBP of 90–99 mmHg, and Stage 2 hypertension is defined as SBP $\geq$ 160 mmHg, and DBP $\geq$ 100 mmHg [4]. Over 90 % of elderly with an elevated BP will have essential hypertension, and the majority with new onset HTN will have systolic hypertension. Because many drugs are known to increase blood pressure, a careful medication review should be performed. The pulse pressure (defined as SBP minus DBP) increases with age and has shown to be a good predictor of cardiovascular disease in the elderly. Nonsteroidal anti-inflammatory drugs including COX-2 inhibitors, erythropoietin, alcohol, corticosteroids, and uncontrolled pain are commonly implicated in elevating BP.

A resident with HTN should be evaluated for comorbid conditions such as diabetes mellitus, chronic kidney disease (CKD), and sleep apnea. Those who present with diastolic HTN or treatment-resistant HTN should be evaluated for renovascular HTN if clinically appropriate. Sleep apnea is common in this population and may cause elevated blood pressure. In addition, elderly with unexplained hypokalemia accompanied by metabolic alkalosis may have primary hyperaldosteronism as a cause of their HTN. Although the incidence of pheochromocytoma is small, it may warrant consideration if a resident's BP is unusually labile and weight loss is present [5].

Treatment Goals

The goals of therapy may differ for each person and need to be defined within the context of their overall clinical condition and comorbidities, as well as its effect on quality of life. Cardiac risk factors should be modified to the extent possible. The elderly should be encouraged to increase physical activity if possible and to stop smoking. The treatment plan should include screening for diabetes and hyperlipidemia, and salt restriction if appropriate. The clinician should be aware that even a relatively simple intervention such as dietary sodium restriction could adversely affect nutritional status and contribute to weight loss.

The JNC 8 *goals for HTN treatment* for those over 60 years of age are a SBP <150 mmHg, and a DBP goal of <90 mmHg. For all adults with diabetes and/or CKD, the recommended goals are SBP <140 mmHg, and DBP <90 mmHg if it can be safely achieved [4]. The following treatment considerations can guide pharmacologic treatment.

- Initiate treatment with lower doses (half the usual dose) to minimize the risk of side effects.
- In the absence of a hypertensive emergency or urgency, lower BP gradually over weeks to months since the elderly have impaired baroreceptor and sympathetic neural responses, and impaired cerebral autoregulation.
- Very frail older persons may not benefit from treatment of HTN.
- Measure supine and standing BP prior to initiating treatment for systolic HTN since 20 % of these individuals have orthostatic and/or postprandial hypotension which increases the risk of falls and hip fracture.
- The degree of blood pressure reduction is the major determinant of cardiovascular risk reduction, not the choice of antihypertensive drug.
- Diuretic therapy is effective in lowering systolic BP and decreases the prevalence of orthostatic hypotension.
- An alternative drug may be selected as the initial agent based on comorbid conditions (DM, HF, CKD).
- If blood pressure goals are not met, add low doses of a second drug chosen from another class depending on comorbidities.
- In Stage 2 hypertension, usually two drugs are required, such as a thiazide diuretic combined with an angiotensin converting enzyme (ACE) inhibitor.
- Combining an ACE inhibitor and an ARB increases the risk of hypotension, syncope, and renal dysfunction without improving cardiovascular outcomes [6].
- When control is poor, or deteriorating, the factors mentioned in Table 1 should be considered (Table 2).

Implications for Long-Term Care

The advantage of lowering blood pressure in the LTC population that are very old (>85 years), frail and have multiple competing comorbidities is not clearly established. At this time there are no data to support lowering of blood pressure to levels recommended by JNC 8 (less than 150/90 mmHg in nondiabetics, and less than 140/90 mmHg in those with diabetes) in persons over 80 years of age. Because the population in long-term care often has a limited life expectancy and is prone to developing orthostatic and post-prandial hypotension, syncope, and falls, the risks of lowering blood pressure with medication are increased and its potential benefit reduced. Data is lacking to help determine how best to treat elevated BP in residents with high-risk conditions such as recent stroke, functional impairment, and aortic aneurysm.

Table 1 Advantages and disadvantages of class of antihypertensive medication

Antihypertensive class	Advantages	Disadvantages	Recommended indications	Cautions
Thiazide diuretics	Greater reduction of systolic BP Daily use Improve bone mineral density	Hypokalemia Urinary frequency	Systolic hypertension	Hyponatremia Gout
ACE inhibitors and angiotensin receptor blockers (ARB)	No CNS side effects Preserve renal function Reduce proteinuria	Cough Hyperkalemia	HF Type 2 Diabetes	Chronic kidney disease Renal artery stenosis Cough, altered taste, and angioneurotic edema with ACE inhibitors (try ARB)
Calcium channel antagonists (CCA)	No CNS side effects No metabolic effects	Constipation Peripheral edema Heart block (Non-dihydropyridine CCAs) HF with amlodipine	Systolic hypertension CAD	Left ventricular dysfunction Avoid short-acting CCAs for HTN
Beta adrenergic receptor blockers	None (not recommended as monotherapy)	CNS (Central Nervous System) side effects Increased glucose and lipids with cardioselective	Post MI CAD HF Atrial fibrillation with rapid rate (*Beneficial in essential tremor, hyperthyroidism*)	COPD (Chronic Obstructive Pulmonary Disease) PAD Heart block Depression Hyper-lipidemia Type 2 DM
Alpha adrenergic receptor blockers	Improved urinary symptoms in Benign Prostatic Hypertrophy (BPH)	Increased CHF hospitalization	Prostatism	Left ventricular dysfunction
Renin inhibitors	Effective without dose-related adverse effects	No outcome data in the elderly Expensive	Systolic hypertension	Diarrhea

Adapted from Geriatric Medicine and Gerontology, Sixth Edition. McGraw-Hill [7]

Table 2 Reasons for poor control of blood pressure	• Inadequate dosing of antihypertensive drugs
	• Inappropriate drug combinations
	• Polypharmacy and increased incidence of adverse drug effects
	• Unrecognized contributing medical conditions or drugs
	• Practitioner inertia and failure to modify treatment

Anemia

Aging predisposes persons to decreased hematopoietic reserve, reduced absorption of essential nutrients, decline in GFR and erythropoietin secretion (EPO), increased concentrations of cytokines; but *anemia is **not** considered a normal part of aging*. Anemia may have an insidious onset with nonspecific symptoms until it is becomes more severe. Mild anemia is often assumed as being benign or attributed to the presence of chronic comorbidities. However, studies in community dwelling elders show that anemia may be an independent risk factor for adverse outcomes when DM, CKD, or cardiovascular disease is present. Anemia has been associated with significant clinical problems and adverse outcomes (Table 3).

Definition and Prevalence of Anemia

There is no uniform definition of anemia. The World Health Organization defines anemia as a hemoglobin (Hb) level less than 12 g/dL in adult women and less than 13 g/dL in adult men. These cutoffs are based on population data that did not include people > 65 years of age, and do not take into account the effect of race and ethnicity. From the NHANES III and the Scripps-Kaiser database, new lower limits of normal for men >59 years and women >49 years have been proposed after excluding those with confounding factors. These values were slightly higher for older white men and women (13.2 and 12.2 g/dL, respectively) and slightly lower for older black men and women (12.7 and 11.5, respectively). However, such levels may not be optimal with regard to morbidity and mortality. For example, in the Women's Health and Aging Study, a risk gradient for adverse outcomes (mortality, frailty, disability) was present with Hb in the "normal range" as was a rise in the erythropoietin level [8]. In a multi-facility study, 56 % of residents were anemic; prior estimates have ranged from 25 to 63 % [9].

Signs and Symptoms

Signs and symptoms in long-term care residents may be nonspecific (Table 4) so staff needs to be aware of their potential significance and report them to the practitioner.

Table 3 Clinical impact
of anemia

Frailty
Falls
Fatigue
Dizziness/syncope
Shortness of breath
Decreased muscle strength
Cognitive impairment
Impaired mobility and physical performance
Heart failure
Increased hospital admissions and mortality

Table 4 Nonspecific signs
and symptoms of anemia

Anorexia, nausea
Bleeding gums
Chest pain, palpitations, tachycardia
Cold intolerance
Dizziness
Decreased activity level or endurance
Dyspnea
Fatigue
Increase in falls
Increased confusion, headache
Jaundice
Melena
Hematuria
Pallor (skin, conjunctivae)

Causes of Anemia

Anemia is generally due to an underlying clinical disorder and warrants an evaluation unless the resident has a reduced life expectancy, is receiving palliative care, or declines further evaluation. A systematic evaluation can help the practitioner make rational treatment decisions. Using empiric iron replacement, for example, can potentially overlook a significant underlying treatable disorder. The causes of anemia may be classified by etiology, bearing in mind that more than one cause may be present in a given person.

- Nutrient deficiency anemia (iron (IDA), folate, B_{12}).
- Blood loss (i.e., gastritis, AV malformation, diverticulosis, bladder tumor)
- Anemia of CKD.
- Anemia of chronic inflammation (ACI).
- Medications (may cause bleeding or marrow suppression).
- Myelodysplastic anemia (affects 5 % of older people).
- Unclassified (may be observed in one-third of LTC residents).

However, an alternative approach to aide clinical decision-making can be more useful in most clinical settings. It includes assessing the resident's medical history, comorbidities, renal function, current and recent medication use, physical findings, and review of laboratory tests. Anemia can then be classified by considering kinetics (decreased production, increased destruction, or blood loss), **or** by considering red cell morphology. The following algorithm (Fig. 1) suggests a diagnostic approach using the corrected reticulocyte count and MCV (as low, normal, or increased) prior to obtaining further tests. Table 5 lists suggested noninvasive diagnostic test for evaluation of anemia [10].

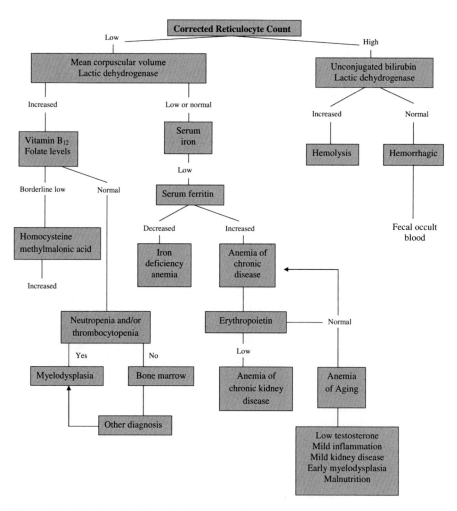

Fig. 1 Algorithm for the diagnosis of anemia (Source: Morley JE. J Am Med Dir Assoc. 13(3):191–4)

Table 5 Noninvasive diagnostic tests

• Complete blood count with reticulocyte count (initial low Hb/Hct may not be evident in volume depletion)
• Examination of peripheral blood smear
• Ferritin, serum iron, total iron-binding capacity (serum soluble transferring receptor)
• Serum folate
• Vitamin B_{12} (methylmalonic acid, homocysteine)
• Renal function (eGFR)
• Liver function
• Sedimentation rate
• Tests for hemolysis (serum LDH, bilirubin, and haptoglobin)
• Serum protein electrophoresis
• Stool for occult blood (endoscopy if appropriate
• Thyroid-stimulating hormone (free T4)
• Total testosterone

Table 6 Lab value differentiation of iron-deficiency anemia from anemia of chronic inflammation

Blood test	ACI	IDA	ACI + IDA
Iron	↓	↓	↓
TIBC	↓	↑	LN or ↓↑
% Transferrin saturation	↓ or N	↓	↓
Ferritin	↑ or N	↓	↓ or N
Soluble transferrin receptor	N	↑	↑ or N

Sometimes it is difficult to differentiate iron deficiency anemia from anemia of chronic inflammation since the typical hematologic abnormalities of advanced iron deficiency occur at a later stage and both types of anemia can coexist. Table 6 will assist in analyzing equivocal results [11]. Measurement of the soluble transferrin receptor in conjunction with iron studies and ferritin, is gaining some acceptance in differentiating iron deficiency anemia from anemia of chronic inflammation.

Anemia of CKD

As renal function declines in people with CKD, the Hb will progressively decline. This drop in Hb is especially noticeable as the GFR trends below 60 mL/min per 1.73 m². The anemia of CKD is typically normochromic and normocytic due primarily to a deficiency of erythropoietin production. About 50 % of nursing facility residents have a GFR below 60 mL/min per 1.73 m² and in one recent study, *60 % of residents with Stage III CKD were anemic.*

Acute or Chronic Immune Activation (ACI)

Acute or chronic immune activation can cause a disturbance of iron homeostasis that limits the availability of iron for erythropoiesis due to the impaired release of iron from macrophages. This disturbance in iron homeostasis is mediated by the proinflammatory cytokine interleukin-6, which increases the production of hepcidin in the liver. Hepcidin decreases duodenal absorption of iron. In addition, erythropoietic cell survival and erythropoietic cell response to EPO is decreased.

Treatment

Treatment of comorbid nutritional deficiencies and hypothyroidism should be undertaken. If anemia is related to medication use, chronic bleeding, CKD, chronic inflammation, malignancy, or hemolysis, then the underlying condition should be stabilized to the extent possible and any offending drugs discontinued. Treatment options for specific types of anemia and cautions to consider are reviewed in Table 7.

Blood transfusions are generally given for acute blood loss associated with hypotension and cardiovascular compromise. For chronic anemia, blood transfusion is recommended if the Hb drops below 7 g/dL, the hematocrit decreases to 21 %, or in the presence of angina, heart failure, dyspnea, tachycardia, or hypotension.

Table 7 Treatment options for anemia based on etiology

Cause of anemia	Treatment options	Cautions
Iron deficiency	• Ferrous sulfate 325 mg daily (65 mg elemental iron) • Ferrous gluconate 300 mg daily (36 mg elemental iron) • Parenteral iron (in cancer, CKD)	• Constipation • GI distress • Consider blood loss
Vitamin B_{12} deficiency	• Vitamin B_{12} 1,000 μg IM weekly × 1 month, then monthly if neurological complications • Oral B_{12} 500–1000 μg daily • Sublingual 2000 μg daily	• Check for concurrent folate deficiency
Folate deficiency	• Folate 1 mg orally, daily for 2–3 weeks, then reevaluate the need for continued therapy	• Check for concurrent B_{12} deficiency
Anemia of chronic inflammation	• Treat or stabilize the underlying disease	• Anemia may persist • Erythropoietin use is not approved
Anemia of chronic kidney disease	• Epoetin alfa or darbepoetin alfa SC • Control diabetes and HTN	• Maintain Hb 10–11 g/dL • Weekly Hb till stable then monthly • Monitor BP
Hemolytic anemia	• Identify underlying cause • Discontinue any contributing medications	

Heart Failure

Cardiovascular disease is the primary diagnosis for 25 % of admissions to nursing facilities. A study sampling of 10 % of skilled nursing facilities (SNFs) during 2003–2004 revealed that 37.4 % of patients had HF. Heart failure is responsible for significant morbidity and readmissions to the hospital. The lifetime risk of HF doubles for BP > 160/90 mmHg. Hypertension is a major risk factor for the development of HF, especially HF with preserved ejection fraction (EF) in long-term care residents. In one study HF with preserved ejection fraction (HFpEF) was present in 50 % of nursing facility residents diagnosed with HF. Heart failure with reduced EF of <45 % is termed HFrEF. Moreover, HF incidence increases significantly in older adults with diabetes and obesity, especially in females. Elderly with HF with either a markedly high or low BP have a worse prognosis as do those with an abnormal LVEF [12]. SNF rehospitalization rates for HF range from 27 to 43 %. Overall, mortality in LTC residents with HF exceeds 45 %, and hospitalization exceeds 50 % annually, although there may be regional differences [13].

Evaluation

The American College of Cardiology/American Heart Association (ACC/AHA) guidelines for the evaluation and management of HF have classified this condition in four stages (A-D) [14]. The first two stages (A, B) are not symptomatic stages of heart failure but defined to help practitioners identify those at risk for developing HF. The NYHA classification can be used to clarify symptom severity (Table 8).

The clinical differentiation between diastolic and systolic dysfunction although challenging, may be helpful in decision-making. A complete history and physical examination should be performed in residents with shortness of breath, reduced exercise tolerance, edema, or other symptoms suggestive of HF. Review of prior records may provide vital information regarding cardiovascular conditions. Current medications, use of alcohol, and/or illicit drugs and alternative therapies, as well as chemotherapy agents should also be considered as contributing factors to HF.

Table 8 New York Heart Association classification

Class	Patient symptoms
Class I	No limitation of physical activity. Ordinary physical activity does not cause undue fatigue, palpitation, or dyspnea (shortness of breath)
Class II (mild)	Slight limitation of physical activity. Comfortable at rest, but ordinary physical activity results in fatigue, palpitation, or dyspnea
Class III (moderate)	Marked limitation of physical activity. Comfortable at rest, but less than ordinary activity causes fatigue, palpitation, or dyspnea
Class IV (severe)	Unable to carry out any physical activity without discomfort. Symptoms of cardiac insufficiency at rest. If any physical activity is undertaken, discomfort is increased

The manifestations of heart failure may be atypical in long-term care residents. Frail elderly may have fatigue, malaise, lethargy, declining function, or neurological symptoms such as confusion, restlessness, or sleep disturbance when they develop an exacerbation of HF. Orthopnea, dyspnea with exertion, cough or edema may be present. Gastrointestinal manifestations of HF may include anorexia, nausea, and abdominal discomfort.

Patients who have HFpEF (i.e., preserved EF) are more often female, have a fourth heart sound, sustained PMI, absence of jugular venous distension, absence of peripheral edema, normal heart size on chest -ray, and left ventricular hypertrophy (LVH) on the electrocardiogram (EKG). By contrast, patients with HFrEF (i.e., reduced EF) are more often male, have a third heart sound, displaced PMI, jugular venous distension, pitting edema, and Q waves on the EKG.

Clinical Diagnosis of HF

- A physical examination is central to the diagnosis of HF and should include the weight (It is important to remember that edema found on physical exam may also be due to non-cardiac causes).
- Electrolytes and renal function (to detect hyponatremia, potassium abnormalities, worsening of renal function, hypomagnesemia).
- A chest X-ray is useful to estimate cardiac size, assess pulmonary congestion, and to detect other pulmonary disease.
- While useful, a comprehensive 2-dimensional echocardiogram with Doppler flow studies (to assess LVEF, the presence of valvular, or pericardial abnormalities) may not be easily available.
- An EKG may indicate the presence of Q waves, LVH, arrhythmias, or conduction disorders.
- Screening for comorbid thyroid disease is also recommended (see section on hypothyroidism).
- Serum assays for natriuretic peptides (BNP and NT-proBNP) are readily available and may lend weight to the suspicion of HF in residents in whom the cause of dyspnea is not clear. However, its use and applicability is unclear in the LTC setting [14].

Electrolytes and renal function should be measured regularly as hypokalemia is a common adverse effect of diuretics and may increase the risk of fatal arrhythmias or digoxin toxicity. Many residents with hypokalemia also have hypomagnesemia, which can result in an inadequate response to potassium supplementation. Hyperkalemia can be associated with ACE inhibitors, angiotensin II receptor blockers, or worsening renal function. The development of hyponatremia may be an indication of disease progression and is associated with reduced survival in the elderly with HF.

Serial chest X-rays are not recommended but monitoring weights 2–3 times a week during an exacerbation of HF is useful practice. The resident's functional status should be monitored in addition to the physical examination with sitting and standing BP.

Table 9 Common factors precipitating HF

Cardiac
Myocardial infarction or ischemia
Poorly controlled hypertension
Excess of dietary sodium
Medication nonadherence
Excess fluid intake (oral or IV)
Arrhythmias—supraventricular (especially atrial fibrillation with rapid rate), bradycardia, sick sinus syndrome
Associated medical conditions—pulmonary embolism, hypoxia due to chronic lung disease, infection (pneumonia, viral illness, sepsis), anemia, hyperthyroidism, chronic kidney disease (eGFR <30 mL/min)
Medications—alcohol, -β adrenergic blockers (including ophthalmic agents), calcium channel-blockers, NSAIDS, glucocorticosteroids, mineralocorticoids, antiarrhythmic drugs
Provider/system problems (e.g., medication reconciliation errors)

Common Precipitants of Heart Failure

In addition to attempting to identify the cause of heart failure, it is also important to be aware of conditions that may precipitate an exacerbation of heart failure in order that the medication regimen and the treatment of these coexisting medical conditions can be optimized. Cardiologist consultation may be required in some instances (Table 9).

Process of Care Considerations

Close observation, and early detection of symptoms and signs may precede an acute HF episode by several days. Timely intervention by the practitioner (with evaluation of weights, chest X-ray, electrolytes and renal function, adjustment of therapy) and regular monitoring by nursing staff may prevent hospitalization. Records of prior cardiac investigations and echocardiograms will assist in better defining the type of HF in terms of LVEF, LVH and valvular dysfunction. A study of 156 episodes of HF in 4693 Medicare nursing facility admissions within the first 90 days of stay, reported that symptom presentation and evaluation by nursing staff at night increased the odds of rehospitalization fourfold. The presence of hypotension and delirium were predictive of death. Residents who received ACE inhibitors and orders for skilled nursing observations more than once a shift decreased the likelihood of dying by 70 % [15]. Residents with anemia (Hb <9.8 g/dL) were twofold more likely, and those with CKD (stage III or greater) were fivefold more likely to be rehospitalized from a nursing facility HF rehabilitation unit.

Management

The following reviews consensus recommendations for the management of HF and should be applied to each resident in an individualized manner [14]. The choice of pharmacologic and non-pharmacologic therapy will depend on the patient's clinical status, goals of care, as well burden of comorbid conditions and prognosis. The suggested treatment paradigm can be based on three broadly identified groups in many facilities: the **Rehabilitation Group** in whom the goal is improved function and discharge; those who are frail with multi-morbidities and have an **Uncertain Prognosis**; and the **Long-term Care Group** who are frail, dependent for care needs, and expected to remain in the facility. Each recommendation should be individualized (Table 10).

Cautions

- Encourage moderate activity and physical therapy if possible.
- Thiazides are ineffective if GFR is <30 ml/min/1.73 m^2; use loop diuretics.
- If symptoms persist and ACEI or ARB cannot be given due to decrease in GFR or hypotension, give isosorbide plus hydralazine, especially in African Americans.
- Avoid calcium channel blockers.

Digoxin

Many residents may receive digoxin (sometimes for years) as a standard part of the treatment regimen for HF despite the presence of sinus rhythm and normal LVEF. The evidence indicates that low dose digoxin (digoxin concentration <1.0 ng/mL) may decrease mortality in HFrEF and NYHA II and III symptoms in elderly who do not have an adequate response to ACE inhibitors, beta-blockers, and diuretics.

The elderly are at increased risk of digoxin toxicity due to renal insufficiency, hypoalbuminemia, hypokalemia with hypomagnesemia, as well as drug–drug interactions. Drug interactions between digoxin and antiarrythmics, erythromycin and tetracycline can be especially problematic. Close monitoring, especially during acute illness causing dehydration, is recommended and serum concentrations should be maintained between 0.5 and 0.8 ng/ml [16].

Refractory HF

HF can have an unpredictable course and a high incidence of sudden death despite intensive medical management. Palliative care should be considered for those with refractory HF and persistence of severe and distressful symptoms such as dyspnea, fatigue, pain, sleep disturbance, and functional decline.

Table 10 Suggested medical management of heart failure based on care goals

Intervention	Rehabilitation group	Uncertain prognosis group	Long-term group
Assessment of LVEF	Yes	Yes	Preferable (individualize)
Sodium restriction	Preferable	Preferable	Preferable, but individualize
Diuretics to treat volume overload	Yes	Yes	Yes
ACEIs/ARBs	Yes for HFrEF (avoid low SBP)	Yes for HFrEF (avoid low SBP)	Yes for HFrEF (avoid low SBP)
β-blocker	Yes for HFrEF as tolerated (BP, HR, fatigue)	Yes for HFrEF as tolerated (BP, HR, fatigue)	Yes for HFrEF as tolerated (BP, HR, fatigue)
Mineralocorticoid receptor antagonist	Yes for HFrEF NYHA II–IV and in NYHA III after MI; avoid in those with eGFR <30 mL/min	Yes for HFrEF NYHA II–IV and in NYHA III after MI; avoid in those with eGFR <30 mL/min	Yes for HFrEF NYHA II–IV and in NYHA III after MI; avoid in those with eGFR <30 mL/min
Hydralazine-nitrates	Yes for HFrEF in black patients with standard therapy; If contraindications to ACEIs or ARBs or as adjunctive therapy for advanced HF	Yes for HFrEF in black patients with standard therapy; If contraindications to ACEIs or ARBs or as adjunctive therapy for advanced HF	Yes for HFrEF in black patients with standard therapy; If contraindications to ACEIs or ARBs or as adjunctive therapy for advanced HF
Digoxin	Yes for HFrEF, only if symptomatic despite treatment with an ACEI or ARB, a β-blocker, and a mineralocorticoid receptor antagonist; low dose (≤0.125 mg/d)	Yes for HFrEF, only if symptomatic despite treatment with an ACEI or ARB, a β-blocker, and a mineralocorticoid receptor antagonist; low dose (≤0.125 mg/d)	Yes for HFrEF, only if symptomatic despite treatment with an ACEI or ARB, a β-blocker, and a mineralocorticoid receptor antagonist; low dose (≤0.125 mg/d)
Implantable cardioverter defibrillator	Stable optimized medications for 3 months, LVEF ≤35 %, NYHA II–III, and expected survival of at least 12 months	Observe until recovery seems likely	Not indicated
Cardiac resynchronization therapy	Persistent symptoms, optimized medications for 3 months, LBBB and LVEF ≤35 % and QRS ≥150 ms and NYHA II–IV	Observe until recovery seems likely	Not indicated
Discuss and identify end-of-life preferences	Yes	Yes	Yes

Adapted from AHA/HFSA Scientific Statement. Circulation. 2015.8(3):655–7

Chronic Obstructive Pulmonary Disease

Chronic obstructive pulmonary disease (COPD) is an insidious, progressive lung disease characterized by airflow obstruction that is not fully reversible. COPD may be difficult to diagnose because persons often gradually modify their lifestyle to compensate for progressive symptoms and dyspnea. COPD may be difficult to differentiate from asthma, HF, or other comorbidities that limit physical activities. COPD is the third leading cause of death in the USA. One in six patients admitted to a nursing facility may have COPD or emphysema, and it is responsible for 1 % of deaths in LTC [17].

Identification of COPD

Smoking (90 % of cases), advanced age, repeated pulmonary infections, prior tuberculosis, occupational or environmental causes, and alpha-1 antitrypsin deficiency are risk factors for COPD. Early identification of COPD is important since 50 % of lung function is lost by the time mild exertional dyspnea occurs and only 30 % of lung function remains when there is dyspnea at rest. All new admissions to LTC and those residents with recurrent pulmonary problems should be screened for COPD utilizing the clinical indicators listed in Table 11 [18].

Diagnosis of COPD

On examination, residents may be barrel-chested, have prolonged expiration or pursed lip breathing, use accessory muscles for respiration, and have wheezing, ronchi, or distant heart sounds. The signs of *cor pulmonale* include jugular venous distension, hepatic congestion, pedal edema, and a loud P2 component of the second heart sound.

   The clinical evaluation and review of past records may be helpful in diagnosing COPD, but the definitive method of diagnosis is by spirometry which usually

Table 11 Clinical indicators of COPD in long-term care	
	Dyspnea (progressive, worse with exertion)
	Cough (may be intermittent and unproductive)
	Chronic sputum production (any pattern)
	Avoidance of activities that lead to dyspnea
	History of smoking
	Recurrent pulmonary infections
	Occupational or environmental exposure to dust particles
	Weight loss, anxiety, or sleep disorders

measures FEV_1 (volume of air exhaled in 1 s) to FVC (forced vital capacity or total volume of air able to be exhaled). Spirometry should be performed in symptomatic individuals and may need to be repeated.

Normal: FEV_1/FVC $\geq$ 70 % or $FEV_1 \geq$ 80 % of predicted

COPD: FEV_1/FVC $\leq$ 70 %

Restrictive lung disease: FEV_1/FVC $\geq$ 90 % (pulmonary fibrosis, severe kyphosis)

COPD is undiagnosed in 80 % of older adults and not all LTC facilities have bed-side spirometers and their use in frail or demented residents is usually not feasible. A screening tool that uses caregivers to rate residents' symptoms was validated in the NF by Zarrowitz et al. They report that a history of asthma, shortness of breath at rest and shortness of breath on exertion, and smoking are likely to be consistent with a diagnosis of COPD.

Other diagnostic tests may provide useful information regarding the presence of COPD or other conditions presenting with similar signs and symptoms. A complete blood count may reveal an abnormally high Hb level due to hypoxia, and a chemistry panel may show a high bicarbonate level (respiratory alkalosis) due to hypercapnea. Even though chest X-rays are not diagnostic, they may reveal HF, bullae, pneumonia, pulmonary scarring; or low flat diaphragms, increased retrosternal airspace and a teardrop shaped heart silhouette are suggestive of COPD. An EKG may show atrial arrhythmias or right heart strain. Pulmonary consultation may be helpful if the cause of dyspnea is not clear or the resident exhibits a poor response to treatment. Clinical judgment is important since the differential diagnosis of COPD can include asthma, heart failure, brochiectasis, recurrent aspiration, ACE-inhibitor induced cough, vocal cord dysfunction, and respiratory tract tumors. The GOLD criteria of COPD severity are shown in Table 12 [19].

Table 12 GOLD spirometry criteria for COPD severity

I:	Mild COPD
	• FEV1/FVC <70 %
	• FEV1 ≥80 % predicted
II:	Moderate COPD
	• FEV1/FVC <70 %
	• 50 % ≤FEV1 <79 % predicted
III:	Severe COPD
	• FEV1/FVC <70 %
	• 30 % ≤ FEV1 < 39 % predicted
IV:	Very severe COPD
	• FEV1/FVC <70 %
	• FEV1 <30 % predicted *or* FEV1 <50 % predicted *plus*
	Chronic respiratory failure[a]

[a]Defined as partial pressure of oxygen less than 60 mmHg with or without partial pressure of carbon dioxide move than 50 mmHg while breathing air at sea level

Management of COPD

Since staging of COPD by spirometry criteria is not usually possible or practical in PA/LTC, clinical presentation and judgment must be utilized to guide treatment [20] (Table 13).

Encouraging smoking cessation is important at any stage of this disease; as are measures to improve nutrition, encourage physical activity and immunization with influenza and pneumococcal vaccines. Complications such as polycythemia, hypoxia, and HF should be treated, and goals of care should be discussed with the resident and family.

Pharmacological treatment should be stepwise and cumulative. Medications can reduce symptoms, increase exercise capacity, and reduce the number and severity of exacerbations; but *no treatment has been shown to modify the progressive decline in lung function*. Three types of bronchodilators are in common clinical use: β-agonists, anticholinergic drugs and inhaled corticosteroids.

- Long-acting bronchodilators are more effective than short-acting bronchodilators or anticholinergics.
- Anticholinergics given four times a day can improve health status.
- A combination of short acting agents (salbutamol/ipratropium) produces a greater change in lung function than either agent alone.

Table 13 Management of COPD

Spirometry	Begin pharmacotherapy if symptomatic		
Pharmacotherapy	• Short-acting bronchodilators PRN • Short-acting bronchodilators (regular and PRN) • Long-acting bronchodilator and PRN short-acting beta-2-agonist • Long-acting bronchodilator + inhaled corticosteroid[a] and PRN short-acting beta-2-agonist • Combination long-acting agents (long-acting beta-2-agonist + long-acting anticholinergic) + inhaled corticosteroids + as needed short-acting beta-2-agonist		
Severe progressive disease	Supplemental oxygen	Noninvasive positive pressure ventilation (patient is conscious, cooperative and without large volumes of sputum)	Theophylline
Other interventions	• Smoking cessation • Influenza and pneumococcal vaccination • Osteopenia/osteoporosis evaluation • Pulmonary rehabilitation • Evaluate for lung-volume reduction surgery		
Plan of care	• End-of-life care directives • Reinforce proper inhaler technique • Depression and anxiety screening		

Adapted from Ref. [20]

[a]If forced expiratory volume <50 % predicted and exacerbations of COPD requiring a course of oral corticosteroid or antibiotic occurred at least once within the last year, consider adding regular inhaled corticosteroid (ICS). If an ICS and a long-acting beta agonist are used, prescribe a combination inhaler

Table 14 Commonly used pharmacologic agents: benefits and cautions

Drug class	Drug example	Dosage	Cautions
Short-acting β agonists	Albuterol MDI	1–2 inhalations every 4–6 h	All four drugs may be used for acute bronchospasm
	Levalbuterol MDI	2 inhalations every 4–6 h PRN	
	Albuterol 2.5 mg for nebulization	3 ml TID-QID	
	Levalbuterol 0.6 mg	3 ml TID	
Long-acting β agonists	Formoterol DPI	1 inhalation (12 mcg) every 12 h	Not for acute bronchospasm. Palpitations, tremor, bronchospasm
	Salmeterol DPI	1 inhalation (50 mcg) every 12 h	
	Arformotero	Nebulization (15 mcg) BID	
Anticholinergics	Ipratropium bromide MDI	2–3 (17 mcg each) inhalations QID	May be used for acute exacerbation
	Ipratropium bromide 500 mcg for nebulization	2.5 ml TID-QID	May be used for acute exacerbation
	Tiotropium DPI	1 inhalation (18 mcg) daily	For maintenance treatment. Not for acute bronchospasm Caution with BPH and glaucoma
	Umecldinium	1 inhalation (62.5 mcg) daily	
	Aclidinium	One inhalation (400 mcg) BID	
Glucocorticoids Inhaled corticosteroids (MDI or DPI)	Beclomethasone diproprionate 40 mcg/ inhalation	1–2 inhalations BID	For severe COPD with repeated exacerbations; added to routine bronchodilator therapy
	Fluticasone DPI	2 inhalations BID	
Oral corticosteroids	Prednisone 5 mg	30–40 mg/d for 10 days	Monitor glucose in patients with DM Osteoporosis, myopathy and cataracts
	Prednisolone 4 mg	24–32 mg/day for 10 days	
Methylxanthines	Theophylline ER	400 mg/day	*Toxicity and multiple drug interactions.* Caution with liver and cardiac disease. Check levels

- Bronchodilators from different classes may improve efficacy, understanding that treatment needs to be long-term.
- An inhaled corticosteroid combined with a long-acting beta-2 agonist is more effective than either agent alone and may reduce the frequency of exacerbations, as well as improve health status.
- The inhaled route of treatment (i.e., use of MDIs) is preferred (Table 14).

The routine use of antibiotics is not recommended other than for acute exacerbations. Mucolytics are not recommended either, but may be considered for patients with viscous mucous. Although cough is troublesome, the regular use of antitussives is only recommended if it impairs daily activities. *The prolonged use of oral glucocorticoids should be avoided.*

Acute Exacerbations

Acute exacerbations are often characterized by an increase in dyspnea and cough, chest tightness, fever, and a change in sputum color, volume, or consistency. The majority of acute exacerbations may be due to tracheobronchitis, while *one third of exacerbations may be non-infectious* in origin. However, an exacerbation may be difficult to distinguish from pneumonia, HF, or thromboembolic disease. *The dose and frequency of inhaled bronchodilators should be increased* and it is advisable to have PRN orders for nursing staff to administer rescue medication. If a resident has difficulty using a metered dose inhaler (MDI), handheld nebulizers should be used. *Oral prednisone* (30–40 mg for 7–10 days) may improve lung function and shorten the course of the acute exacerbation. A *short course (<5 days) of oral antibiotics* (amoxicillin, cephalosporins, doxycycline, or macrolides) may be helpful. Amoxicillin/clavulanate or a respiratory fluoroquinolone should be used if prior antibiotic treatments have failed. Intravenous coverage for *Pseudomonas* is warranted if the resident has moderate or severe COPD, prior hospitalizations, or frequent antibiotic use. Some residents may benefit from suctioning and chest percussion. Ideally oxygen saturation should be checked and supplemental oxygen given to *maintain SaO2 above 90%.* A chest X-ray, CBC, electrolytes, sputum culture, or EKG may provide additional information regarding precipitating causes. A sputum culture is often difficult to obtain.

The decision as to whether to hospitalize a resident should be individualized and based on the LTC setting and its ability to treat the resident. In general, *hospitalization should be considered for any patient who fails to respond to treatment, develops tachypnea (respirations >28 breaths/min), remains hypoxic, develops delirium, has high fever, has significant difficulty sleeping or eating, or has serious comorbidities* (HF, DM, CKD, liver disease) [21]. COPD is a major cause of 30-day readmissions to the hospital.

Non-pulmonary complications of COPD increase morbidity and can reduce functional status. Cardiovascular and skeletal muscle changes contribute to reduced lung and exercise capacity. Residents frequently have a reduced BMI, frailty (which increases mortality), sarcopenia, and male hypogonadism. Vitamin D deficiency, glucocorticoid use, and sedentary lifestyle lead to the development of osteoporosis. In addition, residents often experience anxiety, depression, malnutrition, weight loss, sleep disturbance, decreased awareness of hypoxia and hypercarbia, and cognitive dysfunction. A six-minute walk distance of less than 350 m is predictive of future exacerbations and death. In residents with advanced disease, it is important to have an ongoing discussion with the resident and/or family about realistic expectations and treatment goals [17].

Diabetes

Diabetes affects over 25 % of long-term care residents [22]. Diabetes costs of care accounts for an estimated 32 % of Medicare expenses and is an independent predictor of placement into a LTC facility. Diabetic residents are a heterogeneous group

Table 15 Problems and complications of diabetes in older adults

• Accelerated atherosclerosis with vascular complications (myocardial infarction, stroke)
• Changes in weight (gain or loss)
• Confusion, acceleration of cognitive impairment
• Dehydration
• Depression
• Excessive skin problems (infections, ulcers, delayed wound healing)
• Eye problems (blurred or loss of vision)
• Falls
• Foot ulcers, foot deformities, gangrene, other foot problems
• Frequent infections
• Impaired pain perception, neuropathy
• Nonketotic hyperosmolar coma
• Oral health problems (caries, periodontal disease, tooth loss, dry mouth, burning mouth)
• Polypharmacy
• Urinary frequency, nocturia, urinary incontinence

Adapted with permission from the AMDA Clinical Practice Guideline; Diabetes Management in the Post-Acute and Long-Term, 2015

characterized by a higher degree of cardiovascular comorbidities, infections, lower extremity complications, pain, pressure ulcers, urinary incontinence, injurious falls, oral problems, cognitive dysfunction, as well as functional dependency. The majority of residents who have Type 2 diabetes have little consistency in the management of this condition. There is a paucity of data to guide the practitioner in terms of goals of glycemic control and its impact on clinical outcomes. Many elderly have diabetes-related complications secondary to microvascular and macrovascular disease as well as other comorbidities that require treatment. These potential complications are summarized in Table 15, for which screening and evaluation is recommended [23].

Effective diabetes management is multifaceted and requires a protocol-driven, team-based, individualized approach to care in the nursing facility. Diabetes care that is able to approximate this approach will be more effective. Goals of treatment are affected by life expectancy, patient preferences and values, expected clinical benefit, risks of treatment side effects, particularly hypoglycemia. National organizations have formulated clinical guidelines in an attempt to improve metabolic control and reduce detrimental effects of both hyper and hypoglycemia, and to potentially reduce debilitating complications of DM [23–25]. The challenges of managing diabetes in LTC may be attributed to factors related to the resident and disease, institution, staff and practitioner, and medication management (Table 16).

Abnormal glucose values indicating impaired fasting glucose (fasting plasma glucose (FPG) 100–125 mg/dl, 5.6–6.9 mmol/l), or impaired glucose tolerance (2-h postload or postprandial glucose 140–199 mg/dl, 7.8–11.1 mmol/l) may not be recognized or appropriately followed. *Diabetes is also diagnosed when the A1C is ≥6.5%* and should be repeated to confirm the diagnosis. Those with an A1C below

Table 16 Challenges to managing diabetes in PA/LTC

Resident and disease	Institution	Staff and practitioner	Medication management
Altered pharmacokinetics and pharmacodynamics	Staff turnover and lack of familiarity with residents	Knowledge deficits (disease, complications, selection and modification of therapies)	Multiple and changing treatment approaches
Increased risk of hypoglycemia	Restricted dietary practices	Lack of team communication (hyperglycemia, glucose excursions)	Reliance on sliding scale insulin protocols
Irregular meal consumption	Inadequate review of glucose logs	Therapeutic nihilism	Inappropriate dosing or timing of insulin
Cognitive dysfunction and depression	Lack of facility—specific diabetes treatment algorithms	Failure to individualize care (A1C, BP, lipids)	Hypoglycemia management (delayed recognition or overcorrection)
Psychological insulin resistance	Lack of established blood glucose parameters for physician notification	Failure of timely and stepwise rational advances in therapy	Lack of comfort with newer insulins and injectable agents, and delivery systems
Impaired vision and manual dexterity	Lack of administrative buy-in to promote the role of the Medical Director, the DON and consultant pharmacist		
Greater potential for adverse effects and drug interactions			

the threshold for diabetes, but ≥ 6.0 %, should receive attention to existing cardiovascular risk factors to the extent feasible if clinically appropriate [25].

Elderly with undiagnosed diabetes are at risk of MI, HF, stroke and complications of DM. Low physical activity, some medications and medical conditions such as obesity, pancreatic disorders and hyperthyroidism can all increase the risk of diabetes. Commonly used medications that cause hyperglycemia include glucocorticoids, atypical antipsychotics, β adrenergic agonists, thiazides, and megesterol acetate [23].

Treatment Selection

The general principles for treating diabetes in PA/LTC residents are similar to those used for treating diabetes in the community. While lifestyle changes are effective, dietary restriction is not recommended in LTC since food enjoyment, quality of life,

Table 17 Suggested stepwise approach to diabetic therapy

Monotherapy				
Metformin[a]				
If patient does not reach A1c goal in 3 months, proceed to two-drug combination therapy				
Two-drug combination				
Metformin	Metformin	Metformin		Metformin
+ SU (not glyburide[b])	+ TZD[c]	+ DPP-4 inhibitor	Metformin	+ Insulin (basal)
			+ GLP-1 RA	
If patient does not reach A1c goal in 3 months, proceed to three-drug combination therapy				
Three-drug combination				
Metformin + SU	Metformin + TZD	Metformin +	Metformin +	Metformin
+ TZD	+ SU	DPP-4 inhibitor	GLP-1 RA	+ Insulin (basal)
or + DPP-4 inhibitor	**or** + DPP-4 inhibitor	+ SU	+ SU	+ TZD
or + GLP-1-RA	**or** + GLP-1-RA	**or** + TZD	**or** + TZD	**or** + DPP-4 inhibitor
or + insulin[d]	**or** + insulin	**or** + insulin	**or** + insulin	**or** + GLP-1-RA
If patient does not reach A1C goal after 3 months of three-drug combination therapy, proceed to combination injectable therapy				
Metformin				
+ Basal insulin + meal-time insulin **or** GLP-1-RA				

Source: Adapted from ADA 2015 and AMDA 2015
DPP-4 dipeptyl peptidase 4, *GLP-1 RA* glucagon-like peptide-1 receptor agonist, *SU* sulfonylurea, *TZD* thiazolidinedione, *SGLT-2* sodium-glucose co-transporter 2
[a]Contraindicated in advanced renal disease and alcoholism. Monitor regularly for eGFR < 60 ml/min
[b]Avoid because of elevated risk of prolonged hypoglycemia in older adults
[c]TZD contraindicated in heart failure
[d]Use insulin if A1c greater than 9

and prevention of weight loss take precedence. Ambulation, seated exercise and any physical activity possible should be encouraged. Type 2 diabetes is a progressive disease and combination treatment with oral agents (to take advantage of their respective modes of action) is often required as is the use of insulin secretion in older adults is reduced and delayed. Important considerations in the selection of therapies include the resident's age, functional status, treatment goals (both short and long-term), renal impairment, hepatic impairment, and weight loss. The following algorithm (Table 17) suggested by the American Diabetes Association represents a feasible approach [23, 26].

Medications with the least risk of hypoglycemia are metformin, acarbose, miglitol, DPP-4 inhibitors (e.g., sitagliptan), GLP-1 analogs (e.g., exetanide), short-acting beta-cell enhancers (repaglinide, nateglanide), sodium-glucose co-transporter-2 inhibitors, thiazolidinediones, and long-acting insulin analogs. There are a variety of available injectable glucagon-like peptide agonists, which can be administered once or twice a day or weekly and are efficacious in decreasing A1C levels. Management of blood pressure, lipids, nutritional status, pain control, neuropathic symptoms, lower extremity infections, ulcers, and limb loss, should also be considered in the overall care of the resident.

Insulin

Prolonged severe hyperglycemia leads to glucotoxicity that increases insulin resistance and impairs insulin secretion. The usual course of DM is for the efficacy of oral hypoglycemics to decline with time and the A1C to rise by 0.2–0.3 % per year. Moreover, older adults with type 2 diabetes are known to be more insulinopenic. Timely use of insulin beginning with basal insulin analogs (10 units daily or 0.1–0.2 units/kg/day) with weekly increases of 2–3 units until desired levels of fasting glucose levels are obtained, is simple and effective, especially in the elderly over age 80 with liver or chronic kidney disease. Insulin should be used acutely if there is marked or persistent hyperglycemia despite maximal use of oral agents, or increased insulin requirements resulting from infection, stress, surgery, or injury, significant weight loss, ketonuria, diabetic ketoacidosis or hyperosmolar state. *Sulfonylureas may be discontinued and the dose of thiazolidinediones reduced once the fasting glucose levels have been stabilized.* If the fasting blood glucose levels are adequately controlled, but the A1C remains elevated, the glucose log should be reviewed and prandial insulin (usually a rapid acting insulin analog (4 or 0.1 units/ kg) be added to the main meal). *Basal analog insulins lower the overall risk of hypoglycemia* and possibly nocturnal hypoglycemia, whereas rapid acting analogs allow flexibility for inconsistent mealtimes and erratic intake that is not unusual in PA/LTC residents. *It is important to be aware that these rapid acting insulin analogs should be administered 10–15 min before a meal, while insulin glulisine should be administered up to 20 min after a meal, and insulin lispro can be given immediately after the meal.*

Sliding-Scale Insulin

Sliding-scale insulin (SSI) as a method of glucose control has many disadvantages. Although widely used alone or as an adjunct to oral agents, it provides no basal insulin and is a reactive instead of a proactive approach. Its use is not recommended as a primary or sole method of treatment. SSI uses hyperglycemia as a threshold (e.g., >200) and often involves "one-size-fits-all" dosing and trends in glycemic control and glucose excursions are often not being assessed (e.g., the practitioner only being contacted if glucose is <60 or >300 mg/dL.) On a practical level, SSI results in an increased number of injections, as many as 60 % unnecessary finger-sticks, medication errors, and increased patient discomfort as well as increased nursing time [27]. SSI may be more useful as a correctional scale to be added to scheduled oral and/or insulin therapy if blood glucose levels are highly variable and the patient medically unstable. When using SSI in this manner insulin requirements should be reviewed in 1–2 weeks, and modified.

Suggestions for Adjusting Insulin Therapy Based on Glucose Patterns

Maintaining adequate glucose control in a resident on insulin requires frequent evaluation of targeted glucose levels and adjusting the insulin dose accordingly. Tables 18 and 19 can be used as a guide as to which insulin dose to increase or decrease based on the resident's average glucose levels at various time of the day [23].

Goals of Treatment

Treatment goals should be individualized and take into account the state of the disease, extent of microvascular and macrovascular complications, estimated remaining life expectancy, resident and/or family preferences, functional and cognitive status, presence of a major psychiatric disorder, and risk of hypoglycemia. In one study facility physicians managed diabetes less aggressively in residents who were both cognitively and functionally impaired [28].

Recent evidence from the ACCORD, ADVANCE, and VADT trials, investigated the effects of intensive (goal A1C ≤6.5 %) versus standard glycemic control, and did not show a significant reduction in CVD outcomes during the randomized

Table 18 Standard human insulin therapy: regular and NPH given twice a day

	Regular		NPH	
Average blood glucose	AM	PM	AM	PM
Fasting				
LOW				↓
HIGH[a]				↑
Pre lunch				
LOW	↓		↓	
HIGH	↑			
Pre supper				
LOW[b]			↓	
HIGH			↑	
Bedtime				
LOW		↓		↓
HIGH		↑		

Pre-lunch glucose levels are influenced by both the R and NPH given in the AM
Bedtime glucose levels are influenced by both the R and NPH given at the evening meal
[a]Evaluate 3 a.m. blood glucose level to eliminate possible nocturnal hypoglycemia leading to rebound hyperglycemia
[b]Evaluate 3 PM BG readings for necessity of afternoon snack

Table 19 Analog insulin therapy: basal insulin with rapid acting insulin at each meal

	Basal	Rapid[a]		
Average blood glucose		Breakfast	Lunch	Supper
Fasting				
LOW	↓			
HIGH[b]	↑			
Pre lunch				
LOW		↓		
HIGH		↑		
Pre supper				
LOW			↓	
HIGH[c]			↑	
Bedtime				
LOW				↓
HIGH				↑

Giving rapid acting insulin up to 15 min after eating may be more appropriate if a patient's eating is unpredictable. This allows for not giving the insulin if the patient does not eat

[a]If a correction dose (sliding scale) is routinely being added to the patient's usual rapid insulin dose at meals due to hyperglycemia, the *average correction* dose used for any particular meal can be used as the number of units to increase the rapid acting insulin dose at the *preceding* meal

[b]Evaluate 3 AM BG readings to eliminate possible nocturnal hypoglycemia leading to rebound hyperglycemia

[c]Evaluate 3 PM BG readings for necessity of afternoon snack

periods. However, long-term follow-up of the DCCT and UKPDS cohorts suggests that treatment to A1C targets below or around 7 % in the years soon after the diagnosis of diabetes is associated with long-term reduction in the risk of macrovascular disease [29]. Less stringent A1C goals (7.5–8.5 %), may be more appropriate for many LTC residents who have a history of severe hypoglycemia, limited life expectancy, advanced microvascular or macrovascular complications, or extensive comorbid conditions. The following (Table 20), is consensus framework for establishing treatment goals for glycemic control, blood pressure, and dyslipidemia as proposed by the American Diabetes Association, the American Geriatrics Society, and other stakeholders including AMDA [30]. It stratifies older adults by presence and number of comorbidities, functional impairment and life expectancy.

Hypoglycemia

Symptomatic hypoglycemia is defined by symptoms related to hypoglycemia and confirmed by PG ≤70 mg/dL (≤4.0 mmol/L). This can be problematic since symptoms of hypoglycemia may be atypical such as disorientation, lethargy, weakness, falls, aggression, or altered behavior. These behaviors can mistakenly be attributed to

Table 20 Consensus framework for considering treatment goals in older adults with diabetes

Patient characteristics/ health status	Reasonable A1c goal[a]	Fasting/ preprandial glucose (mg/dL)	Bedtime glucose (mg/dL)	Blood pressure (mm Hg)	Lipids
Healthy[b]	Less than 7.5 %	90–130	90–150	Less than 140/90	Statin unless contraindicated or not tolerated
Complex/ intermediate[c]	Less than 8.0 %	90–150	100–180	Less than 140/90	Statin unless contraindicated or not tolerated
Very complex/ poor health[d]	Less than 8.5 %[‖]	100–180	110–200	Less than 150/90	Consider likelihood of benefit from statin (secondary prevention more than primary)

Source: Adapted from ADA 2015 [26]; Kirkman et al., 2012 [30], AMDA [23]

[a]Lower goals may be set for individuals if achievable without recurrent or severe hypoglycemia or undue treatment burden

[b]Healthy: Few coexisting chronic illnesses, intact cognitive and functional status. Longer remaining life expectancy

[c]Complex/intermediate: Multiple coexisting chronic illnesses (i.e., three or more conditions serious enough to require medications or lifestyle management [e.g., arthritis, cancer, CHF, depression, emphysema, falls, hypertension, incontinence, stage III or worse chronic kidney disease, myocardial infarction, stroke]); or more than two instrumental ADL impairments; **or** mild to moderate cognitive impairment. Intermediate remaining life expectancy, high treatment burden, hypoglycemia vulnerability, fall risk

[d]**Very complex/poor health**: Long-term care or end-stage chronic illnesses (e.g., stage III–IV CHF, oxygen-dependent lung disease, CKD requiring dialysis, uncontrolled metastatic cancer); **or** moderate to severe cognitive impairment; **or** more than two ADL dependencies. Limited remaining life expectancy makes benefit uncertain

dementia, delirium, or other disorders and hypoglycemia overlooked as a potential cause. Moreover, older adults have a lower glucose threshold at which they develop subjective symptoms and repeated episodes of hypoglycemia can lead to worsening of dementia (Table. 21).

Insulin-induced hypoglycemia can result from delayed insulin clearance as in renal failure, erratic absorption by injecting hypertrophic sites, and increased insulin sensitivity due to weight loss or significantly increased physical activity. Frequent use of SSI, improper timing of insulin relative to timing of food intake, low meal consumption, inappropriately tight blood glucose control, injection of wrong type of insulin (e.g., rapid acting instead of long acting), and unawareness of hypoglycemia can all cause insulin-induced hypoglycemia.

*Hypoglycemia may be corrected with ingestion of **15 g** of glucose or carbohydrate*, which is equivalent to 1/2 cup juice, 1/2 cup apple sauce, 1 cup milk, ½ can regular soda, 1 tablespoon sugar or honey, 1 mini candy bar, 1 tube of glucose 15 gel, or 4 glucose tablets. Caregivers should wait **15 min**, recheck blood glucose and if still below the target, give another **15 g** of glucose or carbohydrate. Elderly who are obtunded may be treated with SC or IM glucagon (1 mg or 1 unit) or 50 % dextrose IV (usually 50 mL, on a lesser volume if hypoglycemia is not severe).

Table 21 Risk factors for severe hypoglycemia [31]

• Age
• Unawareness of, or previous severe hypoglycemia
• High doses of insulin or sulfonylureas (associated with unrecognized hypoglycemia)
• Recent hospitalization or intercurrent illness
• Polypharmacy (>5 prescribed meds)
• Poor nutrition or variable oral intake
• Chronic liver, renal, or cardiovascular disease
• Endocrine deficiency (thyroid, adrenal, or pituitary)
• Alcohol use
• Loss of normal counter-regulation

Monitoring

Assessment of Glycemic Control

There is no consensus recommendation regarding the frequency of glucose checks in LTC. The practice of routinely checking pre-meal and bedtime glucose should only be used for those receiving multiple insulin injections or insulin pump therapy and for whom this information will be used to adjust insulin dosing. In residents who are on simpler insulin regimen (1–2 doses a day), then twice daily glucose monitoring for at least 3–4 days a week is suggested. For residents receiving oral agents or less frequent insulin injections, a reasonable approach to glucose monitoring would be twice per day for 1–2 weeks after admission, then once or twice per week and as indicated. Postprandial monitoring may be helpful in situations where the fasting glucose is at goal but the A1C remains elevated.

Expert opinion suggests that A1C should be monitored every 6 months in patients who are achieving their goals and every 3 months in those who are suboptimally controlled.

Facility Management of Diabetes

Successful implementation of facility-wide diabetes evaluation, treatment, and monitoring protocols is possible if there is buy-in from the administration, and effective education and communication with practitioners, nursing staff and medical assistants. In an assisted living facility it may be more difficult to accomplish this due to limited resources. In such situations the resident may be eligible to receive home health services to complement the care provided by the facility staff. The role of each discipline should be defined and a "diabetes nurse" or champion should ensure implementation of any protocols. A quality improvement program could be devised by selecting certain process indicators (e.g., prevalence of sliding-scale insulin use or regularity of foot examinations) or outcome indicators (e.g., incidence of hypoglycemia or A1C levels) for periodic review and performance improvement.

Hypothyroidism

Although thyroid disease is common in the elderly, its presentation is often subtle and varied. Because of its nonspecific presentation, thyroid disease requires screening and interpretation of thyroid function tests in the context of the resident's signs symptoms and medication regimen.

Hypothyroidism is defined as a state of reduced thyroid hormone availability to the peripheral tissues. *Overt hypothyroidism* is present when serum free T4 levels are below the normal range in the presence of hypothyroid symptoms. Mild thyroid failure or *subclinical hypothyroidism* is a condition in which the TSH level is elevated in the presence of a normal free T4 level. Here the presence and severity of symptoms is variable. Despite an increase in fibrosis, lymphocyte infiltration, and nodularity of the thyroid with age, in the vast majority of older adults thyroid function remains normal with no change in total T4 and free T4, a slight decrease in TSH and free T3, and a slight increase in reverse T3.

Screening for Thyroid Dysfunction

The American Thyroid Association recommends screening all individuals after age 35 and every 5 years thereafter [32]. However, the American College of Physicians does not recommend screening, citing a lack of benefit in the treatment of subclinical thyroid disease. In the Colorado Thyroid Disease Prevalence Study, 16 % of women and 21 % of men over age 74 years had elevated TSH levels [33]. Adults over age 60 have a 2.3–10 % prevalence of hypothyroidism, and since symptoms may be nonspecific periodic screening may be justified. Conditions for which screening is suggested are listed in Table 22.

Table 22 Conditions associated with thyroid disease	
	• Biological agents (interferons, growth hormone treatment)
	• Chronic kidney disease
	• Cognitive impairment/psychiatric illness
	• Down's/Turner's syndrome
	• Drug therapy (amiodarone, lithium)
	• Hyperlipidemia
	• Irradiation of head/neck
	• Pituitary surgery irradiation
	• Radical laryngeal/pharyngeal surgery
	• Thyroid disease/surgery in the past, goiter
	• Thyroid nodule
	• Type 1 diabetes
	• Severe head injury
	• Unexplained depression/weight loss

Interpretation of Thyroid Function Tests

In most situations, measurement of serum TSH by immuno-assay is sensitive to distinguish between a normal, low or high value. However, in the elderly with a pituitary or hypothalamic disorder, the TSH may be misleading (subnormal or low-normal). This can also occur in the elderly with acute or chronic illness, hospitalized patients, those with poor adherence to therapy or with drugs that alter thyroid hormone levels (see Tables 23 and 24).

Non-thyroidal illness can cause a low T3 state with normal TSH, FT4 and T4 (due to inhibition of 5' deiodinase and conversion of T4 to T3). Patients who are severely ill may also have a low T4 and low T3. TSH can decline also with severe illness, while *a transient high TSH may be seen during the recovery phase from an acute illness.* There is increasing recognition of *partial hypopituitarism* in frail long-term care residents with cardiovascular disease. Thus when evaluating for

Table 23 Drugs affecting thyroid function [34]

Effect	Drugs
May cause hypothyroidism	Lithium, iodine (all forms, including kelp, contrast media), interferon-alpha
May cause hyperthyroidism	Iodine, interleukins, interferons
Reduce conversion of T4 to T3	Glucocorticoids, iodine, propylthiouracil, beta-blockers, amiodarone
Suppress TSH	Dopamine, dobutamine, glucocorticoids, phenytoin, bromocriptine, octreotide
Increase clearance of T4	Carbamazepine, phenytoin, rifampin, phenobarbital
Reduce binding of T4 to thyroid-binding globulin	Salsalate, salicylates, nonsteroidal anti-inflammatory drugs, furosemide, heparin
Influence absorption of thyroxine	Cholestyramine, aluminum hydroxide, ferrous sulfate, sucralfate, cation exchange resins

Table 24 Interpretations of the TSH and free T4

	Low FT4	Normal FT4	High FT4
High TSH	• Primary hypothyroidism	• Subclinical hypothyroidism	• Intermittent/poor compliance with thyroxine (common) • TSH producing tumor
Normal TSH	• Sick euthyroid • Drug effect • Secondary hypothyroidism	EUTHYROID	• Intermittent/poor compliance with thyroxine • Thyroid hormone resistance
Low TSH	• Secondary hypothyroidism (pituitary or hypothalamic) • Sick euthyroid syndrome	• Subclinical hyperthyroidism • Thyroxine treatment • T3 toxicosis	• Hyperthyroidism

Table 25 Causes of
hypothyroidism in the elderly

Primary hypothyroidism
• Chronic autoimmune hypothyroidism (Hashimoto's thyroiditis)
• Post ^{131}I treatment for hyperthyroidism
• Subtotal or total thyroidectomy
• Radiation therapy for head and neck cancer
• Drugs
Central (secondary) hypothyroidism
• Hypothalamic tumors or infiltrative lesions
• Pituitary tumors or infiltrative lesions
• Pituitary surgery
• Head injury or cranial surgery
• Radiation

thyroid dysfunction a TSH and a free T4 level is more helpful (a "thyroid panel" is usually not necessary). Table 23 provides a guide for the interpretation of TSH and free T4 (FT4) levels [34].

Causes of Hypothyroidism

The majority of residents with hypothyroidism have primary hypothyroidism. Central or secondary hypothyroidism is rare and accounts for less than 1 % of cases. Central hypothyroidism may be due to pituitary or hypothalamic lesions (or dysfunction of the hypothalamic–pituitary axis (Table 25)).

Clinical Evaluation

Clinical signs and symptoms are often nonspecific. Such signs and symptoms include anorexia, cognitive decline, constipation, dry skin, fatigue, slowed reflexes, and weakness. Fatigue has been noted in 68 % and weakness in 53 % [35]. Classical symptoms such as weight gain, cold intolerance, paresthesias and muscle cramps are less frequent in older patients. *Neuropsychiatric symptoms* (e.g., withdrawal, disorientation, delusions or psychosis) may develop gradually and be particularly challenging given the prevalence of dementia and the propensity for developing delirium in the elderly.

Hypothyroidism may also cause bradycardia, diastolic hypertension, dyslipidemia, and increased levels of creatinine phosphokinase. Pericardial effusion can be present in 30–50 % in overt hypothyroidism. Hypothyroidism may mimic symptoms of coronary artery disease due to bradycardia and reduced cardiac contractility. While atypical chest pain, exertional dyspnea and reduced exercise tolerance due to the presence of coronary artery disease may coexist with hypothyroidism.

Treatment of Clinical Hypothyroidism

The goal of treatment is to normalize the thyroid function test (TSH) to achieve a euthyroid state. The dose of thyroid hormone replacement depends on the age and weight of the resident. The average daily requirement for the elderly is 25 % less than that for young adults. Synthetic thyroid hormone preparations (rather than thyroid extracts) are preferred since they have a longer half-life and a more constant serum concentration. Older adults with cardiovascular disease should be started on 12.5–25 µg/day of levothyroxine and the dose adjusted by a similar amount every 6 weeks until the TSH has normalized and then followed every 6–12 months. In primary hypothyroidism, the TSH alone can be used to monitor treatment, but in those with central (secondary) hypothyroidism, a free T4 level should be used. If no residual thyroid function exists the daily replacement dose of levothyroxine is usually 1.6 µg/kg body weight (typically 100–150 µg). After the treatment of Graves' disease, there is often some underlying autonomous thyroid function, necessitating a lower replacement dose (typically 75–125 µg/day).

Dosage adjustments should take into account any worsening condition such as atrial fibrillation, HF or the presence of osteoporosis. In such cases low normal or subnormal TSH levels should be avoided. It is important to note that *linear changes in the concentration of T4 correspond to logarithmic changes in serum TSH*. If a resident has had an abrupt discontinuation or omission of levothyroxine therapy during a care transition, there may be a marked rise in the TSH level. When resumed the dose of levothyroxine should be the prior documented dose.

Subclinical Hypothyroidism

This condition may also be referred as "mild thyroid failure" and is defined by an elevated TSH with a normal free T4 level. Anti-TPO antibodies are positive in 67 % of nursing facility residents with subclinical hypothyroidism. Most elderly are usually asymptomatic. Prevalence of this condition in 80-year-olds ranges from 14 to 20 % and was 14.6 % in one large nursing facility study. The etiology of subclinical hypothyroidism is usually chronic autoimmune thyroiditis, but poor compliance with levothyroxine therapy, suboptimal treatment, recovery from severe illness, thyroiditis, and medications that affect thyroid function should be considered.

The possible effects of subclinical hypothyroidism include progression to overt hypothyroidism, elevation of lipid levels, altered mood and cognition, impaired cardiac function, and increased mortality. A high TSH level (>12 mU/L), presence of autoantibodies, a goiter, advanced age, and a history of radiation history are all risk factors for progression to overt hypothyroidism. In the general population *those age 85 and older* on thyroid replacement with higher levels of TSH may not experience adverse effects and *may have a prolonged life span compared to those with subnormal TSH levels*.

Management of Subclinical Hypothyroidism

Current evidence does not support benefit to routinely treating *subclinical* hypothyroidism to lesson systemic symptoms of hypothyroidism and to improve cardiac function or neuropsychiatric symptoms. The current guidelines for the management of subclinical hypothyroidism are the following [36]:

- If the TS4 is 4.5–10 mU/L in the ***absence*** of symptoms, repeat TSH in 1 month and every 6 months while asymptomatic
- If the TS4 is 4.5–10 mU/L in the ***presence*** of symptoms, consider trial of thyroid hormone replacement
- If the TSH is >10 mU/L, in most circumstances administer thyroid treatment.

Vitamin B_{12} Deficiency

B_{12} deficiency is common in older adults and can lead to hematological abnormalities (though often there is no associated anemia or macrocytosis) as well as serious and irreversible neurological consequences. Population studies show a prevalence of B_{12} deficiency of 10–15 % in older adults, with one study of hospitalized elderly from the community and nursing facilities reporting a prevalence of 5 % with low B_{12} (<200 pg/mL), and 20 % with marginal B_{12} (200–349 pg/mL). The signs and symptoms of B_{12} deficiency are nonspecific and varied and can be attributed to other comorbid disorders or the neurological changes of aging. The elderly may have "subtle B_{12} deficiency" with only a biochemical deficiency. In a population in which the prevalence of dementia and other neurological and neuropsychiatric abnormalities are high, early recognition and treatment of B_{12} deficiency is beneficial [37]. Older age and more established symptoms of B_{12} deficiency are associated with less likelihood of neurologic improvement upon treatment. B_{12} deficiency has also been associated with low bone mineral density and been implicated in pre-frailty.

Risk factors and causes of B_{12} deficiency are listed Table 26. Dietary-cobalamin deficiency is responsible for about 40–50 % of B_{12} deficiency and pernicious anemia

Table 26 Causes of B_{12} deficiency [38]	
	• Atrophic gastritis and hypochlorhydria
	• Chronic proton pump inhibitor use
	• Metformin
	• Gastrectomy (total or partial) or gastric by-pass surgery
	• Ileal resection
	• Small intestine and terminal ileum disorders (Crohn's disease, sprue, malabsorption)
	• H Pylori infection
	• Bacterial overgrowth syndromes
	• Strict vegetarian diet
	• Pernicious anemia (positive anti-intrinsic factor antibodies)
	• AIDS and AIDS treatment (zidovudine)

Table 27 Signs and symptoms of B_{12} deficiency

Hematologic: macrocytosis, anemia, neutrophil hypersegmentation
Neurologic: peripheral neuropathy, paresthesias, spinal column lesions (loss of vibration, position sense, ataxia), extensor plantars, orthostatic, hypotension, limb weakness
Neuropsychiatric: delirium with slow thinking, depression, confusion, memory loss
Other: glossitis, palor

for about 10 %. Achlorhydria and atrophic gastritis is another important contributing factor in older adults. Stomach acid is necessary for the release of vitamin B-12 from food, which then binds to haptocorin, undergoes degradation by pancreatic enzymes, then binds to intrinsic factor and finally absorbed in the terminal ileum. The B-12 intrinsic factor complex then binds to transcobalamin for transport in the blood.

B_{12} deficiency should be suspected in residents with unexplained anemia or neurological symptoms, glossitis, anorexia, diarrhea, or other gastrointestinal disorders as well as the presence of autoimmune diseases such as thyroiditis, vitiligo, and any of the risk factors listed in Table 26. Signs and symptoms of vitamin B_{12} deficiency are listed in Table 27.

Diagnosis

Blood levels of B_{12} and folate are frequently ordered in the elderly with anemia, dementia, and depression. *Falsely low levels of B_{12} may be seen* in AIDS, multiple myeloma, folate deficiency, haptocorin deficiency, and excessive vitamin C intake. *Falsely normal or high levels of B_{12}* may be seen in transcobalamin II deficiency, certain myeloproliferative disorders (CML), liver disease, and intestinal bacterial overgrowth.

Metabolite testing for homocysteine (Hcy) and methyl malonic acid (MMA) is widely available, although the interpretation of these tests may be difficult and affected by other clinical conditions. *MMA elevation is specific for B_{12} deficiency* and indicates tissue deficiency, whereas Hcy levels are elevated in most individuals with B_{12} and folate deficiency. Holotranscobalamin (holoTC) represents B_{12} bound to transcobalamin and is the fraction available for tissue uptake. This test is not widely available and may be equivalent to total B_{12} in its ability to discriminate between people with or without B_{12} deficiency.

The elderly may have a tissue deficiency of B_{12} with levels as high as 400 pg/mL. Conversely, some subnormal B_{12} levels have normal Hyc and MMA levels. Falsely elevated levels of MMA may be seen in hypovolemia and both MMA and Hcy may be falsely elevated in renal insufficiency. Hence there is no clear recommendation for the diagnosis of B_{12} deficiency, but Hyc and MMA levels may be useful if B_{12} levels are borderline (100–350 pg/mL) and symptoms are nonspecific [39]. No further evaluation is usually required once the diagnosis of B12 deficiency is made with first-line blood tests. The Shilling test or other tests of gastric function are rarely performed. Bone marrow examination is rarely needed and only to rule out malignancy.

Treatment

In symptomatic patients a common treatment is to replace B_{12} in the form of 1000 μg cyanocobalamin by intramuscular injection weekly (for 3–4 weeks), then monthly, though intervals can be extended to every 3 months. For residents in whom B_{12} was discovered incidentally it may be replaced orally. Crystalline B_{12} is well absorbed and at least 500–1000 μg/day is required to reverse the biochemical signs of B_{12} deficiency. Sublingual and intranasal forms of B_{12} are more costly and have been less rigorously tested.

Monitoring recommendations vary and depend on the manifestation and severity of B_{12} deficiency. Elderly with anemia due to B_{12} deficiency should have a reticulocyte count in one week and hemoglobin levels in 1–2 months. Biochemical monitoring is not required in those receiving parenteral replacement, but B_{12}, MMA or Hcy may be measured to assess absorption and compliance in patients receiving oral supplementation. Treatment of B_{12} deficiency may unmask underlying folate and iron deficiency. Thus as red cell production increases folate and iron supplementation may be needed.

Skin Disorders

Scabies

Scabies is a contagious parasitic infestation of the skin caused by the human itch mite *Sarcoptes scabei*. It can cause large outbreaks among residents and staff unless timely treated and systematic infection control protocols followed. The severity of the scabies infection depends on the number of mites infesting the skin. *Norwegian scabies* is a severe atypical infection characterized by extremely pruritic crusty skin lesions with thousands to millions of live mites. Mental retardation, dementia, immunodeficiency states, renal failure, malnutrition, HIV, insulin-treated diabetes, and administration of topical and systemic corticosteroids can increase the severity of scabies.

Transmission and Diagnosis

The incubation period of scabies is 3–6 weeks. Healthy individuals without prior infestation may be asymptomatic during this period. Those with previous infestation often develop pruritis within 48 h of reinfection as the itching originates from an allergic reaction to the mite. The itching is often severe, and can be particularly problematic at night. Skin areas typically affect the web spaces between the fingers, breast folds, buttocks, genitalia, and flexor surfaces of the wrists, elbows, and axillae. The differential diagnosis will include eczema, folliculitis, tinea, psoriasis, insect bites, or dermatitis herpetiformis.

An outbreak is be defined as one or more confirmed cases within a finite period of time and in a defined facility location (e.g., a nursing unit or ward). Norwegian scabies causes on extremely high rate of transmission. Transmission of scabies occurs from person to person skin contact or from infested clothing. Chair covers and bed linens play a smaller role in transmission.

Skin scrapings that show the presence of mites, eggs, or fecal pellets on microscopic exam will confirm scabies. Scrapings should be performed in areas that are typically infested by the mite. However, in recently exposed persons, skin scrapings can be negative on multiple occasions and the Burrows Ink Test may provide clues to infestation. The Burrows Ink Test is performed by running a black or green felt tip pen over the waxy red raised burrows, and then wiping the skin off with alcohol to reveal a black or green zigzag line under magnification [40]. An eczematous eruption can frequently be seen covering the trunk of elderly infected with scabies, but this is usually an allergic reaction to the mite and may shown little evidence of mite infestation. Skin biopsies are not recommended due to low yield. Hence empiric treatment based on symptoms may be necessary. A dermatology consultation may be considered for indeterminate rashes.

Controlling the Outbreak

Barrier precautions using gowns and gloves should be used until the diagnosis of scabies has been eliminated as a possibility. The medical director should be notified and treatment ordered and other practitioners also notified. The infection control nurse should track cases and contacts as well as implement barrier precautions. The staff needs to treat all residents in an area if multiple cases are found. Staff education should be reinforced and work assignments should restrict care areas in order to limit transmission. Any exposed visitors and volunteers should be treated as well. The local health department or the state regulatory agency should also be notified.

Contact precautions should be used for at least 24 h after initiating treatment. Residents with crusted scabies will require several treatments and may be contagious for several weeks. *In the case of crusted scabies contact isolation in a single room should be continued until three consecutive skin scrapings are negative.* Clothing, pillows, blankets, wheelchair pads can be washed, sealed in plastic for 5–7 days, or placed in a hot dryer. Environmental surfaces, beds, assistive devices, diagnostic and therapy equipment should be cleaned with an Environmental Protection Agency (EPA)-registered cleaning product. Furniture with fabric upholstery will need to be removed for 5–7 days, topical creams and lotions discarded, all carpets vacuumed and the vacuum bag disposed of immediately.

Treatment of Scabies [40]

- Gamma-hexachlorocyclohexane (Lindane) *is no longer recommended due to resistance of the mites* and *neurotoxicity* concerns.
- Permethrin 5 % (Elimite) cream is 90 % effective after the first application. In some patients, *a second application after 7–10 days may be necessary,*
- All symptomatic patients, and close contacts including staff should be treated with permethrin in the same 24–48 h period.
- Health care workers and their household contacts should be treated at the end of the work shift. *Leave permethrin cream on and shower after 8–12 h.*
- Permethrin should be applied on the *entire area of skin from the hairline to the feet*, including the palms and soles, under the fingernails and toenails; the scalp may rarely need treatment unless infested.
- Topical steroid creams or antihistamines to treat pruritis *should not be applied until the scabicide has been removed.*
- Oral ivermectin (Stromectol) is an effective and cost-comparable alternative to topical scabicides although it is not FDA approved for use in scabies. It may be particularly useful in demented patients, in large outbreaks, and in the treatment of severely crusted scabies in immunocompromised residents or when topical therapy has failed. A single dose of 200 µg/kg is effective or a standard dose of 6 mg for a 70 kg adult.

Herpes Zoster

The prevalence of herpes zoster (HZ) in LTC residents is unknown, but has been reported to be 1.4 % in the elderly with 50 % developing post-herpetic neuralgia (PHN). This can be a devastating complication requiring prolonged pharmacotherapy and other pain management interventions, as well as lead to depression and a decline in function. Herpes zoster is characterized by a pruritic, maculopapular vesicular rash that evolves into noninfectious dried crusts over a 5–6-day period. It is triggered by a decline in cell-mediated immunity that facilitates the reactivation of latent varicella virus in the sensory ganglia of the spinal cord. Long-term care residents are at greater risk because of age-related decline in cell-medicated immunity, malnutrition, multiple comorbidities, frailty, and functional impairment. They also have diminished reserves to respond to stressors related to an episode of HZ.

The lesions of HZ are often described as a "dew drops on a rose petal" which are clustered in a dermatomal distribution, not crossing the midline. Most often, HZ is diagnosed clinically, but the laboratory diagnosis can be made by isolation of the varicella virus from a lesion. Rapid varicella virus identification using PCR is preferred if available, but direct fluorescent antibody (DFA) testing or a significant rise in varicella IgG can be used to make the diagnosis as well.

General Measures

The nursing leadership and medical staff should educate the resident and direct caregivers regarding the nature of the infection and the risk of viral transmission to individuals who have not had chickenpox. HZ is not contagious for those who have a history of chicken pox or adequate titers of IgG to varicella. Skin lesions should be kept clean and dry to avoid bacterial superinfection. Antibiotic ointments and adhesive dressings should be avoided since healing and drying of the lesions will be delayed. Shingles in immunocompromised individuals and those with ophthalmic zoster should be treated with antiviral agents [41].

Vaccination

The Advisory Committee on Immunization Practices (ACIP) recommends a single dose of zoster vaccine for persons 60 years and older, regardless of prior history of HZ. People with a chronic medical condition may be vaccinated unless a contraindication or precaution exists. It is not recommended for pregnant or immunocompromised individuals [42]. *Although zoster vaccine (Zostavax) in general has been associated with 51% fewer episodes of HZ, and 66% less PHN, the figures were only 18% and 26% respectively in those 80 and over.* Also, the Shingles Prevention Study did not include cognitively impaired, nonambulatory residents with less than 5 years expected survival. Hence response to the vaccine in LTC residents cannot reliably be predicted and currently widespread facility immunization programs for herpes zoster are not currently recommended [43].

Treatment

- Topical antiviral treatment is not efficacious.
- Systemic antiviral treatment recommended if ≥ 50year age, moderate to severe pain or rash; or have non-truncal involvement within 72 h of rash onset. Begin immediately or even after 72 h if neurologic or ocular signs, or severe pain and/ or rash.

  - Acyclovir 800 mg, five times daily (every 4–5 h) for 7–10 days
  - Famciclovir 500 mg, three times daily for 7 days
  - Valacyclovir 1000 mg, three times daily 7 days

- Adjuncts to antiviral therapy consider:

  - Analgesics (acetaminophen, opiods, tramadol)
  - Gabapentin (up to 3600 mg daily), pregabalin (75 mg twice daily), or a tricyclic antidepressant (nortriptyline 25 mg at bedtime, up to 150 mg daily), if no improvement in pain

– Oral corticosteroid (e.g., prednisone 60 mg daily for 7 days) for moderate to severe pain, polyneuropathy, cranial nerve paralysis, or CNS dysfunction

- Referral to a pain specialist is recommended to evaluate for neural blockade if analgesics, adjunct therapies, and corticosteroids are not effective in relieving post-herpetic neuralgia.
- Psychosocial evaluation to avoid isolation and severe depression
- Attention to nutrition and maintenance of functional status

Clostridium difficile Infection

Clostridium difficile (*C. difficile*) infections are a serious cause of morbidity and mortality in the post-acute and long-term setting. Nationwide, 500,000 infections and 30,000 deaths occurred in 2011 [44]. *C. difficile* colonizes the gut after normal flora has been altered by antibiotic treatment. Three quarters of these infections present in the PA/LTC setting and more than 90 % of deaths occur in those over 65 years. Over half of PA/LTC residents are thought to be carriers and the infection is transmitted in health care facilities from environmental surface contamination and hand carriage by staff members and infected patients (Table 28).

Clinical features

Older adults may be asymptomatic, have mild diarrhea, colitis, or pseudomembranous colitis. *Symptoms may begin during antibiotic treatment or up to 8 weeks after completion*, and the most common incriminating antibiotics are clindamycin, cephalosporins, and fluoroquinolones. In PA/LTC residents, diarrhea may be not be the initial problem, but fever, confusion, abdominal pain, anorexia, nausea, leukocytosis, and hypoalbuminemia. *Diagnosis should be made by testing diarrheal stool.* Testing options are as follows:

- *C. diff* toxin testing by EIA for toxins A and B is of inferior sensitivity (75 %) but low cost
- Real time PCR testing for toxins A and B is superior and can be available in 1 h. Beware of false positives.

Table 28 Risk factors for *C. difficile*	
	• Advanced age
	• Frequent need for hospitalization
	• Recurrent exposure to antibiotics
	• Presence of comorbid medical conditions
	• Gastrointestinal surgery
	• Use of acid suppressant medications (proton-pump inhibitors)
	• Age-related effects on host defense mechanisms

- EIA testing for *C. difficile* glutamate dehydrogenase (GDH), but it cannot distinguish between toxigenic and nontoxigenic strains; results available in 1 h and may be a screening test
- *Repeat testing to confirm cure is not recommended*
- Discontinue the use of any inciting antibiotics and avoid the use of anti-peristaltic agents. Consider discontinuing PPI's.

Management

- *For mild to moderate disease* (diarrhea plus other symptoms not meeting severe or complicated criteria);

  - Metronidazole 500 mg po TID for 10–14 days
  - Vancomycin 125 mg po QID if unable to take metronidazole or no improvement in 5–7 days

- *For severe disease* (albumin <3 g/dL **and** one of the following: WBC >15,000, or abdominal tenderness);

  - Vancomycin 125 mg po QID

- *For severe and complicated disease* (ICU admission, hypotension, fever, ileus or abdominal distension, confusion, WBC >35,000 or <2000), lactate >2 mmol/L)

  - Vancomycin 500 mg po QID
  - Vancomycin by enema (500 mg in 500 ml normal saline QID **and** metronidazole 500 mg IV q 8 h if oral therapy is not tolerated

- *For recurrent C. Diff infection* (10–20 % recur within 8 weeks)

  - Confirm diagnosis
  - Conservative treatment for mild symptoms
  - Same regimen as for the initial episode
  - "Pulsed vancomycin" regimen
  - Fidaxomycin 200 mg BID for 10 days (questionable efficacy)
  - Fecal bacteriotherapy (fecal microbiota transplant)

Antibiotic stewardship is crucial as is *hand hygiene* and the maintenance of *contact precautions*. Environmental surfaces should be disinfected using an approved sporicidal agent. Proton pump inhibitors should be used judiciously or discontinued. Moreover, there is no conclusive evidence supporting the use of probiotics though commonly prescribed during *C. difficile* treatment or as preventive therapy when antibiotics are prescribed for other infections.

Multidrug Resistant Organisms (MDROs)

The occurrence and transmission of MDROs most commonly occurs in acute care facilities. MDROs are defined as microorganisms, predominantly bacteria, that are resistant to one or more classes of antimicrobial drugs. Clinical manifestations of infection by MDROs are similar to those caused by susceptible pathogens; however, the choice of antibiotics is limited. MDROs include the following:

- MRSA
- VRE
- ESBL producing K. pneumonia
- ESBL producing *E. coli*
- MDR *Acinetobacter baumannii*
- CRE carbapenem-resistant bacterobacteriaceae
- MDR S. pneumonia
- Vancomycin-resistant *S. aureus*.

Management of these infections is beyond the scope of this chapter. Refer to the 2006 CDC report: Management of Multi-Drug Resistant Organism in Healthcare Settings and the website for the Healthcare Infection Central Practices Advisory Committee (HICPAC).

Prevention of transmission of MDROs within the nursing facility is critical. This includes strict adherence to hand hygiene (standard precautions) and donning of gown and glove use (contact precautions). There is uncertainty as to when to discontinue standard and contact precautions, partially due to the difficulty determining whether a positive culture of a MDRO is a true infection or colonization. Antibiotic stewardship to evaluate and optimize antibiotic use in the facility is essential. It is highly recommended to identify community experts who can provide consultation.

Conclusion

The management of medical conditions in patients and residents in the long-term care continuum is challenging due to patient complicity, multi-morbidities, guarded prognosis, individual advance directives for health care, goals of care and the healthcare setting in which care is provided by an interprofessional team, under the scrutiny of government and survey agencies.

It is essential to determine the risks and benefits to patients as it relates to the identification, assessment, treatment and monitoring when managing of multiple clinical conditions. This chapter has reviewed common clinical conditions encountered by practitioners. However, practitioners need not forget *less common conditions* that can afflict residents such as cancer, Parkinson's disease, polymyalgia rheumatic, traumatic brain injury, and abuse and neglect.

Peals for the Practitioner

- Studies have shown that the treatment of HTN in those over age 80 has resulted in a significant reduction in fatal and nonfatal stroke and all-cause mortality within 1–2 years of starting antihypertensive treatment.
- Once diagnosed with anemia, residents should be evaluated for possible comorbid conditions such as impaired physical performance, risk for falls, and cognitive impairment.
- Residents with HF have a 74 or 92 % 5-year mortality with either a normal or reduced LVEF, respectively. HF is a major cause of hospital admissions and readmissions.
- COPD, the third leading cause of US deaths, is present in one in six people admitted to nursing facilities and yet remains either unrecognized or suboptimally treated.
- Effective management of diabetes requires an approach that is multifaceted, protocol-driven, interdisciplinary, and individualized. If used, sliding-scale insulin is best utilized as a supplement to scheduled oral hypoglycemic agents and/or basal insulin therapy and not as a primary means to control blood glucose.
- Subclinical hypothyroidism is both common and not associated with the classic signs and symptoms of hypothyroidism often seen in younger adults. Subclinical hypothyroidism is not uncommon in those already diagnosed with DM or vitamin B_{12} deficiency.
- Vitamin B_{12} deficiency in older age is commonly not associated with anemia or macrocytosis, so a high index of suspicion is warranted as to its possible presence.
- For scabies, permethrin 5 % cream has a 90 % effective cure rate after its first application. A second application may be necessary 7–10 days after initial treatment.
- In those 80 years and older, zoster vaccine (Zostavax®) is associated with only 18 % fewer attacks of shingles and 26 % less occurrence of PHN, while more effective in those age 60 and over (51 and 66 %, respectively)
- Clinical practice guidelines related to PA/LTC for are available for ordering at ww.amda.com (e.g., Anemia, Heart Failure, COPD, and Common Infections).

Websites

- AMDA-The Society of Post-Acute and Long-Term Care Medicine www.amda.com.
- National Guideline Clearing House www.guideline.gov.
- AHA www.americanheart.org.
- American College of cardiology www.acc.org.
- The Global Initiative for Chronic Obstructive Lung Disease www.goldcopd.com.
- American Diabetes Association www.diabetes.org.
- American Thyroid Association Professional Guidelines www.thyroidguidelines.net.
- Center for Disease Control and Prevention www.cdc.gov.

References

Hypertension

1. Koka M, Josph J, Aronow WS. Adequacy of control of hypertension in an academic nursing home. J Am Med Dir Assoc. 2007;8(8):538–40.
2. Musini, Vijaya M, Tejani, et al. Pharmacotherapy for hypertension in the elderly. Cochrane Database Syst Rev. 2009, 4. Art. No.: CD000028. DOI: 10.1002/14651858.CD000028.pub2.
3. Beckett NS, Peters R, Fletcher AE, et al. Treatment of hypertension in patients 80 years of age or older. N Engl J Med. 2008;358(18):1887–98.
4. James PA, Oparil S, Carter BL, et al. 2014 Evidence-based guideline for the management of high blood pressure in adults: Report from the panel members appointed to the Eighth Joint National Committee (JNC 8). JAMA. 2014;311:507.
5. Vongpatanasin WL. Resistant hypertension: a review of diagnosis and management. JAMA. 2014;311(21):2216–24.
6. Rosendorff C et al. Treatment of hypertension in the prevention and management of ischemic heart disease: a scientific statement from the American Heart Association Council for high blood pressure research and the councils on clinical cardiology and epidemiology and prevention. Circulation. 2007;115:2761–88.
7. Jeffrey B. Halter, Joseph G. Ouslander, Mary E. Tinetti, Stephanie Studenski, Kevin P. High, Sanjay Asthana. Hazzard's geriatric medicine and gerontology, 6th edn. Chapter 81. McGraw Hill.

Anemia

8. Chaves P, Ashar T, Guralnik JM, et al. Looking at the relationship between hemoglobin concentration and previous mobility difficulty in older women: Should the criteria used to define anemia in older people be changed? J Am Geriatr Soc. 2002;50:1257–64.
9. Pandya N et al. Study of anemia in long-term care (SALT): prevalence of anemia and its relationship with the risk of falls in nursing home residents. Curr Med Res Opin. 2008;24(8): 2139–49.
10. American Medical Directors Association (AMDA). Anemia in the long-term care setting. Clinical practice guideline. Columbia, MD: American Medical Directors Association (AMDA); 2007.
11. Weiss G, Goodnough L. Anemia of chronic disease. N Engl J Med. 2005;352:1011–23.

Heart Failure

12. Aronow WS. Treatment of systolic and diastolic heart failure in the elderly. J Am Med Dir Assoc. 2006;7(1):29–36.
13. Hutt E, Elder SJ, Fish R, Min S. Regional variation in mortality and subsequent hospitalization of nursing residents with heart failure. J Am Med Dir Assoc. 2003;12(8):595–601.
14. A scientific statement from the American Heart Association and the Heart Failure Society of America: Heart failure. Circulation. 2015;8: 655–87.
15. Hutt E, Frederickson E, Ecord M, Kramer AM. Associations among processes and outcomes of care for Medicare nursing home residents with acute heart failure. J Am Med Dir Assoc. 2003;4(4):195–9.
16. Chun J, Chodosh J. Controversy in heart failure management: digoxin use in the elderly. J Am Med Dir Assoc. 2006;7(9):581–6.

COPD

17. American Medical Director's Association. COPD management in the long-term care setting. Clinical practice guideline. Columbia, MD: American Medical Director's Association; 2003. Revision in process.
18. Doherty DE. Identification and assessment of chronic obstructive pulmonary disease in the elderly. J Am Med Dir Assoc. 2003;4(5):S116–20.
19. Global strategy for the diagnosis, management, and prevention of chronic obstructive pulmonary disease: Revised 2014. Global Initiative for Chronic Obstructive Lung Disease (GOLD). www.goldcopd.org. Accessed 21 Jun 2015.
20. Gooneratne NS, Patel NP, Corcoran A. Chronic obstructive pulmonary disease diagnosis and management in older adults. J Am Geriatr Soc. 2010;58(6):1153–62.
21. Ziment I, Yick D. Treatment of chronic obstructive pulmonary disease. J Am Med Dir Assoc. 2003;4(5):S121–6.

Diabetes

22. Resnick HE, Heineman J, Stone R, Shorr RI. Diabetes in U.S. nursing homes, 2004. Diabetes Care. 2008;31:287–8. doi:10.2337/dc07-1425.
23. American Medical Directors Association (AMDA). Diabetes management in the post-acute and long-term care setting. Clinical practice guideline. Columbia, MD: American Medical Directors Association (AMDA); 2015.
24. Guidelines abstracted from the American Geriatrics Society guidelines for improving the care of older adults with diabetes mellitus: 2013 update. J Am Geriatr Soc. 2013;61:2020–6.
25. International Expert Committee Report on the role of the A1C assay in the diagnosis of diabetes. Diabetes Care 2009;32(7):1–8.
26. American Diabetes Association. Approaches to glycemic treatment. Sec. 7 in: Standards of Medical Care in Diabetes–2015. Diabetes Care. 2015; 38:S41–8. doi: 10.2337/dc15-S010 44.
27. Pandya N, Wei W, Meyers JL, et al. Burden of sliding scale insulin use in elderly long-term care residents with type 2 diabetes mellitus. J Am Geriatr Soc. 2013;61:2103–10. doi:10.1111/jgs.12547.
28. McNabney M, Pandya N, Iwuagwu C, et al. Differences in diabetes management of nursing home patients based on functional and cognitive status. J Am Med Dir Assoc. 2005;6:375–82.
29. Intensive glycemic control and the prevention of cardiovascular events: Implications of the ACCORD, ADVANCE, and VA diabetes trials: a position statement of the American Diabetes Association and a scientific statement of the American College of Cardiology Foundation and the American Heart Association Diabetes Care. 2009; 32:187–192.
30. Kirkman MS, Briscoe VJ, Clark N, et al. Diabetes in older adults. Diabetes Care. 2012;35:2650–64. doi:10.2337/dc12-1801.
31. Chelliah A, Burge MR. Hypoglycaemia in elderly patients with diabetes mellitus: causes and strategies for prevention. Drugs & Aging. 2004;21(8):511–30.

Thyroid Disease

32. Ladenson PW et al. American Thyroid Association Guidelines for detection of thyroid dysfunction. Arch Intern Med. 2000;160:1573–5.
33. Canaris GJ, Manowitz NR, Mayor G, Ridgway EC. The Colorado thyroid disease prevalence study. Arch Intern Med. 2000;160:526–34.

34. Finucane P et al. Thyroid function tests in elderly patients with and without an acute illness. Age Ageing. 1989;18:398–402.
35. Mohandas R. Managing thyroid dysfunction in the elderly. Postgrad Med. 2003;113(5):54–6; 65–8; 100.
36. Surks MI et al. Subclinical thyroid disease: scientific review and guidelines for diagnosis and management. JAMA. 2004;291:228–38.

Vitamin B$_{12}$ Deficiency

37. Malouf R, Evans GJ. Folic acid with or without vitamin B12 for the prevention and treatment of healthy elderly and demented people [update of Cochrane Database Syst Rev. 2003;(4):CD004514;PMID: 14584018][Review][121 refs]. Cochrane Database Syst Rev. 2008;(4):CD004514.
38. Smith RL. Evaluation of vitamin B12 and folate status in the nursing home. J Am Med Dir Assoc. 2001;2(5):230–8.
39. Hvas AM, Nexo E. Diagnosis and treatment of vitamin B12 deficiency- an update. Haematologica. 2006;91:1506–12.

Scabies

40. Cahill CK et al. Scabies surveillance, prevention, and control. Ann Long Term Care Clin Care Aging. 2009;17(4):31–5.

Zoster

41. Dworkin RH, Johnson RW, Breuer J, Gann JW. Recommendations for management of herpes zoster. Clin Infect Dis. 2007;44(Suppl l):S1–26.
42. Update on recommendations for use of Herpes Zoster vaccine. Morbidity and Mortality Weekly. 2014;63(33);729–7.
43. Drinka PJ. How should nursing homes use vaccine to prevent Zoster? J Am Med Dir Assoc. 2007;8(7):419–20.

Clostridium difficile

44. Lessa FC et al. Burden of Clostridium Difficile Infection in the United States. N Engl J Med. 2015;372:825–32.

Preventing Hospital Admissions and Readmissions

J. Kenneth Brubaker

Introduction

During the past several years there has been attention focused on the high number of hospital admissions and 30-day readmissions from nursing facilities (NF) and skilled nursing facilities (SNF) especially among dually eligible patients (Medicare and Medicaid).

Geriatricians agree that hospitals serve an important function for frail adults residing at NFs/SNFs. However, many adverse events can occur when admitted to hospital, which likely would not have occurred had the hospitalization been avoided. Dr. Ouslander has described many adverse hospital events and reminded patients, families, and NF providers that the hospital might not be the safest place for frail adults. Adverse hospital outcomes include [1]:

- Distress and discomfort for the resident and family.
- Delirium at least partially related to a change in environment.
- Polypharmacy and drug errors during transitions between care settings.
- Falls/fractures.
- Incontinence and catheter use.
- Hospital acquired infections (HAI).
- Unintentional weight loss and poor nutrition.
- Immobility, deconditioning, and pressure wounds.

J.K. Brubaker, MD, CMD (✉)
Masonic Villages, Elizabethtown, PA, USA

Lancaster General Health, 2112 Harrisburg Pike, Suite 312, Lancaster, PA 17601, USA
e-mail: jkbrubak@lghealth.org; jkbrubak@masonicvillages.org

© Springer International Publishing Switzerland 2016
P.A. Fenstemacher, P. Winn (eds.), *Post-Acute and Long-Term Medicine*,
Current Clinical Practice, DOI 10.1007/978-3-319-16979-8_9

In 2009, Dr. Gawande wrote a sentinel article in The New Republic that was disturbing to many health care providers. When 2006 Medicare data was reviewed, he found that the cost of care for Medicare recipients varied from $6500 to more than $15,000. What was even more surprising was the fact that some health care systems such as Mayo Clinic demonstrated consistently high quality of care at a cost that was less than half of other health care systems. Furthermore, many of those health systems that had higher costs had quality measures that were below average [2].

Attendees at the 2013 AMDA Annual Symposium were reminded by Dr. Paul McGann, Director of Medicare and Medicaid Innovations at CMS that the cause of America's poor quality and costly care is not due to insufficient federal and state funding. The USA spends nearly twice as much of Gross National Product (GNP) on health care when compared with many western countries; yet do poorly in quality measures (QM) as defined by the World Health Organization (WHO) [3]. So what do the other countries know that we do not know when it comes to providing high quality cost-effective care?

There are a growing number of physicians providing care in nursing homes who have demonstrated significant success in reducing *avoidable hospitalizations* from long-term care facilities (LTCF) and post-acute care (PAC). This chapter reviews strategies and tools in preventing avoidable hospital admissions and readmissions. The topics to be covered include the following:

- Transitions of care
- Accountable Care Organizations (ACOs) and their impact on NFs/SNFs
- Acute change in condition
- Antibiotic stewardship
- OPTUM system of care and INTERACT tool
- Physician Orders for Life-Sustaining Treatment (POLST) and goals of care

Transitions of Care

Care transitioning into and out of the NF impacts three systems of care that have the potential to reduce avoidable hospitalizations and improve the quality of patient care: the NF, the hospital and primary care in the community. These transfers of care include: from *hospitals to NF*, from *NF to hospital*, and from *NF to the community*. While each setting is unique, and under various state and federal regulations, the key elements needed for successful transfers include the following:

1. Patient-centered and family-oriented care
2. Effective communication between all systems that provide care to patients

Most health care providers believe their care is already person-centered when in fact it usually is not. What is frequently forgotten is an advocate for the frail adult. Among the many tasks required of an advocate, listening, asking questions, and requesting clarification of instructions are the most important. Many patients experience various degrees of memory, hearing, and visual loss. Thus, it is not surprising to learn that most discharge instructions are not remembered, heard, or read. For these reasons, it is imperative to review the plan of care with the healthcare proxy, power of attorney (POA)/or family member as well as the patient whenever possible.

Whether the patient transitions to the hospital, NF, or home in the community, it is critical that *goals of care* be reviewed with the patient, assuming he/she has the capacity to understand and appreciate the goals of care. If the patient has memory loss, future goals should be discussed and clarified with the patient's proxy decision maker.

During a care transition *important opportunities arise to talk about the "what ifs" that may occur in the future. What if* you are unable to care for yourself? *What if* you have CHF again for the fifth time in 4 months? *What if* palliative care would be the most reasonable and decided upon next step in providing care for a patient who is experiencing progressive weight loss and decline in ADLs? It may be an opportunity to discern the patient's wishes for future hospitalizations, emergency room visits, and NF care. Goals of care should include a discussion regarding orders on cardiopulmonary resuscitation (CPR), do not resuscitate (DNR), and if appropriate, to not transfer to the ER or to not admit to hospital.

Effective Communication

Effective communication with the patient, the POA, and the receiving health care provider should be the gold standard of health care. Written communication is most effective when transferring patients from one system of care to another. Ideally, a discharge or transfer summary should be sent with the patient at the time of discharge. Another copy should be sent/e-mailed/faxed to the primary care physician. A discharge summary should be succinct and include the following information [4]:

- Up-to-date discharge medication list.
- Discharge instructions from the facility's primary provider.
- Medical conditions to be monitored (e.g., daily weights for CHF, fall prevention interventions if high fall risk).
- Contact person at the discharging facility for answering any care questions.
- Pertinent consultations, emergency room visits, and needed follow-up visits with the primary care provider and any consultants.
- Copies of any advanced directives and goals of care.

More recently hospitals and NFs are taking the additional steps of calling discharged patients or their caregiver the following day to ensure the patient has experienced a safe transition back to home. The follow-up phone call discussion should include:

- Medication related issues
- Planned follow-up visits (primary care physician, consultants)
- Follow-up laboratory work and testing that has been recommended

If NFs/SNFs are committed to improving transitions of care and reducing avoidable hospital admissions, there are two very important elements of care that cannot be sacrificed:

1. Practitioners must acquire and maintain *geriatric competencies* in caring for frail adults.
2. The NF/SNF must *have the patient seen by the practitioner as soon as possible* upon admission or when an acute change in condition occurs.

Practitioners must be knowledgeable about the diagnosis and treatment of complex geriatric syndromes such as dysphagia associated with aspiration pneumonitis, fever, difficult behaviors (not responding to behavioral interventions), and delirium. Despite patients being transferred from the hospital with frequent drug errors, inappropriate drugs, without discharge summaries, or goals of care identified, many NF/SNF practitioners have been able to decrease avoidable hospitalizations. Figure 1 is an example of one institution in south central Pennsylvania that has maintained very low hospital admissions and readmission rates by applying principles of good geriatric medicine.

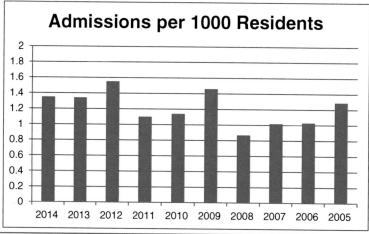

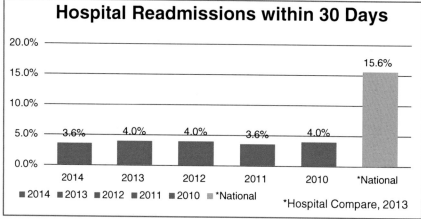

Fig. 1 Following the Principles of Geriatric Medicine and Preventing Hospital Admissions and Readmissions

Accountable Care Organizations (ACO)

Over the past several years population Health Management (PHM) and ACOs have become initiatives of the Centers for Medicare and Medicaid Services (CMS). Most health care planners agree that the present health system has failed to provide *health care value* (HCV) to American consumers. Dr. Dan Berwick has defined HCV as quality (quality measures and patient satisfaction scores) divided by the cost of care.

HCV = Quality / Cost

Future health care must develop healthcare delivery systems that make healthcare more clinically effective and safe at less cost.

One of the high cost drivers of the current system of care is the inducement to NFs to admit and readmit their patients to hospital. Having a three night hospital stay creates more opportunities for the NF to receive higher per diem reimbursement for those patients returning on SNF Medicare A services. In 2013, CMS initiated a hospital reimbursement system that penalizes hospitals that have a higher than expected 30-day readmission rate. Penalizing hospitals became a game changer for the many NFs that previously had benefited financially as a result of repeated hospitalizations.

ACOs were created by CMS in an attempt to emphasize prevention and early treatment of serious medical illness. *Medicare decided to incentivize the ACOs by allowing the ACO to share with Medicare any cost savings but at the same time placing them at risk for financial losses.* In the future, a successful ACO will be defined by *low occupancy hospital bed rates* and a system of care that is able to diagnose and treat chronic medical conditions before crises occur, thus preventing hospitalization.

How will ACOs impact those who care for the frail adults? There is growing evidence that NF physicians and management will have be prepared to work collaboratively and successfully with others in the health care system in order to be successful in the ACO market. If a NF is considering involvement with an ACO there are at least three questions on readiness that need to be addressed:

1. Can the NF/SNF promote a culture of early assessment, diagnosis, and *treatment in place* for a patient's change of condition?
2. Is the NF/SNF prepared to develop better educational programs to train staff and providers?
3. Is the practitioner readily available to assess patients when a change in condition occurs?

Medicare data demonstrates three diagnoses that consistently show up on its yearly reports on *Common Reasons for Hospitalization*: pneumonia; congestive heart failure; and urinary tract infections. Medicare data published in 2014 demonstrated that of all causes for NF/SNF admissions to the hospital: 9 % are due to pneumonia, 6 % due to CHF, and 4 % due to urosepsis.

It has been suggested that 30 % of pneumonia, 17 % of CHF, and 13 % of admissions for urosepsis could possibly have been avoided and successfully treated at the NF/SNF [5]. There are a number of opinions published in the medical literature stating that perhaps up to 75 % of the hospital admissions for these three illnesses could possibly have been avoided.

ACOs will also impact NFs/SNFs by referring frail adults suffering from an acute illness directly to the NFs/SNFs rather than admitting them to the hospital. Frail adults who are medially stable but unable to care for themselves during an acute illness, could more appropriately be directly referred to a NF/SNF from the hospital emergency room. *Licensed ACO provider groups that take both upside and downside Medicare and Medicaid risks will have incentive to place patients directly into the NF/SNF.* Patients in commercially insured mature ACOs are already being directly admitted to NFs/SNFs. Nursing facilities that are prepared to receive admissions 24 h/7, including holidays, and which demonstrate good HCV (i.e., outcomes at less cost) will be role models in defining how future care will be provided for the elderly. These successful nursing facilities will be attractive partners for ACOs because they will help to ensure the ACOs success.

Responding to Acute Change in Condition

When nursing facilities make a commitment to reduce preventable hospital admissions and readmissions, attention needs to be given to appropriate training of licensed staff in the early recognition and assessment of patients experiencing an acute change in condition. There are many excellent training materials available. One of the best educational and user-friendly tools is the Know-It-All tool available at the AMDA.com website. It is a thorough assessment tool for many common symptoms and geriatric conditions, is easy to use, and has been shown to improve the skills of licensed staff. Dr. Ouslander has also developed an excellent tool, INTERACT II, which when used has demonstrated improvements in quality of care and reduction of avoidable hospitalizations [6].

In addition to a well-trained staff, it is equally important to have physicians, nurse practitioners, and physician assistants available to assess patients with an acute change in condition within 24–48 h. While the 48-h guideline may be a hardship in rural areas, frequent contact with well-trained licensed staff is very important. Timely communication needs to occur until the change in condition is accurately assessed, treatment initiated, stabilization obtained, and improvement has begun to occur. Currently there are entrepreneurs developing a telemedicine model to fill this void, offering emergency physician care on nights and weekends via telecommunication.

While the list for acute changes in condition is extensive, included here are some of the more commons conditions with which licensed staff should be knowledgeable. They include the following:

- Change in mental status
- Chest pain
- Dehydration
- Acute onset of physical or verbal aggressive behavior
- Congestive heart failure

- Fever of unknown origin
- Asymptomatic bacteriuria and urinary tract infection
- Pneumonia.

Change in Mental Status

An acute change in mental status is commonly observed among frail older adults. There are many possible reasons that a NF resident/patient can have a change in mental status. Commonly seen triggers include medication, infection, and/or pain. Research suggests that the prevalence of memory loss in NF patients varies between 50 % and 80 %, therefore it is critical to get a baseline cognitive assessment completed within the first few days after admission. If a recently admitted patient is diagnosed with delirium and/or depression, their cognition should be reevaluated after successful treatment of their acute change in mental status (see chapter "Dementia, Delirium, and Depression" for further discussion of Depression and Delirium).

Many clinicians have heard staff report, "the patient seems more confused". When this occurs, use the opportunity to educate staff that an increase in confusion is more appropriately called delirium and reinforce the importance of recognizing such a change in mental status and notifying the PCP. After recognizing a change in mental status and obtaining vital signs, staff should contact the PCP. The patient's complaints and any significant physical findings on nurse assessment need to be conveyed to the PCP. The PCP should then inquire about the patient's medical history, medications and recent laboratory studies. Vital signs should be monitored each shift for at least 3 days. When reviewing the patient's medications, it is important to look for any problematic medications (see chapter "Medication Management in Long Term Care" on Medication Management for further discussion) and recent medication changes. Recent laboratory studies should be reviewed for any evidence of disease including but not limited to hematologic, liver or renal abnormalities. Some laboratory studies may need to be repeated. Nursing facilities should have established systems of care that facilitate licensed staff assessing any resident's acute change in condition in a timely manner. Early recognition, diagnosis, and treatment of an acute change of condition plays an important role in preventing avoidable hospitalizations.

Chest Pain

In most settings chest pain is viewed as a potential 911 call. However, 911 may not always be appropriate in the nursing facility setting. If the PCP has had a previous conversation with the resident/POA regarding goals of care and the risks and benefits of hospitalization, many residents prefer treatment in the NF whenever possible.

This is especially true for patients who have established "comfort" as their goal of care at which time the primary treatment of chest pain is usually focused on pain relief. Then treating chest pain with aspirin, nitroglycerin, and morphine sulfate would be appropriate.

Dehydration

Dehydration is frequently caused by acute onset of protracted vomiting and/or diarrhea without adequate fluid replacement. Early diagnosis and intervention can potentially prevent an avoidable hospitalization. Early interventions include adding medication to treat the symptoms, holding or reducing any medications that may cause further adverse effects (such as warfarin, digoxin, diuretics, iron, bowel medications) and administering intravenous (IV) fluids or giving careful attention to oral fluid intake. Intravenous fluids may not be appropriate in patients who have multi-morbidities associated with progressive unavoidable weight loss (see chapter "Weight and Nutrition" for further discussion).

If goals of care have previously been addressed, the decision to withhold artificial hydration or to not hospitalize is usually less difficult for the patient/ POA. Occasionally, if the problem is acute, some patients/POAs request IV therapy. Since more than 60 % of long-term care facilities (LTCF) residents have significant cognitive impairment, it is appropriate to request that a family member be present when administering IV therapy. This family member can calm a delirious patient and prevent the accidental removal of the IV line.

Behavioral Problems

Acute onset of physically or verbally aggressive behavior is common among NF residents in memory loss specialty units. The PCP should have a conversation with the POA regarding physical or verbal abusive behaviors that are unresponsive to behavioral interventions. This is especially important when a patient is attempting to physically harm staff or other patients. Residents that are subjected to verbally aggressive speech from another resident may manifest distress by becoming abusive to the offender.

Hospitalizing residents with serious behavioral problems has little benefit other than temporarily removing them from the NF until the staff can successfully de-escalate the behaviors of the remaining patients. Consequently, successful memory loss units have experienced staff and PCPs who use creative behavioral interventions to de-escalate most physically or verbally aggressive behavior. Maintaining educated and consistent caregivers and staff that are familiar with the nuances of the unit residents is extremely important. Administrators frequently find preventing high staff turnover very challenging as they work to maintain consistency and quality of care in memory loss units.

Because of the lack of psychiatrists trained in geriatrics, many NF PCPs use psychiatrists trained in adult psychiatry to assist with residents who have challenging behaviors. Unfortunately these psychiatrists often are not trained in evaluating and treating behavioral problems in residents with memory loss. There are no psychotropic medications approved by the FDA or proven effective in treating behavioral symptoms of dementia as of 2015. Although there are no medications that have been shown to improve the behaviors of residents with dementia, many clinicians and facilities have found the advice of psychologists who are interested in helping staff manage the behaviors of these cognitively impaired residents to be extremely helpful.

As a last resort, medications can be used off-label to attempt improvement of disruptive resident behaviors. Before resorting to using any off-labeled medications, a family member or the resident's POA may want to assist with de-escalating their family member's behavior by phone contact or by a visit to the NF. If a PCP is considering using an off-label medication for behavioral problems, it is important that staff or preferably the PCP to share with the POA the risks and benefits of using these medications.

Congestive Heart Failure (CHF)

Unexpected weight gain that occurs either very rapidly or is not due to high calorie intake is usually congestive heart failure until proven otherwise. CHF is the second most common diagnosis for which residents are hospitalized, and the hospitalization is often avoidable. During monthly or bimonthly visits the residents' weights should be reviewed. Except for very rare situations (e.g., ruptured heart valve), PCPs should be able to treat CHF at the faculty and avoid hospitalization unless refractory pulmonary edema develops. The management of heart failure is thoroughly reviewed in AMDA's clinical practice guideline on *Heart Failure in the Post-Acute and Long-Term Settings*.

Acute Onset of Fever

One of the most commonly overlooked vital signs is a slightly elevated temperature among frail older adults. It is not uncommon for fevers in NF residents to be symptomatically treated like they are in younger and healthier people. Standing orders for antipyretics in NFs should be avoided. Giving medication for a fever without identifying the underlying cause can lead to poor outcomes. Castle et al. have reported that repeated oral temperatures greater than 99 °F (37.2 °C) has a sensitivity of 80 % and specificity of 89 % for fever. In addition, Castle advised that either *a single oral temperature greater than 100 °F (37.8 °C) or*, a single temperature 2 °F (1.1 °C) above a patient's baseline, *or* repeated oral temperatures greater than 99 °F (37.2 °C) are significant for infection and need to be addressed by the PCP [7]. CMS has indicated that pneumonia and urosepsis are two common diagnoses among NF/SNF residents that lead to potentially avoidable hospitalizations. It is reasonable to suspect that many of these potentially avoidable hospitalizations resulted from poor monitoring of vital signs, lack of licensed staff adequately assessing the ill resident, and lack of timely notification of the PCP.

Asymptomatic Bacteriuria and Urinary Tract Infections

Guidelines for Diagnosing Urinary Tract Infection or Urosepsis

Whether to initiate treatment or not for an abnormal urinalysis is common dilemma faced when caring for frail older adults. However, knowing when to order a urinalysis is the greater challenge for the clinician. Often when cognitively impaired resident demonstrates disruptive behavior, an order for a urinalysis is requested from the PCP. However over 40 % of all urine specimens of frail older adult females residing in nursing facilities will have bacteriuria. If a resident solely has a mental status change and no other symptoms or signs to suggest a UTI, it has been found that only 11 % of these residents will have a UTI [8]. *Unless a resident meets the criteria for a UTI/urosepsis with or without an indwelling catheter (see criteria below), the clinician should refrain from diagnosing a UTI or urosepsis.*

New criteria have recently been developed for LTC facility-acquired infections by *the Society for Healthcare Epidemiology of America (SHEA)* [9]. These criteria for a urinary tract infection address residents with and without a urinary catheter.

1. **For residents *without* an indwelling urinary catheter** (both criteria 1 and 2 must be present)

   Criteria 1 At least one of the following sign or symptom subcriteria:

   - Acute dysuria or acute pain, swelling, or tenderness of the testes, epididymis, or prostate.
   - *Fever or leukocytosis* (neutrophilia >14,000 or left shift >6 % bands or 1500 or more bands/mm^3) and *at least one of the following localizing urinary tract* subcriteria:

     - Acute costovertebral angle pain or tenderness
     - Suprapubic pain
     - Gross hematuria

- New or marked increase in urgency
- New or marked increase in incontinence
- New or marked increase in frequency

Criteria 1a *In the absence fever or leukocytosis, then 2 or more of the following* localizing urinary tract subcriteria:

- Suprapubic pain
- Gross hematuria
- New or marked increase in incontinence
- New or marked increase in urgency
- New or marked increase in frequency

Criteria 2 One of the following microbiologic subcriteria:
- At least 100,000 cfu/ml of *no more than two species* of microorganism in a voided urine sample
- *At least 100 cfu/ml* if any number of organism in a specimen collected by in-and-out catheter

2. **For residents *with* an indwelling catheter** (*both criteria 1 and 2 must be present*)

Criteria 1 At least one of the following sign or symptom subcriteria:

- Fever, rigors, or new-onset hypotension, with no alternate site of infection
- Either acute change in mental status or acute functional decline, with no alternate diagnosis and leukocytosis
- New-onset suprapubic pain or costovertebral angle pain or tenderness
- Purulent discharge from around the catheter or acute pain, swelling, or tenderness of the testes, epididymis, or prostate

Criteria 2 Urinary catheter specimen culture with at least 100,000 cfu/ml of any organism(s)

If the resident has an indwelling catheter, the Infectious Disease Society of America (IDSA) recommends *changing the catheter before collecting a urine specimen for a culture and sensitivity (C&S).* However, even with a catheter change, it is common to culture two or three organisms. The clinician must then decide which, if any of these organisms, are responsible for the resident's illness. When identifying an organism(s) in a catheterized resident with urosepsis (fever, shaking chills, hypotension and/or delirium), it is considered reasonable to obtain a urine culture. But will this help the clinician decide which organism(s) is responsible for the illness? *In addition to urine for culture and sensitivities in a catheterized resident paired blood cultures may be very useful.* While waiting for the results of the blood cultures, aggressive treatment with a broad-spectrum antibiotic is recommended.

A helpful rule of thumb is that *within a month of inserting an indwelling catheter, a resident has 75–95 % chance of developing bacteriuria,* while the risk of bacteriuria is reduced to between 18 and 40 % 1 month after replacement of a suprapubic catheter. A condom catheter reduces the risk of bacteriuria even lower (12 %). Finally, the risk of bacteriuria is lowest with proper hygiene and self-catheterization, which reduces it to 1–3 % in 1 month [10].

Nursing Home Acquired Pneumonia

Pneumonia is a common infection seen in PA/ LTC. Some studies have shown that lower respiratory infections are more common than UTIs, since many so-called UTIs are actually treated cases of asymptomatic bacteriuria. The incidence rates of pneumonia in the nursing facility setting range from 0.3 to 2.5 infections/1000 resident care-days [11]. These numbers may vary depending upon the availability and quality of chest X-rays used to make the diagnosis of pneumonia. In addition, a number of residents may be inappropriately diagnosed with pneumonia when in fact the resident has experienced aspiration (chemical) pneumonitis.

There is a tenfold increase in the incidence of pneumonia in LTC residents compared to age-matched persons living in the community [12]. LTC residents are predisposed to lower respiratory infections because they have a decreased ability to clear mucus from the airways, are more prone to swallowing difficulties due to decreased oral and pharyngeal reflexes, and thus are more prone to aspiration. Residents with dementia are often uncooperative with oral care and recent research has demonstrated that the increased bacterial load in the mouth with poor oral care to be associated with an increased risk of pneumonia.

The criteria for diagnosing pneumonia in the NF/SNF setting were recently revised by SHEA. The following criteria are the most current guidelines for LTCFs:

Pneumonia Criterion (All Three Criteria Must Be Met)

1. Interpretation of a chest radiograph as demonstrating pneumonia or the presence of a new infiltrate
2. At least one of the following respiratory subcriteria

   (a) New or increased cough
   (b) New or increased sputum production
   (c) Oxygen saturation <94 % on room air or a reduction in oxygen saturation of 3 % from baseline
   (d) New or changed lung examination abnormalities
   (e) Pleuritic chest pain
   (f) Respiratory rate of 25 or greater breaths/min

3. At least one of the constitutional criteria in residents of LTCFs are included in the following list: (Constitutional Criteria in Residents of LTC Facilities)

- Fever

  - Single oral temperature >37.8 °C (>100 °F) or
  - Repeated oral temperatures >37.2 °C (99 °F) or rectal temp.
  - >37.5 °C (99.4 °F) or
  - Single temperature >1.1 °C (2 °F) over baseline form any site (Oral, tympanic, axillary)

- Leukocytosis

  - Neutrophilia (>14,000 leukocytes/mm^3) or
  - Left shift (6 % bands or 1500 or more bands/mm^3)

- Acute change in mental status from baseline (criteria for delirium assessment, Confusion Assessment Method {CAM}, must be present—see chapter "Dementia, Delirium and Depression" for further discussion of delirium)

  - Acute onset
  - Fluctuating course
  - Inattention
  - And
  - Either disorganized thinking or altered level of consciousness

- Acute functional decline

  - A new three-point increase in total activities of daily living (ADL) score (range 0–28) from baseline based on the following seven ADL items. Each scored form 0 (independent) to 4 (total dependence)

  Bed mobility
  Transfer
  Locomotion within LTCF
  Dressing
  Toilet use
  Personal hygiene
  Eating

Where to Treat Residents with Pneumonia?

Use of diagnostic criteria is critical if one wants to prevent a potentially avoidable hospitalization for pneumonia. Rapid diagnosis and early treatment with antibiotics is very important, so much so that it is a quality measure hospitals have utilized in determining ER quality of care. Early diagnosis and treatment is also an important component of care in the PA/LTC setting.

There are many factors that contribute to determining the most appropriate setting for the treatment of pneumonia. If the resident is stable with acceptable oxygen saturations (with or without O_2), and the staff is skilled at treating pneumonia and closely monitoring the resident's condition, then most clinicians are comfortable treating pneumonia in the NF/SNF setting as long as the resident and/or the health care proxy are comfortable with this decision as well. If the resident and/or health care proxy want aggressive treatment including respiratory ventilation if needed, then hospitalization would be more appropriate. On the other hand, many request their pneumonia be treated in place, have no interest in artificial respiratory ventilation, and have DNR status.

Dosa reviewed the literature for criteria regarding the treatment of LTCF residents with pneumonia in place versus hospitalizing the residents [13]. The literature review suggested that *residents with respiratory rates over 40/min benefit most by hospitalization*. Mortality rates have been shown to be similar or even reduced when residents were treated in place as compared to those who were hospitalized. Cost savings are also significant. Other risks to the resident that increase with hospitalization include:

- Development of pressure ulcers
- Colonization with highly virulent or drug-resistant organisms
- Delirium, especially in residents with dementia
- Difficult-to-manage behaviors from being in a strange environment, especially among residents with an underlying memory disorder.

Antibiotic Stewardship in the NH

Over the past several decades a number of published studies have demonstrated that multiple drug resistant organisms (MDRO) are frequently found in NF/SNFs patients *upon admission to the hospital*. When screening cultures were obtained among a fixed NF population over an extended period of time, 72 % of the 82 NF residents (59 residents) had one or more antibiotic resistant organisms and that 53 % of those same 59 residents developed facility-acquired antibiotic resistance when tracked for several months [14].

Because of the high number of resistant organisms found in NF patients, PCPs need to work towards reducing the use of antibiotics in the NF. Inappropriate use of antibiotics is seen with the treatment of asymptomatic bacteriuria, especially in patients with chronic indwelling urinary catheters. Expectations that antibiotics will be prescribed whenever a patient has increased confusion or behavioral problems, increases the chance that antibiotics will be inappropriately prescribed. Even consultants occasionally inappropriately prescribe antibiotics (e.g., urologists recommending long-term antibiotic prophylaxis for asymptomatic bacteriuria).

Nursing facilities committed to reducing the prevalence of MDROs such as *Clostridium difficile*, Enterococcus, and Staphylococcus, benefit from medical director leadership and assistance with developing an antibiotic stewardship program. Resources and strategies that a medical director can recommend include:

- Use the recently updated SHEA criteria for LTCF acquired infections before ordering a urinalysis.
- Avoid antibiotics for viral upper respiratory infections
- Use topical (rather than oral) antibiotics for superficial skin infections whenever possible
- Treat infected cysts with I&D and appropriate packing before adding a systemic antibiotic (most infected cysts heal very quickly without antibiotics).
- Avoid antibiotics for aspiration pneumonitis without pneumonia.
- Have an antibiotic czar who can give guidance in the selection of the most appropriate antibiotic and length of treatment.

Using the most recently established criteria to determine Nursing Home Acquired Infections (NHAIs), medical directors can begin to collect data regarding antibiotic treatment of one or two common infections such as urinary tract infections and upper or lower respiratory infections. Medical directors are often surprised at how many patients in their NF were given antibiotics for symptoms that do not meet the established criteria for NHAIs. Medical directors have the opportunity to initiate a process improvement project (PIP) for Quality Assurance and Process Improvement (QAPI). QAPI can track antibiotics used per 1000 patient days and/or number of antibiotic days given/1000 patient days. Not only can antibiotic usage data help the NF evaluate the effectiveness of antibiotic stewardship, but it can also be used to compare results with other facilities or state and federal benchmarks. Antibiotic stewardship will eventually become an expectation by payer systems and survey agencies. In 2008 Pennsylvania passed a law that required all NFs in the state to report NHAIs, a topic of great interest to CMS. Being proactive is better than being reactive and antibiotic stewardship is all about improving the quality of patient care and safety while reducing avoidable hospitalizations.

Optum and Interact II

The OPTUM system of care developed through United Health Care and the INTERACT tool have both demonstrated a significant reduction in admissions from NFs to hospitals. The original model of NF care developed for United (by several nurse practitioners from Minnesota) incorporated the idea of having certified registered nurse practitioners (CRNP) available for resident care at least 5 days a week. OPTUM's effective continuity of medical care system utilizes electronic medical records (EMR) to make needed information accessible to the on-call CRNPs during nights and weekends. The OPTUM intervention has prevented many potential admissions and readmissions to hospital and at the same time improved the quality of medical care in the SNFs and NFs.

INTERACT II is a system for collecting meaningful information that licensed staff can share with the PCP and the facility QAPI committee. The information has been shown to significantly improve the quality of NF care and reduce inappropriate hospital admissions and readmissions. As Dr Ouslander's states, "Interact includes evidence and expert-recommended clinical practice tools, strategies to implement them, and related educational resources." The INTERACT II program is available at their website [15].

Both OPTUM and INTERACT II have had a major impact on improving the quality of health care in PA/LTC and have significantly reduced avoidable hospitalizations but it is important to remember there is no perfect system or tool of care to achieve quality of care. Rather, well trained staff (physicians, CRNPs, PAs, CNAs, LPNs, and RNs) who consistently apply the principles of geriatric care, will always supersede whatever tools or systems of care that have been developed for institutional and non-institutional LTC.

Physician Order for Life Sustaining Treatment (POLST) and Advance Directives

For the practitioner committed to providing quality geriatric care and reducing avoidable hospital admissions, it is difficult to achieve success without addressing resident goals of care. Experienced practitioners who take the time to have these discussions with patients and family members usually find that it is uncommon for families to expect aggressive interventions in a frail resident with advanced, life-limiting illness near the end-of-life. Unfortunately, many patients/families have never had a conversation with their primary provider regarding goals of care until a crisis occurs such as stroke, aspiration pneumonia, or a serious injury due to a fall. Having a conversation regarding goals of care in the midst of a crisis is not an ideal time. *During a crisis, there are three fundamental questions that are usually asked by the patient* [16]. What is happening to me and why? What does this mean for my future? What can be done about it and how will it change my future? Having a conversation regarding goals of care, though requiring extra time, will help the practitioner build a trusting relationship. Trusting relationships are not only key ingredients needed for providing quality patient care but also for reducing avoidable hospitalizations.

In a Pennsylvania community the hospital systems, emergency medical staff, and nursing facilities have adopted the Physician Orders for Life Sustaining Treatment (POLST). While the POLST does not change a person's Advance Directive it helps to clarify the wishes of patients who are experiencing serious and/or chronic illness. It is important that the PCP have a conversation with the patient/POA *upon every admission to the SNF/NF*. Most families desire the highest quality of life possible for their ill family member and have less interest in maintaining life as long as possible. Accordingly, one can shift the conversation from clarification of DNR status to future expectations when an acute change in condition occurs. When families learn that a NF prefers to treat frail adults in place rather than in the hospital setting, it is frequently easy for the patient or POA to agree to "NO HOSPITALIZATION" and "NO EMERGENCY ROOM VISIT". The resident should only be hospitalized when the NF/SNF is unable to provide sufficient treatment and comfort to meet the resident's needs.

Summary

Preventing avoidable hospital admissions and readmissions is challenging. If the nursing home is committed to reducing avoidable hospitalizations, its culture should reflect the following practices:

- PCPs must acquire and maintain skills to care for frail adults with complex multi-morbidities.
- Regular educational activities are a priority.
- The management team should work closely with local hospitals and home health care agencies to develop transitions of care that are person-centered and have clearly defined expectations
- GOALS OF CARE are discussed with all resident/patients (POAs when appropriate)
- Expectations of care should be discussed by the PCP in advance of an acute change in condition (e.g., DNR/CPR, ER visits, hospitalizations).
- Newly admitted residents are seen within 2–5 days of admission or when a significant change in condition occurs.
- The management team is committed and able to treat residents in place when appropriate and congruent with the wishes of the patient/POA.
- PCPs and licensed nursing staff provide timely and frequent communication with the patient/POA whenever a significant change in condition occurs.
- Have an effective antibiotic stewardship program that uses the updated LTCF criteria by SHEA in defining LTCF-acquired infections.

Pearls for the Practitioner

- Preventing avoidable hospitalizations requires accurate and early resident assessment whenever a resident experiences a change in condition.
- Preventing avoidable admissions requires a conversation between the patient and/or proxy decision maker and the PCP regarding goals of care.
- When a resident with memory loss demonstrates increase behavioral problems without meeting other criteria for a UTI, the medical literature indicates only 11 % will have a UTI.
- Avoid standing orders to treat elevated temperatures without notifying the practitioner, because treating a fever of unknown origin without an adequate evaluation and workup is considered substandard care.
- Do not treat residents with urinary catheters for a UTI unless they meet the SHEA criteria for a UTI/urosepsis.
- If a clinician suspects urosepsis, blood cultures should be drawn before initiation of broad spectrum antibiotics, which is often more helpful in determining appropriate antibiotic treatment than the results of a urine C & S.
- Aspiration pneumonitis without pneumonia does not require antibiotic treatment.

PCP Fax Transitional Care Summary: SNF to Home

PCP FAX Transitional Care Summary: SNF to Home

Clinical Course	**Hospitalization:** _____ Dates: _____to_____ Diagnoses: _____ Summary: _____ _____ – _____ **_SNF:**_____ Dates: _____to_____ Diagnoses: _____ Summary: _____ _____ _____ — _____ **_Recent VS Trends BP:** **Weights:** **Follow-up Issues:** _____ _____ _____ –
LABS	**Recent Labs** - -or attach-
ID	Vax dates if known: Influenza:_____ Pneumococcal:_____ Tetanus:_____ Recent Infections ☐ MRSA ☐ C-diff ☐ VRE Other:
MS	☐ Alert ☐ Oriented ☐ Confused ☐ Comatose ☐ Depressed ☐ Forgetful☐ Withdrawn ☐ Wanderer ☐ Climbs out of bed ☐ Follows directions ☐ Other
Function (ADL s)	Bathing: ☐ Independent ☐ Needs assistance ☐ Dependent Dressing: ☐ Independent ☐ Needs assistance ☐ Dependent Feeding: ☐ Independent ☐ Needs assistance ☐ Dependent **Diet:** Toileting: ☐ Independent ☐ Needs assistance ☐ Dependent Bowel: Bladder: Transfer: ☐ Independent ☐ 1 assist ☐ 2 assist ☐ Total lift Ambulation: ☐ Independent ☐ 1 assist ☐ 2 assist ☐ N/A (does not ambulate) **Caregiver Plan:**
Assistive Devices	☐ Cane ☐ Crutches ☐ Walker ☐ Wheelchair ☐ Prosthesis ☐ Braces ☐ Specialty Bed ☐ Hearing aide(s) ☐ R ☐ L ☐ Glasses ☐ Dentures ☐ N/A
	☐ POLST ☐ Advanced directive/ living will ☐ **CPR** ☐ **DNR** ☐ **Home Care Referral** ATTACHMENTS: ☐ Medication List (required) ☐ H&P ☐ Discharge Summary ☐ List of Referrals and Appointments **SNF Physician:** **SNF Contact:**
	PMDA / The Pennsylvania Society for Post-Acute and Long-Term Care Medicine 2015

Guidance

- The nursing facility discharge summary frequently is not completed by the day of discharge and may not reach the PCP in a timely fashion thereby causing a delay in information transfer.
- Many NF discharge summaries lack complete clinical information that the PCP requires to assume care coordination for the patient.
- The PCP Fax Summary ensures timely communication of critical clinical information to the PCP on the day of discharge from the facility.
- The PCP Fax is a collaborative document that is to be completed prior to discharge from the facility. Elements of the form may be completed by the Attending Physician, other providers, and the nursing staff.

Instructions for Use

1. The PCP Fax Summary should be completed and faxed on the day of discharge to the patients PCP—the physician who will be assuming the care of the patient.
2. The Summary should not be faxed prior to the day of transfer as it may be incomplete. It should not be faxed after the day of transfer as the task may be dropped by the nursing facility staff.
3. The name and contact number of the Attending Physician and SNF staff contact person should be written on the form.
4. The form does not require a signature as this would delay its completion.
5. Additional documents such as the medication list, list of referrals, admission history and physical exam, should be faxed along with the form for completeness and to avoid redundancy.
6. Do not provide a copy of the form to the patient in lieu of faxing, as it may not reliably reach the PCP in a timely way, remembering that the PCP may begin to receive phone calls regarding the patient's care as early as the day of discharge.

References

1. Transitions and long-term care: reducing preventable hospital readmissions among hospital readmissions among nursing facility residents, CMS. 2012. http://www.aoa.gov/Aging_Statistics/docs/AoA_ACA_Slides_032712.pdf
2. Gawande A. The cost conundrum. 2009. http://www.newyorker.com/magazine/2009/06/01/the-cost-conundrum
3. World Health Organization. http://www.who.int/countries/en/
4. Improving care transitions between the nursing facility and the acute-care hospital settings, AMDA White Paper H10. http://www.amda.com/governance/whitepapers/H10.cfm
5. Crecelius C. Reducing hospitalizations of nursing home residents. Caring for the ages. 2014. http://www.caringfortheages.com/issues/february-2014/single-view/reducing-hospitalizations-of-nursing-home-residents/13c73583c360eb7527126ac21c573a81.html

6. Ouslander J. Overview of the INTERACT, Program and Curriculum. 2011. http://medicaring. org/wp-content/uploads/2011/09/INTERACT-short-overview-Ouslander-for-Sept-22.pdf

7. Castle SC, Yeh M, Norman DC, et al. Lowering the temperature criterion improves detection of infections in nursing home residents. Aging Immunol Infect Dis. 1993;4:67–76.

8. Noelle LE. SHEA Long-Term-Care Committee. Urinary tract infections in long-term care facilities. Infect Control Hosp Epidemiol. 2001;22:167–75.

9. Stone ND, Ashraf MS, Calder J, et al. Surveillance definitions of infections in long term care facilities: reviewing the McGeer criteria. Infect Control Hosp Epidemiol. 2012;33(10): 965–77.

10. Saint S, Lipsky BA. Preventing catheter-related bacteriuria: should we? Can we? How? Arch Intern Med. 1999;159(8):800–8.

11. Loeb M, Mcgeer A, McArthur M, et al. Risk factors for pneumonia and other lower respiratory tract infections in elderly residents of long-term care facilities. Arch Intern Med. 1999;159: 2058–64.

12. Muder RR. Pneumonia in residents of long-term care facilities: epidemiology, etiology, management, and prevention. Am J Med. 1998;105(4):319–30.

13. Dosa D. Should I, hospitalize my resident with nursing home-acquired Pneumonia? J Am Med Dir Assoc. 2005;6:327–33.

14. Fisch J, Lansing B, Wang L, et al. New acquisition of antibiotic-resistant organism in skilled nursing facilities. J Clin Microbiol. 2013;50(5):1698–703.

15. Oslander J. Perloe M. INTERACT: interventions to reduce acute care transfers https://interact2. net/index.aspx

16. LeBlond RF, Brown DD, DeGowin RL. DeGowin's diagnostic examination. 9 (electronic)th ed. New York: McGraw-Hill; 2008.

Goals of Care and Prevention

Cynthia Kuttner

Introduction

Your nursing facility (NF) resident has diabetes, hypertension, chronic renal insufficiency, and peripheral arterial disease. Interventions such as aspirin to prevent a cardiac event or stroke, meticulous foot care to prevent infection and subsequent amputation, and tightly controlled diabetes and hypertension can be instituted. But how do these interventions reflect the resident's goals of care? Does the resident have days, months or years to live? Consider that the resident is a frail 97-year-old female with dementia who frequently refuses her medications and care, and who now has unavoidable weight loss. Her goals of care need to be considered with every intervention. How are her goals of care to be determined?

This chapter will discuss goals of care and aspects of health promotion and disease prevention in post-acute and long-term care (PA/LTC), particularly as it relates to fall prevention, immunizations, nutrition, screening tests, and exercise. Most residents and patients in PA/LTC are challenging to practitioners because they have a long list of diagnoses from multi-morbidities. When developing the plan of care for these multi-morbidities it is important to partner with the patient and/or proxy health care decision maker who can help determine the benefit verses burden of diagnostic testing, treatment, as well as the desired outcomes. *Any recommendations for health promotion or disease prevention should be based on goals of care.* Once goals of care are decided upon, it is prudent to succinctly document the discussion with the practitioner's plan of care. If issues arise with the family or during a state survey or ombudsman visit, this *documentation can be extremely helpful.*

C. Kuttner, MD, CMD (✉)
Department Chair and Assistant Professor, Department of Geriatrics and Gerontology,
Ohio University Heritage College of Osteopathic Medicine, 250 Grosvenor Hall, Athens,
Ohio 45701, USA
e-mail: kuttner@ohio.edu

© Springer International Publishing Switzerland 2016
P.A. Fenstemacher, P. Winn (eds.), *Post-Acute and Long-Term Medicine,*
Current Clinical Practice, DOI 10.1007/978-3-319-16979-8_10

Goals of Care

Determining a resident's goals of care and understanding their wishes and preferences for care is an entrusted responsibility of all practitioners. Anticipating that goals of care frequently change over an illness trajectory is crucial. These changes need to be acknowledged and incorporated into the plan of care to ensure that care is patient centered. Currently there is no nation-wide or state database for persons to document their wishes or preferences for care. At this time many states have the *POLST* (Physician Orders for Life-Sustaining Treatment) [1] or the *MOLST* (Medical Orders for Life-Sustaining Treatment) [2] that can be used to document patient wishes on the use (or not) of CPR, intubation, feeding tubes, IV therapy and antibiotics. Most states also have laws pertaining to the use of advance directives on health care such as a living will or durable power of attorney, which can further enable patients to document their wishes and preferences for care (see Chapter "Ethical and Legal Issues" for further discussion).

Providing quality medical and nursing care is more complex than writing a "do not resuscitate" or "full code" order. Practitioners and staff should meet with patients and family to review their expectations on admission to a facility or program and to establish goals of care. *Periodic follow-up meetings are often necessary as illness progresses and crises occur that will necessitate modification of the goals of care.* For example, if a patient has dysphagia and needs an altered diet with thickened liquids, a discussion about aspiration and feeding tubes is vital (see Chapter "Weight and Nutrition" for further discussion). If a patient is admitted with severe COPD, then a discussion on CPR and respirators is needed.

Most people appreciate the opportunity to discuss end-of-life care and have often had previous experiences with friends or other family members that will influence their thoughts and decisions. Listening to the stories of the resident and their family can provide that health care team invaluable information on their beliefs and values, which will assist the team with providing the care that they desire. Suggesting a palliative care approach can often help facilitate difficult conversations focusing on goals of care and treatment at end of life. Documenting these conversations in the resident's medical record will support the staff in providing goal directed patient-centered care as the patient's condition progresses.

Fall Prevention

Falls are an all too common event in long-term care. Falls are potentially life threatening and can result in fractures, particularly of the hip or pelvis, as well as brain trauma. An increasing percentage of residents are taking anticoagulants and their risk of serious bleeding (especially intracranial) is increased when a fall occurs. Between 50 and 75 % of residents in NFs fall each year, and many fall more than once ("frequent fallers"). Ten to twenty percent of NF falls cause serious injuries and up to 6 % of these falls result in fractures. The CDC reports that nursing home residents account for 20 % of deaths from falls in the over 65 age group, even though only 5 % of people over 65 live in nursing facilities. In the USA alone about 1800 people living in NFs die each year from a fall [3].

The 2010 AGS Clinical Practice Guideline: "Prevention of Falls in Older Persons" has excellent recommendations on the screening and assessment of patients at increased risk of falls or who have fallen [4]. All patients should be questioned about a history of falls and the circumstances surrounding those falls. A multifactorial risk assessment should be completed as well as a physical exam that includes a gait and balance evaluation. A *focused history* about falls, all medications being taken (including OTC medications), and relevant risk factors should be included in a multifactorial fall risk assessment. Relevant risk factors include: diabetic neuropathy, urinary urge incontinence, multiple antihypertensive medications, and depression on psychotropic medications.

When performing the *Physical Examination* assessing gait, balance, mobility, and lower extremity joint stability and function is important. Neurologic function including cognition, peripheral nerves, proprioception, reflexes, cortical, extrapyramidal and cerebellar function, as well as muscle strength of the lower extremities should all be included. Cardiovascular assessment should include heart rate and rhythm, orthostatic blood pressure and peripheral pulses, and possibly carotid sinus stimulation. Test visual acuity and check feet and footwear. The *Functional Assessment* should include an assessment of ADLs and adaptive equipment including mobility aids. Query about fear of falling and any self-imposed limitations due to that fear. An *Environmental Assessment* should be done to check for lighting, obstacles, uneven surfaces, and other hazards, especially in community dwelling elderly.

Recommendations to decrease fall risk include:

- Consider exercise programs to maintain strength and mobility and decrease risk of falls.
- Supplement residents with at least 800 IU of vitamin D daily for those with vitamin D deficiency and/or impaired balance.
- Consider dose reduction of medications that can cause orthostasis or increase risk of falls (such as psychotropic medications particularly benzodiazepines and anxiolytics) or use of multiple antihypertensives (see Chapter "Medication Management in Long-Term Care" for further discussion).
- Consider treatment of osteoporosis in residents who can tolerate pharmacologic therapy and have a life expectancy of several years, particularly for those who have had prior fracture(s).

Residents with cognitive impairment may be impulsive and unable to remember information they are taught on fall prevention. Frequent monitoring and regular toileting may decrease but not eliminate their risk of falls.

Bed and chair alarms do not prevent falls; they only alert staff to a resident who is trying to stand or get out of bed. Restraints should be avoided at all times (both chemical and physical) because they do not prevent falls [7]. The use of side rails is controversial, with double rails considered a restraint. Many side rail injuries are linked to older beds, which allowed entrapment of the patient in the rails. There is a risk that a patient will climb over the side rail and fall from a higher height and thus suffer an even more severe impact injury than without the rail [5]. Not only are hip pads usually not acceptable to patients, but also they have been shown to have minimal efficacy [6]. Most nursing facilities now have "fall teams" or a falls protocol to evaluate each fall and to determine what preventive interventions to initiate like the use of low bed. Input by the practitioner can be vital due to the practitioner's ability to take into account risk factors (intrinsic and extrinsic), patient multi-morbidities, and guide the interdisciplinary term to create a plan of care to lessen fall risk. *The medication review performed by the practitioner often plays a critical role in reducing falls* [8].

Immunizations

Currently recommended vaccines for the elderly population include the influenza vaccine, pneumococcal vaccine (Pneumovax and Prevnar 13), and herpes zoster vaccine (Zostavax). The Prevnar 13 had only been administered to children, but as of 2015 it has been recommended and covered (by Medicare) for adults age 65 and older. Because immunosenescence can diminish the antibody response to vaccines and thus vaccine efficacy, research continues on the development of vaccines with higher efficacy [15].

Influenza

Efficacy of influenza vaccine varies on a yearly basis, depending upon the strains selected for the vaccine and the ultimate strains that infect the population. *It is paramount to vaccinate residents, staff, and visiting family members while discouraging sick visitors from coming into the facility during influenza season.* If unvaccinated staff become ill with influenza, they can spread the virus to residents, patients, and staff, causing absenteeism and increased workload on remaining staff. Influenza can be a life threatening illness, so practitioners and staff should be vigilant watching for evidence that an influenza outbreak might have occurred [9]. In 2014, a study reported by Nace et al. showed that the high dose influenza vaccine produced higher antibody titers than the standard dose vaccine among frail nursing facility residents, except for the H1N1 strain that showed no substantial increase [10].

The Medical director is often called upon to assess an outbreak of influenza and decide if and when to provide prophylaxis to all residents in a facility. CDC.gov provides an excellent "Toolkit for Long-term Care Employers" that describes all aspects of influenza prophylaxis and treatment [11]. *Vaccination of residents and staff with the trivalent influenza vaccine should start as soon as the vaccine is available* (usually in September). Having standing orders to vaccinate residents and vaccinating all staff unless there is a medical contraindication or personal choice not to receive the vaccine can increase compliance.

An outbreak in a nursing facility is defined when 2 residents are sick with flu-like symptoms within a 72-h period and one has confirmed Influenza by viral testing. When this occurs, all residents should be treated or prophylaxed with either oseltamivir or zanamivir for 5 days. Transit between facility units by staff and residents should be limited. Standard and droplet precautions should be followed for all residents with suspected or confirmed influenza. To help prevent further spread, dining and activities may need to occur in patient rooms rather than in common areas. Note that amantadine and rimantadine are no longer considered to be effective due to the development of resistance and should not be used for treatment or prophylaxis.

Pneumococcus

Currently there are two recommended vaccines to help prevent pneumococcal disease in older adults: the *Pneumovax 23* and the *Prevnar 13*. The most common presentations of pneumococcal disease are pneumonia, sepsis, and meningitis. *In 2014, the Advisory Committee on Immunization Practices (ACIP) recommended that the Prevnar 13 be used as a first-line immunization in person's age 65 and older who had not previously been vaccinated against pneumococcal disease, to be followed 12 months later by the Pneumovax 23.* Similarly, if a patient has previously been vaccinated with Pneumovax 23, it is recommended to administer the Prevnar 13. The Prevnar 13 should be given no sooner than 6–12 months after the Pneumovax 23. The Prevnar 13 has been reported to be 45 % effective in preventing invasive pneumococcal disease in patients over 65 [12].

Prevnar 13 is a conjugate vaccine while Pneumovax 23 is a polysaccharide vaccine. Prevnar 13 protects against the 13 strains of pneumococcus that are most frequently seen in the elderly population. The Pneumovax 23 protects against 23 strains, but seems more effective when given in a series with the Prevnar 13. *The main contraindication to vaccination with Prevnar 13 is an allergy to diphtheria vaccine.* Contraindication to Pneumovax is an allergic reaction to prior Pneumovax vaccination. Both vaccines can cause some swelling, redness and tenderness at the injection site that usually resolves within a week.

Shingles (Herpes Zoster)

Herpes Zoster vaccine (Zostavax) is approved to decrease the risk of shingles and post-herpetic neuralgia [13]. *The vaccine is most effective in ages 60–69*, which is younger than many of our NF residents. It decreases the risk of shingles by 50 % and the risk of post-herpetic neuralgia by 67 %. Unlike Influenza and pneumococcal vaccines that are covered by Medicare Part B, Zostavax is covered by Medicare D. Because the vaccine is covered by Medicare D residents often have significant co-pay or no coverage for this vaccination. The Zostavax is known to provide protection for up to 5 years after vaccination before immunity wanes. Other shingles vaccines are being studied which may provide longer protection [14]. *Contraindications to using the Zostavax* are allergies to gelatin or neomycin, and having weakened immune systems due to steroids or other immunosuppressants, HIV/AIDS, cancer treatment, leukemia, or lymphoma. Antiviral agents can decrease the duration and severity of symptoms if given within 48 h of the development of shingles.

Nutrition and Vitamin and Mineral Supplementation

"We are what we eat," continues to be true in the LTC setting. There are consequences to being underweight and overweight. Being *underweight* increases risk for infections, pressure ulcers, physical decline, cognitive decline, and death. Malnutrition and dehydration are common in the NF setting, with a recent article identifying the prevalence of malnutrition as high as 30 % [16]. Being *overweight* increases risks of developing metabolic syndrome, HTN, DM, and the personal need for more physical assistance from staff for daily task of living (ADLs).

A nutritional and dietary plan is necessary for all residents in order to ensure that nutrient and calorie needs are being met. Goals of care are paramount. *Resident rights* allow patients to decline a prescribed diet and to eat what they choose, even if it compromises their medical condition. This can complicate the treatment of diabetes, CHF, and renal disease, and raise conflict between the health care providers and the resident/patient. However, the nursing facility is their "home" and just like community dwelling persons, they are entitled to make informed decisions on food preferences. For most residents, however, the goal is to maintain adequate nourishment as long as possible (see Chapter "Weight and Nutrition" for further discussion).

Poor dentition is often an issue with residents and can be a barrier to adequate nutrition. Encouraging the nursing staff to provide routine and thorough mouth care can be helpful. Engaging a dentist with an interest in geriatrics to come to the facility can be invaluable.

Another common problem seen in the NF is swallowing dysfunction (*dysphagia*), either due to presbyesophagus or neurologic conditions such as Parkinson's or cerebrovascular disease. Dysphagia may affect the texture of food and liquids that can be tolerated. A visit to the dining room at mealtime to observe how the patient is eating can be informative. Is staff assistance needed? How is the food texture and liquid consistency being tolerated? Such a visit can provide insight into why your resident is losing weight and suggest possible therapeutic interventions. If a resident has end stage dementia and chooses comfort care, hand feeding to the best of the staff's ability is the best option for nutrition. Choosing Wisely guidelines from AGS and AMDA strongly advise against insertion of feeding tubes in those with dementia (see Chapter "Weight and Nutrition" for further discussion) [17–19].

A multivitamin is thought to be beneficial for NF residents, as well as a diet balanced with protein, carbohydrates, and fats. Fresh fruit and vegetables, often absent in dietary plans, should be encouraged in order to provide natural nutrients, hydration, and fiber. The medical director can encourage the nursing facility administration and dietary departments to supply more fresh fruit and vegetables on the meal plan as well as healthy snacks.

Many residents are deficient in vitamin D, which has been associated with falls, fractures, musculoskeletal pain, and muscle weakness. Routine testing of 25-hydroxyvitamin D levels is not usually needed if a vitamin D supplement is being given. However, if checked, a level of at least 40–50 is optimal. Different organizations recommend differing doses of vitamin D supplements, ranging from 800 to 4000 IU a day. Residents at highest risk of vitamin D deficiency are those with dark pigmented skin, obesity, malabsorption, and who take medications that accelerate the breakdown of vitamin D (such as phenytoin and phenobarbital) or bind oral vitamin D (such as cholestyramine) [20]. Also consider calcium supplements of 1000–1200 mg daily with vitamin D if dietary intake is poor and supplementation is consistent with goals of care. Calcium supplements enhance the benefit of vitamin D on bone mineral density. However, you need to keep in mind the constipating effect of supplementary calcium.

Magnesium is often deficient, particularly in patients on diuretics or proton pump inhibitors for an extended period of time and those with diabetes mellitus [21]. Oral Zinc replacement has been found to be beneficial in patients who have zinc deficiency and a wound; the optimal amount of supplementation and duration of therapy is currently being studied. A recent study has shown that there is a correlation between adequate zinc levels, cognition and depression in nursing facility residents as well [22].

Screening Tests

Screening for Osteoporosis

The US Preventive Services Task Force has *not made a specific recommendation about resident screening for osteoporosis*. However, they do recommend consideration of screening in women over age 65. There is currently inadequate evidence to recommend screening in men. On the other hand, the National Osteoporosis Foundation recommends screening in women over 65 and men over 70 [23]. This may be done with *DEXA scanning* of the spine and hip, quantitative ultrasound of the calcaneum or by *FRAX risk calculation* [24]. For many residents, they may have already sustained an osteoporotic fracture or have an elevated T-score. Optimal intervals for screening are undefined. Life expectancy, prognosis, and clinical judgment should determine which residents would be most appropriate for screening.

For many, treatment with bisphosphonates or other agents may be tolerated and desired; for others, it is burdensome, and inconvenient and has potential adverse side effects.

Tuberculosis Screening

Tuberculosis screening is routinely done in nursing facilities with a *2-step tuberculin skin test* (TST). However, many older people are anergic due to immunosenescence and may not to respond to testing (manifest as a false negative). Symptoms of active or reactivated TB should be aggressively pursued. Fortunately, this situation is infrequent in most US NFs. Some NFs (especially those at low risk) use an annual "symptom screen" rather than repeating the TST every year.

Cancer Screening

Cancer screening of residents in NFs is central to resident goals of care. Depending on the age, prognosis, and physical/cognitive function of the patient, decisions about whether or not to screen should be made in concert with the patient/family [25, 26].

Cervical Cancer screening should *rarely if ever be needed* and *Breast Cancer screening* can be considered if the patient is able to participate in mammography. AGS suggests that patients undergoing mammography *should have a life expectancy of at least 4 years*, and be willing to undergo surgery and other treatments if a cancer is found. Physical exam can detect most significant breast cancers in elderly residents. Workup and treatment of any breast mass should be discussed with the patient/family. Periodic clinical breast exams by the practitioner are reasonable.

Colon cancer screening is *not recommended over the age of 75 by the USPSTF*, and should only be undertaken if the patient is willing and able to undergo major surgery.

Screening for lung cancer with low dose CT scan is limited to select patient populations who are under the age of 75 and have smoked at least 40 pack years and would be willing/able to undergo treatment if a cancer is found. This CT screening recommendation was *intended for otherwise healthy patients in the community; not for frail elderly in a nursing* facility.

Prostate Cancer screening is *NOT recommended* with PSA testing for almost any facility resident, as there is no mortality benefit and there may actually be increased morbidity and mortality resulting from screening and unnecessary treatment.

Exercise

Exercise is a low risk with high benefit intervention to prevent physical decline in residents. It has been shown to have positive effects on mood in patients with Alzheimer's disease as well as maintaining physical function [27]. The best interventions involve an exercise program that includes walking, strength training, balance, and flexibility exercises [28]. Unfortunately, not all residents are able to walk, but restorative programs can keep many residents ambulatory for longer than expected. Exercise programs for people who are wheelchair-dependent or bedbound are also encouraged, although they are less well developed. Novel ideas include the use of robots in Japan and Finland to conduct exercise sessions when staff is not available [29]. Exercise combined with music has also been shown to be very effective in patients with Parkinson's disease [30]. Further research on best practices is needed to avert increased frailty and sarcopenia.

Peals for the Practitioner

- Discuss, revisit, and then document patient's revised goals of care when a change in condition occurs.
- Preventive health interventions and treatments are guided by patients' multimorbidities, prognosis, advance directives and goals of care.
- Fall prevention should always include a medication review and attempts to discontinue medications that potentially increase fall risk.
- Vaccination of residents and staff is vital to maintaining personal health and preventing outbreaks of infectious disease in the facility.
- Good nutrition is key to the maintenance of physical and cognitive health. Observation of residents at mealtime may help determine interventions in those with weight loss.
- Liberal diets are appropriate for most frail older patients. Restrictive diets should be avoided unless medically necessary.
- Screening for cancer should be individualized.
- Exercise programs can improve quality of life of residents; meeting the exercise needs of individual residents requires thought, teamwork, and creativity.

References

1. What is POLST? POLST, physician orders for life-sustaining treatment paradigm®. http://www.polst.org. Accessed 14 Jun 2015.
2. Medical orders for life-sustaining treatment—professionals. Compassion and support at the end of life. http://www.compassionandsupport.org/index.php/for_professionals/molst_training_center. Accessed 14 Jun 2015.

3. Centers for Disease Control and Prevention, National Center for Injury Prevention and Control, Division of Unintentional Injury Prevention. Falls in nursing homes. http://www.cdc.gov/HomeandRecreationalSafety/Falls/nursing.html. Last updated 19 Mar 2015.
4. The American Geriatrics Society. AGS/BGS clinical practice guideline: prevention of falls in older persons, summary of recommendations. http://www.americangeriatrics.org/health_care_professionals/clinical_practice/clinical_guidelines_recommendations/prevention_of_falls_summary_of_recommendations. Accessed 14 Jun 2015.
5. Healy F, Oliver D, Milne A, Connelly JB. The effect of bedrails on falls and injury: a systemic review of clinical studies. Age Ageing. 2008;37(4):368–78.
6. Santesso N, Carrasco-Labra A, Brignardello-Petersen R. Hip protectors for preventing hip fractures in older people. Cochrane Database Syst Rev. 2014;3, CD001255. doi:10.1002/14651858.CD001255.pub5.
7. Castle NG, Engberg J. The health consequences of using physical restraints in nursing homes. MedCare. 2009;47:1164–73.
8. Quigley P, Bulat T, Kurtzman E, et al. Fall prevention and injury protection for nursing home residents. J Am Med Dir Assoc. 2010;11:284–93.
9. Centers for Disease Control and Prevention. Interim guidance for influenza outbreak management in long-term care facilities. http://www.cdc.gov/flu/professionals/infectioncontrol/ltc-facility-guidance.htm. Last updated 19 Dec 2011.
10. Nace DA, Lin CJ, Ross TM, et al. Randomized, controlled trial of high-dose influenza vaccine among frail residents of long-term care facilities. J Infect Dis. 2015;211(12):1915–24.
11. Centers for Disease Control and Prevention. Influenza (Flu), a toolkit for long-term-care employers. http://www.cdc.gov/flu/toolkit/long-term-care/index.htm. Last updated 11 Jun 2015.
12. Tomczyk S, Bennett NM, Stoecker C, et al. Use of 13-valent pneumococcal conjugate vaccine and 23-valent pneumococcal polysaccharide vaccine among adults aged ≥65 years: recommendations of the Advisory Committee on Immunization Practices (ACIP). MMWR Morb Mortal Wkly Rep. 2014;63(37):822–5.
13. Lal H, Cunningham AL, Godeaux O, et al. Efficacy of an adjuvanted herpes zoster subunit vaccine in older adults. N Engl J Med. 2015;372(22):2087–96.
14. Cohen JI. A new vaccine to prevent herpes zoster. N Engl J Med. 2015;372(22):2149–50. See comment in PubMed Commons below.
15. Fulop T, Pawelec G, Castle S, Loeb M. Immunosenescence and vaccination in nursing home residents. Clin Infect Dis. 2009;48(4):443–8.
16. Torma J, Winblad U, Cederholm T, Saletti A. Does undernutrition still prevail among nursing home residents? Clin Nutr. 2013;32(4):562–8.
17. AMDA releases list of potentially unnecessary medical tests, procedures as part of the ABIM Foundation's Choosing Wisely Campaign. Choosing Wisely, ABIM Foundation. http://www.choosingwisely.org/amda-releases-list-of-potentially-unnecessary-medical-tests-procedures-as-part-of-the-abim-foundations-choosing-wisely-campaign. Accessed 4 Sep 2013.
18. AMDA releases second round of potentially unnecessary medical tests, procedures as part of the ABIM Foundation's Choosing Wisely Campaign. Choosing Wisely, ABIM Foundation. http://www.choosingwisely.org/amda-releases-second-round-of-potentially-unnecessary-medical-tests-procedures-as-part-of-the-abim-foundations-choosing-wisely-campaign. Accessed 20 Mar 2013.
19. American Geriatrics Society releases second choosing wisely list: identifies 5 more tests and treatments that older patients and providers should question. Choosing Wisely, ABIM Foundation. http://www.choosingwisely.org/american-geriatrics-society-releases-second-choosing-wisely-list-identifies-5-more-tests-and-treatments-that-older-patients-and-providers-should-question. Accessed 27 Feb 2014.
20. Judge J, Birge S, Gloth 3rd F, et al. Recommendations abstracted from the American Geriatrics Society Consensus Statement on vitamin D for prevention of falls and their consequences. J Am Geriatr Soc. 2014;62(1):147–52.

21. Arinzon Z, Peisakh A, Schrire S, Berner YN. Prevalence of hypomagnesemia (HM) in a geriatric long-term care (LTC) setting. Arch Gerontol Geriatr. 2010;51(1):36–40.
22. Markiewicz-Żukowska R, Gutowska A, Borawska MH. Serum zinc concentrations correlate with mental and physical status of nursing home residents. PLoS One. 2015;10(1), e0117257.
23. Cosman F, de Beur SJ, Le Boff MS, et al. Clinician's guide to prevention and treatment of osteoporosis. Osteoporos Int. 2014;25:2794. doi:10.1007/S00198-014-2794-2.
24. Welcome to FRAX®. FRAX® WHO fracture risk assessment tool. http://www.shef.ac.uk/FRAX. Accessed June 14, 2015.
25. AGS unveils revised list of topics to talk about with older adults as part of Choosing Wisely Campaign. Choosing Wisely, ABIM Foundation. http://www.choosingwisely.org/ags-unveils-revised-list-of-topics-to-talk-about-with-older-adults-as-part-of-choosing-wisely-campaign. Accessed 23 Apr 2015.
26. The guide to clinical preventive services 2014: recommendations of the U.S. Preventive Services Task Force. uspreventiveservicestaskforce.org. Accessed 15 Jun 2015.
27. Rolland Y, Pillard F, Klapouszczak A, et al. Exercise program for nursing home residents with Alzheimer's disease: a 1-year randomized, controlled trial. J Am Geriatr Soc. 2007; 55(2):158–65.
28. Williams CL, Tappen RM. Effect of exercise on mood in nursing home residents with Alzheimer's disease. Am J Alzheimers Dis Other Demen. 2007;22(5):389–97.
29. Iivari Bäck, Kari Makela, Jouko Kallio. Robot-guided exercise program for the rehabilitation of older nursing home residents. Ann Longterm Care 2013;21(6). http://www.annalsoflongtermcare.com/article/robot-guided-exercise-program-rehabilitation-older-nursing-home-residents. Accessed 14 Jun 2015.
30. de Dreu MJ, van der Wilk AS, Poppe E. Rehabilitation, exercise therapy and music in patients with Parkinson's disease: a meta-analysis of the effects of music-based movement therapy on walking ability, balance and quality of life. Parkinsonism Relat Disord. 2012;18 Suppl 1: S114–9.

Integrating Palliative Care into Practice

Peter Winn and Deborah Way

Introduction

Practitioners in post-acute and long-term care medicine are seeing an ever-increasing number of persons with chronic progressive illness who reside either at home or in an LTC setting (nursing facility, SNF, assisted living or residential care). Currently 46 % of all deaths in the USA occur in these settings. In 2008, a report by the Center to Advance Palliative Care (CAPC) concluded that up to 80 % of residents in nursing facilities could benefit from palliative care irrespective of prognosis. Despite the lack of formal palliative care consultation services in such settings, practitioners must apply and integrate the principals of palliative care into practice [1]. Others have promoted the need for a multidimensional model of *successful aging* (despite chronic illness) where disease and its physiological and functional limitations are countered by compensatory psycho-emotional and social interventions that result in emotional vitality, well-being, and engagement with life and spirituality [2].

Palliative care can complement traditional care, where disease-modifying treatments are not necessarily abandoned if appropriate and congruent with patients' goals of care. Such an approach to care embodies the true philosophy of palliative care. Such "total care" should be safe, effective, patient-centered, timely, efficient, and equitable, all consistent with the six aims of the Institute of Medicine 2001 report to improve health care in the USA.

F tag 309 of the State Operations Manual now contains guidance to surveyors on residents at or approaching end of life, those receiving hospice services, the

P. Winn
Department of Family and Preventive Medicine, Geriatric Assessment Clinic, OUHSC
Family Medicine Center, University of Oklahoma, Oklahoma, OK, USA

D. Way, MD (✉)
Department of Palliative Care, Corporal Michael J. Crescenz VA Medical Center,
3900 Woodland Avenue, Philadelphia, PA 19104, USA
e-mail: Deborah.Way@va.gov

© Springer International Publishing Switzerland 2016
P.A. Fenstemacher, P. Winn (eds.), *Post-Acute and Long-Term Medicine*,
Current Clinical Practice, DOI 10.1007/978-3-319-16979-8_11

recognition and management of pain, and the management of behavioral and psychological symptoms of dementia. All of these are both critical and relevant to providing timely and effective palliative care in post-acute and LTC.

Illness Trajectories and Prognostication

Irrespective of the place of residence heart disease, cancer, stroke, lung disease, Alzheimer's disease, influenza, pneumonia, and kidney disease are among the top 10 leading causes of death in the USA (in addition to unintentional injuries, diabetes, and septicemia). These diseases commonly afflict patients/residents in the LTC continuum who can benefit from the integration of effective palliative care into traditional medical treatment, whether it is during the early, middle, late, or terminal phase of their illness trajectory.

For persons who reside in nursing facilities, common causes of death are [3, 4]:

- 30–60 % cardiovascular (includes sudden cardiac death, myocardial infarction, heart failure, and stroke).
- 1–23 % pulmonary (COPD, pneumonia, lung cancer).
- 36 % Alzheimer's disease and other dementia (10 % of all dementia deaths occur in nursing facilities).
- 7–9 % cancer.
- 2–3 % end stage renal disease.

Generally, *illness trajectories* that lead to subsequent death can manifest in *one of three ways:*

- *A short period of rapid decline* (usually a few weeks or months) as often seen in cancer.
- *Prolonged dwindling over 6–8 years* as seen in dementia, frailty, and generalized debility or
- *Long term functional decline over 2–5 years*, with intermittent serious episodes of illness, often associated with multiple ER visits and hospitalizations, with only partial recovery after each episode, and eventual death. This is most often seen in heart and respiratory failure.

Timely recognition of a patient's illness trajectory together with a poor prognosis should serve as a trigger to discuss advance care planning that reviews *goals of life* and establishes appropriate *goals of care* for patients and their families.

Though challenging to prognosticate in the chronically ill the Flacker Mortality Score can provide a percentage probability of death in 1 year, while other patient characteristics (available from the MDS) can also assist in prognostication (e.g., significant weight loss, swallowing problems, BMI < 22, age > 88, CHF, shortness of breath, male sex). Another prognostic tool is the Palliative Prognostic Score that may predict 30-day survival.

Principles of Palliative Care

Irrespective of the age of the patient, the clinical setting, place of residence/care or whether the person is suffering from chronic progressive illness or an acute life threatening illness, the *core principles ofpalliative care* are the same:

- Reduce the symptom burden from pain and other distressful symptoms, including the relief of suffering.
- Recognize and address the physical, psycho-emotional, social and spiritual needs, and dimensions of pain and other symptoms experienced by both the *patient and family*.
- Provide medical treatment congruent with the wishes, values, preferences, beliefs, culture, and concerns of the patient and family.
- Provide care that is interdisciplinary.
- Assist the patient, family, facility staff, and practitioners with ethical and legal issues, and advanced care planning.

Practitioners must be committed to the highest quality (palliative) care that is both timely and comprehensive. To do so, requires regular clinical assessment, diagnosis, care planning, interventions, and monitoring the patient's response to these interventions while recognizing the natural trajectory of the disease. Also practitioners should anticipate and prevent/alleviate distressful symptoms, and suffering. Care should be *patient-centered* and *family-focused*. Practitioners and the interdisciplinary team are challenged on many levels to provide seamless transitions in care between institutional, hospital, and home care settings where effective communication skills are essential.

For the patient and family the primary goals of palliative care include:

- Strive for the highest practical quality of life, despite late stage illness.
- Be in control (autonomy) and maintain one's dignity.
- Relieve distressful symptoms and suffering (social, spiritual).
- Alleviate family burden (can be psycho-emotional, financial, practical).
- Lessen spiritual distress and if possible mend relationships.

In LTC medicine, the goals of palliative care are similar whether patients are at end-of-life on hospice or not. Medical care should be delivered in accordance within the ethical principles of heath care, its legal framework (State and Federal), the practitioner's scope of practice, and provided with cultural sensitivity and competency (see Chaps. on "Ethical and Legal Issues" and "Caring for Families").

Symptom Assessment and Management

In persons with advanced illness, appropriate assessment is often challenging due to patient cognitive impairment, fatigue, and multimorbidities. Non-pain symptoms are prevalent, often greater than pain even in persons diagnosed with cancer (see Table 1).

Table 1 Symptom prevalence in advanced illness

Symptom	Cancer (%) [16, 19]	Non-cancer (%) [18]	Cancer, AIDS, COPD, heart and renal disease (%) [17]
Fatigue	72–74	76	32–90
Pain	71–74	67	34–96
Lack of energy	69		
Weakness	60		
Appetite loss	53–70	55	
Breathlessness	36	36	60–95
Anxiety/depression	40	57	

For *any* symptom experienced by patients, a quasi-stepped approach can enable practitioners to intervene in a timely and effective manner.

First, recognize the presence of each symptom, then proceed to:

- Establish its intensity, temporal pattern, any exacerbating/relieving factors, location, and effect on function and cognition.
- Determine whether the symptom is acute, chronic or intermittent.
- Identify any associated symptoms.
- Assess its impact on quality of life, ADLs, cognition, decisional capacity, sleep, mood, and dignity.
- Review previous and current treatment for the symptom.
- Perform an appropriate, timely, and *symptom focused* physical exam.
- Ascertain if possible, the likely pathophysiology underlying the symptom.
- Consider whether any medication could be causing or aggravating the symptom.
- Identify potentially reversible causes.
- If necessary, use the least invasive diagnostic testing, if any, to minimize patient pain, discomfort, or suffering.
- Given the above steps determine the most likely diagnosis, (if possible).
- Always evaluate for the presence of any psycho-emotional, spiritual, social, or practical factors to the symptom.
- Initiate palliative and traditional treatment based upon the primary illness, phase of illness, prognosis, comorbidities, patient/family preferences for care, and care setting.
- Consider complementary and alternative therapies especially if requested by patients and families.

Any symptom can be complex and multifaceted, thus an *interdisciplinary* and *transdisciplinary* approach, and treatment plan is more likely to be successful. Foremost, consider nonpharmacologic and practical interventions in an attempt to alleviate each symptom, i.e., change in body position, room temperature or ventilation, patient/family and staff education. Then consider pharmacologic interventions to primarily palliate each symptom. Finally, consider medical and/or pharmacologic treatments directed at the *underlying cause of the symptom* (if known).

Response to the treatment and its outcomes, benefits, and burdens must be carefully monitored with the treatment adjusted accordingly, acknowledging that the *goals of care can change over time* where advanced care planning transitions to *terminal care planning.*

Keep in mind that interventions to relieve distressful symptoms can lead to unintended consequences (concept of *double effect*). For example the use of opioids to treat pain can result in constipation and/ or nausea, which in turn will require treatment. In such a situation, it is reasonable to continue the first treatment while initiating another treatment to alleviate its adverse effects. In the rare case of severe and intractable symptoms, including intolerable existential or psychological distress, the use of *palliative sedation* may be a consideration (NHPCO Position Statement 2010).

At the practitioner and systems level, use of unidimensional or multidimensional tools may be helpful to assess a variety of symptoms (refer to Table 2) dependent upon ease of use and evidence-based palliative care. The Edmonton Symptom Assessment Survey (ESAS) is a scale that assesses for the presence and intensity of multiple symptoms.

Several reviews have more thoroughly detailed the management of pain and other symptoms that occur in patients with advanced illness who reside in long-term care facilities [5, 6] and in general practice [7]. Other excellent resources include the "UNIPAC" Series, a publication of the American Academy of Hospice and Palliative Medicine [8], Fast Facts and Concepts (available at the Center to Advance Palliative Care website), the American Medical Directors Association

Table 2 Symptom assessment scales

Symptom	Assessment scales to consider
Anorexia	Functional Assessment Anorexia/Cachexia Therapy Scale
Anxiety	Hamilton Anxiety Rating Scale (HAM-A)
Cognition	Folstein MMSE, COGNISTAT
Constipation	Modified Constipation Assessment Scale, Patient Assessment of Constipation tool
Delirium	Confusion Assessment Method (CAM), Delirium Rating Scale
Depression	Beck Depression Inventory, Short Form Geriatric Depression Scale, Zung Depression Scale, Cornell Scale for Depression in Dementia, CES-D Boston Short Form
Dyspnea	Numerical Analog Scale (i.e., 0–10), Visual Analog Scale (VAS)
Fatigue	NAS, VAS, Fatigue Symptom Inventory
Nausea	VAS
Pain	Numerical Analog Scales (NAS), Visual Analog Scales (VAS), Verbal Descriptive Scale, Wong-Baker FACES Scale, FLACC Scale, Brief Pain Inventory (BPI)
Spiritual pain	FICA spiritual assessment tool, Herth hope index

Resources
City of Hope Pain and Palliative Care Resource Center. http://www.cityofhope.org/prc
UNIPAC Series. American Academy of Hospice and Palliative Medicine, 4th edn. 2012

Clinical Practice Guideline (CPG) on "Pain Management in the Long-Term Care Setting" [9] and its respective CPG implementation manual, ePOCRATES Online [10], and ref. [11].

It should be noted that many medications used to palliate distressful symptoms are not FDA-approved for the treatment of these symptoms.

Anorexia

Anorexia is defined as a loss of appetite that may be associated with cachexia, the latter a catabolic state characterized by severe weight loss. Either may occur in the late stages of any severe progressive illness.

Management of anorexia includes the following:

- Assess anorexigenic effects of medications such as chemotherapy, antidepressants, NSAIDs, opioids.
- Evaluate whether it could be caused by or related to other symptoms such as nausea, constipation, or pain.
- Assess for any potentially reversible medical condition such as rectal fecal impaction, urinary retention, oral candidiasis or other treatable causes such as GER, gastritis, or gastroparesis.
- Initiate practical interventions: small, frequent meals; administer medications separate from or with meals; encourage good mouth care; try a variety of foods; improve the social and environmental aspects of eating.

Consider treating the primary symptom (i.e., anorexia) with an appetite stimulant such as:

- A corticosteroid: prednisone 5–20 mg/day; dexamethasone 4–8 mg/day.
- A progestin: megestrol 400–800 mg/day (trial 4–8 weeks).
- If anorexia is concomitant with depression, it may be reasonable to prescribe mirtazapine as an appetite stimulant and mood enhancer that can also improve sleep.

Note that the appetite stimulant effect of corticosteroids often decrease after several weeks. Megestrol is associated with lower limb edema and an increased risk of thromboembolism. Consider oral nutritional supplements, though subsequent decreased intake at meals can occur as a result of their use. Giving smaller amounts of a high Calorie supplement throughout the day, with medication administration, may result in less decrease of intake at meals. If used, it is preferable to use nutritional supplements that are lactose free, especially in the elderly or African Americans who have a higher prevalence of lactose intolerance. There is insufficient evidence to recommend the use of cannabinoids (dronabinol), cyproheptadine, an androgenic steroid (oxandrolone) or thalidomide, though a therapeutic trial may be worthwhile in refractory anorexia. A patient's advance directive for health care may either *request* or *preclude* artificially administered nutrition and hydration.

Dyspnea

Dyspnea is defined as discomfort in breathing that includes the sensation of breathlessness, shortness of breath or an increased work of breathing. Often it is **not** associated with tachypnea or hypoxemia. Its management includes the following:

- Initiate practical interventions such as the use of a fan, ensure a comfortable ambient room temperature, eliminate respiratory irritants, reposition the person, encourage purse-lip breathing.
- Assess for potentially reversible causes: pneumonia, pleural effusion, pulmonary embolus, heart failure, anemia, bronchospasm.
- Identify any associated symptoms such as aspiration, excessive respiratory secretions, anxiety, social or financial problems, and spiritual suffering.
- *First-line pharmacotherapy for palliation of dyspnea is an opioid* administered every 3–4 h. For mild dyspnea and to minimize the risk of respiratory depression in an *opioid-naïve* patient, start with morphine sulfate 2.5–5 mg PO or the oral morphine equivalent (OME) of another opioid, (refer to OME interconversion Table 12 later in this chapter). Titrate the opioid dose upward 25–50 % every 12–24 h to attain sufficient relief of dyspnea. Note that an *opioid-tolerant* patient is one who has been taking a daily oral morphine equivalent dose of 60 mg or more for 7–10 days.
- Optimize medical treatment of the primary respiratory or cardiac condition (i.e., COPD, heart failure).
- Consider addition of a low dose benzodiazepine for breakthrough or refractory dyspnea as anxiety can be a contributing factor.
- Consider other medical treatments based upon their benefits and burdens, phase of illness, patient preferences, and advance health care directives.
- Remember that patients with dyspnea often do better with a *scheduled* dose of an opioid (and a benzodiazepine) rather than as needed (PRN) dosing. Opioids are effective in treating dyspnea in patients with COPD, though may be less effective in patients with cancer or heart failure. There is poor evidence as to the effectiveness of nebulized opioids, though it may warrant a therapeutic trial in refractory dyspnea. Though the use of oxygen may reverse hypoxemia, dyspnea may not improve. Be aware of the potential for oxygen therapy to cause hypercapnia and subsequent obtundation or respiratory arrest. When using an opioid for dyspnea it is prudent to aim for a respiratory rate between 14 and 20.
- Initiation or continuation of noninvasive ventilatory support (e.g., CPAP, BiPAP) may be warranted in special circumstances such as late stage COPD or ALS.

Not infrequently a family member may request the use of oxygen for non-hypoxemic dyspnea. While there is no evidence to support this, many times it may alleviate the discomfort of breathing that patients may feel as well as the emotional distress that families may experience when observing their dyspneic family member.

Table 3 Major mechanisms of nausea/vomiting

Cause	Pharmacologic management
Cortical:	
• Tumor, increased intracranial pressure	Dexamethasone
• Anxiety, situational stressors	Benzodiazepine
• Pain response	Opioid, other pain medication/adjuvants
Vestibular:	
	Meclizine
	Scopolamine
	Dimenhydrinate
Chemoreceptor trigger zone:	
• Medications	Decrease dose or discontinue, if possible
• Metabolic (e.g., kidney/liver failure)	Haloperidol, olanzapine
• Hyponatremia	Sodium chloride, demeclocycline
• Hypercalcemia	Bisphosphonate, dexamethasone
Gastrointestinal:	
• Drug related	Stop drug, consider PPI
• Tumor	Promethazine, metoclopramide, octreotide
• Constipation	Bowel regimen
• Cough-induced	Opioid, anticholinergic

Adapted from UNIPAC Four, 4th edn., 2012, AAHPM

Nausea and Vomiting

The most rational approach to managing nausea and/or vomiting is to understand the four main pathophysiologic mechanisms and the neurotransmitters that mediate the emetic reflex in the brain (refer to Table 3). This will allow for a more rational and effective choice of antiemetic drugs (i.e., antihistaminic, anticholinergic, antiserotinergic, or antidopaminergic).

Management of nausea/vomiting includes:

- Determine whether any medications are emetogenic such as chemotherapeutic agents, some antibiotics, bowel stimulants, opioids, NSAIDs.
- Identify potentially reversible causes such as GER, gastroparesis, constipation, urinary retention, adynamic ileus, UTI.
- Consider emotional and spiritual factors, including *anticipatory anxiety* related to medical treatments.
- Initiate practical, non-pharmacologic interventions such as offering smaller, more frequent meals of blander food, relaxation techniques, appropriate body positioning while eating or when being fed orally or by PEG tube.
- Prescribe pharmacologic treatment based on the major cause(s) of nausea/vomiting (refer to Table 3).

Combination pharmacotherapy based on each medication's different antiemetic physiologic mechanism may be necessary especially if nausea/vomiting has multiple etiologies or is refractory. Dexamethasone, metoclopramide, and low-dose antipsychotics have central antiemetic effects.

Be aware of the likely side effects of serotonin receptor antagonists such as ondansetron (headache, constipation, fatigue, xerostomia), as well as anticholinergics and antihistamines (drowsiness, fatigue, confusion, dry mouth, constipation, urinary retention, blurred vision). Metoclopramide can induce EPS, dystonia and tardive dyskinesia. Low dose haloperidol (0.5–2 mg) or olanzapine (2.5–7.5 mg) may be useful in alleviating nausea/vomiting.

Dronabinol can have an antiemetic effect though poor evidence of efficacy (start at 2.5 mg twice a day to a maximum of 20 mg/day). Common adverse effects include somnolence, asthenia, paranoia, nausea, and vomiting. Opioid-induced nausea/vomiting may require either a dose reduction of the opioid or rotation to another opioid.

Constipation

Many patients who reside in a long term care setting experience constipation, especially if terminally ill. Constipation can occur because of a combination of poor fluid intake, low dietary fiber, impaired mobility and constipating drugs such as opioids, anticholinergics, iron, calcium preparations, and antihypertensives such as calcium channel blockers, diuretics, and clonidine.

Management of constipation includes the following:

- *Prevention* is paramount.
- Identify potentially reversible causes, including medication-induced and medical conditions such as a fecal impaction; metabolic disturbances (hypercalcemia, hypothyroidism); GI causes (especially be aware if obstruction is present); and neurologic causes (such as nerve root or spinal cord compression or visceral neuropathy that may occur in Parkinson's disease).
- Identify life-threatening causes such as a bowel obstruction or narcotic bowel syndrome.
- Practical interventions include making toilets accessible, establishing a bowel routine, and encouraging increased fluid intake (if tolerated).
- Reduce the anticholinergic medication load if possible.
- Establish an individualized bowel regimen according to each laxative's mechanism of action (refer to Table 4). Combination therapy is often required.
- Monitor for side effects of laxatives that can include bloating, cramping, nausea, and diarrhea.
- Bulk-forming laxatives are usually *not* recommended because they can exacerbate constipation in underhydrated and less mobile patients and often cause or worsen bloating, nausea or vomiting.

Table 4 Stepwise regimen to prevent or treat constipation "The Sixth Vital Sign"

1. Begin with:	Senna with/without docusate	1–2 tabs/cap qd-bid
2. Titrate up to:	Senna	3–4 tabs bid
3. If needed *add*:	Sorbitol or lactulose	30 cc qd-bid
	or	
	Polyethylene glycol	17 g in 8 oz water qd-bid
4. Consider, *in addition*:	Glycerin rectal suppository with/ without bisacodyl rectal suppository	Scheduled qd-qod
5. If needed:	Mineral oil or soapsuds enema	
6. If rectal impaction:	May need digital disimpaction	

Remember to prevent opioid-induced constipation: *as the dose of the opioid is increased, so must the laxative regimen also be increased.* Stimulant laxatives such as senna are most effective for opioid-induced constipation. In severe constipation, consider oral lubiprostone or methylnaltrexone sc, though they are expensive.

Stool softeners are considered to have poor effectiveness but can be initially prescribed in some patients when initiating their bowel regimen, i.e., the "laxative ladder". Remember that some patients may also require use of a rectally administered lubricating agent (glycerin) and/or stimulant (bisacodyl) to ensure adequate defecation in combination with oral agents. Noted that rectal fecal impaction can cause "paradoxical" diarrhea or urinary retention, either of which may not be evident. This often requires manual disimpaction, though a polyethylene glycol solution taken orally may be effective.

Delirium

Delirium is an acute confusional state that is characterized by a fluctuating course through the day/night, inattention, and disorganized thinking and speech. Delirium can be hyperactive, hypoactive, or mixed. A good caveat to remember is that any acute illness or any medication regardless of when it was started, can precipitate delirium especially in patients with advanced illness.

Management of delirium in patients with advanced, serious illness includes the following:

- Identify potentially reversible causes, especially whether it may be medication-induced.
- Discontinue nonessential medications and reduce anticholinergic load.
- Initiate practical interventions: familiarize the patient to the environment, improve sleep and the sleep–wake cycle, reduce environmental stimuli, optimize hearing and eyesight (i.e., hearing aids "in," eyeglasses "on"), and ensure adequate hydration.

- Reduce immobility by removing/minimizing use of any physical restraints, including Foley catheters.
- Determine whether pain could be contributing to the delirium, and if so, treat it appropriately.
- If delirium persists consider first line medication therapy with low-dose haloperidol (no more than 2–3 mg/day), often in divided doses.
- Second line medication may include a low-dose benzodiazepine, usually lorazepam 0.5–1 mg PO/SL every 6–8 h, more frequent if necessary; or valproic acid 125–250 mg every 12 h or upon awaking in the morning and at bedtime.

Remember that opioids and steroids can cause delirium. Both haloperidol and lorazepam can cause paradoxical agitation or restlessness in which case their dose should be decreased (not increased) or discontinued. It is not uncommon to use combination therapy with both haloperidol and lorazepam. Be aware that patients with dementia are more sensitive to the adverse effects of antipsychotic medications that include sedation and EPS, and that antipsychotics have also been associated with an increased risk of sudden death and cerebrovascular events. Communication with the patient and their family about these risks and benefits must occur. Overall, judicious medication management as well as social, environmental, and practical interventions must all be implemented in an attempt to prevent and treat delirium. For further information refer to the Chap. "Dementia, Delirium, and Depression," which discusses delirium.

Pain Management

Effective pain management is essential to high quality palliative care in post-acute and LTC medicine. Given that there is a high prevalence of potentially pain-producing medical conditions in this patient population. The goals of pain control include:

- Relieve pain
- Relieve suffering
- Prevent/minimize disability
- Preserve decision-making capacity

It is necessary for practitioners to assess each patient for the presence of pain and for "total pain"; that is, the physical, psycho-emotional, social, and spiritual components of pain and how each can affect the other. Successful pain management entails evaluation and interventions that address each component of a patient's total pain. As with any distressful symptom, pain is more optimally managed if its cause and pathophysiologic mechanisms can be determined. Using an interdisciplinary approach with multiple treatment modalities, including both nonpharmacologic and pharmacologic treatments, will also optimize pain management. The most recent AMDA Clinical Practice Guideline on pain management [9] and the AGS publication, *Geriatrics at Your Fingertips* [12] are excellent up-to-date resources that provide more in depth content than permits in this chapter. Also, the AGS guidelines on the pharmacologic management of persistent pain in older persons is another noteworthy resource [13].

Key components to the *evaluation* of pain include the following:

- If possible, *prevent*the occurrence of pain or a painful condition. For example, advanced osteoarthritis of one knee may result in contralateral hip pain: a total knee arthroplasty may prevent this from happening. Another example is prescribing medication in an attempt to prevent the occurrence of postherpetic neuralgia.
- *Anticipate* the occurrence of pain. For example, postsurgical incision pain; the pain associated with the onset of peripheral neuropathy in diabetics; or onset of bone pain in cancer patients with known bone metastases.
- Identify the presence of pain or a painful condition. Remember to look for nonverbal cues of pain such as guarding on movement or on transfers, rubbing and grimacing, or other behaviors such as agitation, restlessness, withdrawn behavior, and insomnia.
- Establish the pain's location, intensity, temporal pattern, any exacerbating and relieving factors and effect on (loss of) function and cognition. Consider using a pain assessment scale.
- Determine whether the pain is acute, chronic (duration of 1 month or more), recent onset, intermittent, incidental (i.e., related to movement), breakthrough pain, and whether multiple causes of pain are present.
- Try to determine whether the pain is **nociceptive** (either somatic or visceral), **neuropathic**, or **inflammatory**, according to the patient's description of the pain (see Table 5).
- Identify associated signs and/or symptoms such as headache, dizziness, nausea/vomiting, constipation, decreased urination, a swollen joint or extremity.
- Review previous and current pharmacologic and nonpharmacologic treatments and their effectiveness, and any complementary and alternative medicine interventions.
- Assess "total pain" by elucidating any psycho-emotional, social, and spiritual dimensions to the physical pain, as well as the person's cultural beliefs as to the meaning of pain and manner of expressing pain.

Table 5 Classification of pain

Type of pain	Descriptors
Nociceptive	
• Somatic pain	Sharp, tender
• Visceral pain	Dull, cramping
• Bone pain	Throbbing, aching
Neuropathic	Burning, tingling, stabbing shooting
Inflammatory	e.g., Pleuritic, abdominal rebound, inflamed joints

Von Roenn JH et al. Current Diagnosis and Treatment of Pain, Lange Series McGraw-Hill. 2006

- Perform a detailed physical exam, with particular attention to those body regions or organs systems that appear to be related to or contributing to the pain.
- Assess the need for diagnostic testing, if likely to be helpful in determining a diagnosis, always considering the potential pain or discomfort these tests may cause.
- Determine the probable cause of the pain. Remember persons may have multiple and different types of pain. Always evaluate for reversible causes of pain. For example, abdominal pain may be due to urinary retention, constipation, and rectal/fecal impaction or caused by medications such as a bowel stimulant or bulk forming laxative.
- Remember that conditions such as bladder spasms, contractures, improper positioning, pressure ulcers, muscle strain, oral thrush, urinary retention, fecal impaction, or a DVT can all cause pain.

Key components to the ***treatment*** of pain include the following:

- Consider treatment options taking into account the patient's health status, prognosis, and known advance directives for health care. Also conduct a thorough discussion to ensure informed choice by the patient and family or proxy decision maker.
- Promote an interdisciplinary treatment plan, part of which will be determined by the disciplines available at the patient's care setting (i.e., nursing facility, SNF, residential/assisted living, home, or hospital).
- Set goals for pain relief. For example, the desired or accepted level of pain reduction that promotes the achievement of positive functional outcomes in self-care, participation in desired personal and recreational activities, improved sleep, mood, and cognition. Also, it is important to assess whether a certain level of sedation is acceptable to both patient and family in order to achieve effective pain control.

In up to 90 % of persons with pain, practitioners can adequately control pain with orally administered medications guided by the World Health Organization (WHO) three-stepped analgesic ladder (see Table 6). The WHO recommends administering analgesic and co-analgesic (i.e., adjuvant) medications as follows:

- By mouth: whenever possible prescribe an oral analgesic. Avoid IM injections as they can be painful; subcutaneous injections are less painful. Opioids in a concentrated liquid form can be administered sublingually or transbuccally.
- Around-the-clock: scheduled dosing for continuous pain and to minimize breakthrough pain.
- According to the ladder: the initial choice of analgesic and use of adjuvants is based on the severity of the pain. Using numerical pain scale, 1–3 can be considered mild pain; 4–6 moderate pain; 7–9 severe pain; and 10 excruciating pain.
- Adapted to the individual: the choice of analgesic should be based upon the patient's condition, comorbidities (such as liver and kidney failure; coexistent dementia or delirium), drug safety and toxicity profile, ease of administration, and goals of both pain relief and the overall desired outcome.

Table 6 The WHO 3-step analgesic ladder

		3. Severe
	2. Moderate	Morphine
1. Mild	A/Codeine	Hydromorphone
ASA	A/Hydrocodone	Methadone
Acetaminophen	A/Oxycodone	Levorphanol
NSAIDs	A/Dihydrocodeine	Fentanyl
	Tramadol/apap	Oxycodone
±Adjuvants	±Adjuvants	±Adjuvants

Adapted from: Technical Report Series 804. Geneva: WHO. 1990

Table 7 Select first and second line analgesics based on type of pain

Type of pain	Consider First line	Consider Second Line
Nociceptive pain	WHO step 1 or 2 drug	WHO step 3 drug
Neuropathic pain	TCAs, anticonvulsants	WHO step 2 or 3 drug
Bone pain	NSAIDs, corticosteroids	WHO step 2 or 3 drug
Intracranial pain	Corticosteroids	WHO step 2 or 3 drug
Visceral pain	Anticholinergic, opioid	Steroids, opioids

Source: UNIPAC Three. AAHPM. 2012

- With attention to detail: ensure correct dosing: consider drug pharmokinetics and pharmacodynamics; make appropriate dose adjustments in timely manner: always monitor benefit verses potential harm and adverse effects.

Optimal pain management entails the choice of the most appropriate analgesic(s) based upon the primary and secondary diagnoses, the physiologic mechanism underlying the pain (see Table 7), pain severity, diagnosis, the potential adverse effects of each medication and/or treatment modality and the patient's individual characteristics that can alter each drug's pharmacokinetics and pharmacodynamics.

Caveats for pain management include:

- In most patients, prescribe at least one analgesic as scheduled, i.e., administered routinely, rather than just as needed (i.e., PRN).
- Choose an appropriate analgesic and dose for breakthrough pain.
- Most types of pain respond, at least partially, to an opioid.
- The maximum dose of acetaminophen is 3000–4000 mg/day, but 2000 mg/day may be prudent if renal or hepatic insufficiency is present.
- Care must be used when prescribing opioid/acetaminophen combinations as the ceiling dose of acetaminophen may be reached before pain is controlled.
- The maximum dose of tramadol is 300 mg/24 h; it may precipitate confusion, seizures, and serotonin syndrome.
- Conventional nonselective NSAIDs (e.g., ibuprofen, naproxen) should only be used short term, that is days to 3–4 weeks; precautions include risk for gastrointestinal

bleeding, renal impairment, platelet dysfunction and exacerbation of edema, increased blood pressure, and worsened heart failure.

- Selective COX-2 inhibitors (e.g., celecoxib) can still have a significant risk of GI bleeding and renal insufficiency.
- Consider holding or discontinuing ASA chemoprophylaxis when administering a conventional or COX-2 NSAID.
- Consider concomitant proton pump inhibitor therapy in patients at increased risk for GI bleeding when prescribing a NSAID.
- Never prescribe a NSAID if the patient is taking warfarin as the risk for GI bleeding is too high.
- Consider use of a topical analgesic such as capsaicin cream, diclofenac gel or a lidocaine patch for persons with one or two localized areas of musculoskeletal, arthritic or neuropathic pain.
- Remember use of the lidocaine patch is noncontinuous, that it is to be applied for only 12 h each 24-h period, off the remaining 12 h, applying no more than three patches at a time.
- Avoid use of meperidine due to its potential for causing undesirable CNS side effects such as confusion or seizures.
- Partial opioid agents such as butorphanol, pentazocine, buprenorphine and nalbuphine are not recommended because of their analgesic ceiling effects and ability to counteract the analgesic effect of pure agonist opioids, as these medications can either precipitate an opioid-withdrawal pain crisis, or lessen other opioid analgesic effects.

Opioid Analgesics

Opioids are both appropriate and effective for the treatment of moderate to severe acute or chronic pain not relieved by other analgesics or modalities. Judicious prescribing can provide effective pain management in patients in post-acute and LTC with a low likelihood of psychological dependency or addiction. Scheduled low doses of opioids can be very effective in the treatment of chronic pain associated with various chronic musculoskeletal conditions that afflict the elderly. Note that physical dependency, characterized by withdrawal symptoms, can occur when regularly scheduled opioids are abruptly discontinued. Gradual dose reduction can prevent this if an opioid is to be discontinued.

General guidelines to the use of opioids include:

- *For acute pain:* start by prescribing an immediate-release opioid preparation (see Table 8 for suggested equianalgesic starting doses).
- *For chronic pain:* consider starting a *sustained-released* opioid, with a sufficient dose of an *immediate release* opioid for breakthrough pain.
- Remember that the total dose of a mixed opioid (i.e., an opioid with acetaminophen) is limited by its 24 h dose of acetaminophen.

Table 8 Suggested equianalgesic starting doses for selected oral opioids

Frail or elderly opioid-naïve patients	
The practitioner may choose from the following suggested starting doses:	
Morphine 2 mg PO or SL	0.1 cc morphine 20 mg/cc (Roxanol®)
Oxycodone liquid 2 mg PO or SL	0.1 cc oxycodone 20 mg/cc (Oxyfast®)
Oxycodone 2.5 mg	• ½ tablet 5 mg oxycodone • ½ tablet oxycodone 5 mg/acetaminophen 325 mg (Percocet®)
Hydromorphone 0.5 mg PO	0.5 cc hydromorphone 1 mg/cc (Dilaudid®)
Hydrocodone 2.5 mg PO	½ tablet hydrocodone 5 mg/acetaminophen 500 mg (Vicodin®)
Adult-opioid-naive patients	
The practitioner may choose from the following suggested starting doses:	
Morphine 5 mg PO or SL	0.25 cc morphine 20 mg/cc (Roxanol®)
Oxycodone liquid 5 mg PO or SL	0.25 cc oxycodone 20 mg/cc (Oxyfast®)
Oxycodone 5 mg	• 5 mg oxycodone • 1 tablet oxycodone 5 mg/acetaminophen 325 mg (Percocet®)
Hydromorphone 1 mg	• ½ of 2 mg tablet PO (Dilaudid®) • 1 cc of hydromorphone 1 mg/cc SL
Hydrocodone 5 mg	1 tablet (Vicodin®) 5/500

Source: Permission granted by American Medical Directors Association. Palliative Care in the Long-Term Care Setting (LTC Physician Information Tool Kit Series). Columbia, MD. 2012

Table 9 Available formulations of sustained-release oral opioids

Morphine sulfate ER (MS Contin®)[a]	q 8 h–12 h	15, 30, 60, 100, 200 mg ER
Morphine sulfate ER (Kadian®) [a, b]	q 12–24 h	10, 20, 30, 50, 60, 80, 100, 200 ER
Morphine sulfate ER (Avinza®) [a, b, c]	q 24 h	30, 45, 60, 75, 90, 120 ER
Oxycodone ER (Oxycontin®)[a]	q 8–2 h	10, 15, 20, 30, 40, 60, 80 ER
Oxymorphone (Opana ER®)[a]	q 12 h	5, 7.5, 10, 15, 20, 30, 40 ER

[a] Formulation not to be crushed
[b] Capsules can be opened and contents administered per PEG
[c] Formulation components: 90 % ER and 10 % immediate release

- Once the total daily dose of an immediate release opioid has been able to adequately control the patient's pain, consider converting it to an equivalent dose of a sustained-release opioid (see Table 9 on the different formulizations of sustained-release opioids that are available).
- Note that the duration of analgesic action for all immediate-release morphine preparations is 3–4 h whether administered PO, SL, SC, or IV. Though the onset of action and peak analgesic effect do vary (see Table 10).
- The opioid dose for breakthrough pain is 10–15 % of the total daily opioid dose, administered as often as every 1–2 h *if* needed.
- One can usually safely uptitrate the total 24 h dose of an opioid 25–50 % for mild to moderate pain and 50–100 % for moderate to severe pain.

Table 10 Pharmacodynamics of immediate release morphine

Administered	Peak analgesic effect (min)	Duration of analgesia (h)
Oral/sublingual	45–60	3–4
Subcutaneous	15–30	3–4
Intravenous	5–15	3–4

Table 11 Common and less common side effects of opioids

Common	Less common
Constipation (almost always)	Hypotension
Somnolescence	Diaphoresis
Nausea/vomiting	Urinary retention
Dizziness	Confusion, delirium
Sweating	Bradycardia
Dry mouth	Seizures
Asthenia	Respiratory depression, apnea
Dysesthesias	Paralytic ileus
Pruritus	Paresthesia, hyperesthesia
	Shock, cardiac arrest

- When starting a patient on an opioid, *ALWAYS start the patient on a prophylactic bowel regimen to prevent constipation.* A stimulant and/or osmotic agent are preferable.
- The use of an *adjuvant* analgesic can often allow a lower dose of an opioid to be used and thus lessen the likelihood of opioid adverse effects.

In contrast to non-opioids and NSAIDs, those opioids commonly used for the treatment of pain have no analgesic ceiling. However, adverse drug effects may limit further dose increases (see Table 11) or require "rotating" to another opioid, especially if adequate pain relief is not achieved (see below).

As already noted, meperidine should be avoided because of its high potential for CNS toxicities. Codeine is too constipating in relation to the dose required for an adequate analgesic effect. It is NOT recommended to use three or more different opioids because of the potential for adverse drug–drug or opioid–receptor interactions (either unknown or unrecognized by clinicians). Different opioids interact to different degrees at the mu, delta and kappa opioid receptors. For a patient on transdermal fentanyl patch an immediate release opioid such as morphine or oxycodone needs to be prescribed for breakthrough pain. Transmucosal oral fentanyl (i.e., Actiq®) is only indicated for severe breakthrough cancer pain and its use should be *avoided* in the LTC setting.

When changing from one opioid to another, whether because of inadequate pain relief or unmanageable adverse effects of the opioid, use *oral morphine equivalents.* Oral morphine equivalents are used as a common denominator for opioid dose conversion to avoid either underdosing or overdosing and to maintain or obtain effective pain relief (see Table 12 on oral morphine equivalents). In order to adjust for

Table 12 Oralmorphine
equivalents (mg)

	Oral	Parenteral
Morphine	30	10 (1/3 oral dose)
Oxycodone	20–30	N/A
Oxymorphone	10	1 (1/10 oral dose)
Hydromorphone	7.5	1.5 (1/5 oral dose)
Meperidine	300	75 (1/4 oral dose)
Hydrocodone	30	N/A
Codeine	180–200	N/A

25 µg fentanyl patch=50 mg oral morphine/24 h);
N/A no parenteral formulation available
Source: Adapted from American Pain Society.
Principles of analgesic use in the treatment of acute
pain and cancer pain. 6th edn. 2008

incomplete cross-tolerance the relative (conversion) total daily dosage of the new opioid should be decreased by 25–50 %. When converting from one opioid to another it is prudent to do so over 2 or 3 days, with downward titration of the opioid being discontinued, coupled with the upward titration of the newly prescribed opioid. This gradual titration is especially important if the patient is on a high dose of opioid and can avoid a pain withdrawal crisis.

Caution is warranted when prescribing opioids in an *opioid-naïve* patient where the dictum, "start low and go slow" is advisable. The suggested starting dose of oral morphine is 0.2–0.5 mg every 3–4 h or the equianalgesic dose of another opioid. The use of a fentanyl patch when initiating opioid treatment in the frail elderly opioid-naïve patient is not advisable as the lower strength patches of 12 and 25 mcg/h provide an oral morphine equivalent (OME) approximate dose of 25 and 50 mg respectively *every 24 h*. Such doses can cause excess fatigue or sedation. Though expensive, the fentanyl patch has an ease of use and can provide excellent analgesia in some patients. The fentanyl patch is frequently ineffective in thin patients and those who weigh less than 105 lbs, due to inadequate subcutaneous fat depot necessary for fentanyl absorption through the skin into the blood.

Morphine, oxycodone, and hydromorphone should be used cautiously in patients with moderate to severe renal failure (GFR 30–50 ml/min or less) because of the risk of neurotoxic metabolite accumulation. Methadone and fentanyl are safe to use for patients with advanced renal failure or on dialysis, though neither is dialyzable. Non-opioid medications that are safe to use for patients with renal failure include acetaminophen and tramadol, though the maximal daily dose of tramadol should be reduced to no more than 50–100 mg twice a day.

Morphine and codeine doses may need to be reduced in patients with liver disease, especially those with cirrhosis. Fentanyl may be easier to use in such patients, unless there is inadequate subcutaneous tissue.

Methadone is gaining popularity in the treatment of chronic musculoskeletal pain and clinicians are prescribing it more frequently for the treatment of cancer pain and neuropathic pain. Other indications for its use include refractory pain, intolerance to other opioids, or clinician concerns that the patient is diverting opioids.

Methadone has several mechanisms of action, is extensively metabolized in the liver, is minimally renally excreted, and is cheap. However, its prolonged and variable metabolism (half-life may vary from 45 to 180 h) is such that its steady state plasma concentration is not reached for up to 10 days. It has complex medication interactions, has been associated with prolongation of the QT interval, and an increasingly more common cause of opioid related deaths. Thus, methadone should only be used by (or in consultation with) a clinician who is experienced with its use. When treating frail elders, starting at a low dose of methadone between 2.5 and 5 mg, two or three times a day would be prudent. *Methadone should never be used for the treatment of acute or breakthrough pain,* as the risk of respiratory depression is too high. For more complete information on methadone use in long-term care, refer to Appendix 4 of the AMDA Clinical Practice Guideline on Pain Management in the Long Term Care Setting [9]. For guidelines on the use of patient controlled analgesia (PCA), refer to refs. 8 (UNIPAC Three) and 14.

Eligibility Guidelines for Hospice

Practitioners in post-acute and LTC must consider, offer and facilitate resident access to hospice care as residents transition into the terminal phase of advanced illness. Most residents will be eligible for the Medicare Hospice Benefit (MHB). Hospice is an underutilized benefit with many patients being referred too late in their illness to be able to fully benefit from its services. The National Hospice and Palliative Care Origination (NHPCO) reports that the proportion of hospice stays of 7 days or less to be 35 % of hospice admissions, while longer stays greater than 180 days account for 10 % of admissions.

Practitioner knowledge of the *general eligibility guidelines* and *disease-specific guidelines* (see Table 13) for hospice can help prognosticate whether a resident with advanced illness may have less than 6 months to live. Such a determination can prompt a frank discussion with the resident and family on advance care planning, which can lead to a more palliative approach to care whether or not the resident and family opt for life-sustaining treatment.

General indicators (i.e., general eligibility guidelines for hospice) that a chronic illness may have progressed to its *terminal phase* include the following:

- Frequent transfers to the ER.
- More frequent hospitalizations.
- Significant weight loss (5 % in 1 month; 10 % in the past 6 months).
- Multiple stage 3 or 4 decubitus ulcers.
- Serum albumin less that 2.5 g/dl.
- Recurrent life-threatening infections such as pneumonia, pyelonephritis, or sepsis.
- Declining functional status as determined by either a Karnofsky Performance status of <70 % or increasing dependency in 2 or more of 6 Basic Activities of Daily Living.

Table 13 Disease specific eligibility criteria/guidelines for hospice

Cancer
Widespread metastatic disease
Palliative Performance Scale (PPS) ≤ 70 %
No longer seeking curative care
Dementia (Alzheimer's Disease)
Inability to ambulate due to dementia (FAST 7c)
No consistent meaningful speech
Life threatening infections, multiple stage 3 or 4 skin ulcers
Inability to maintain sufficient fluid and calorie intake
Heart disease
Poor response or intolerant to optimal medical treatment
NYHA class IV CHF
EF ≤ 20 % (helpful, not required)
HIV/AIDS
CD 4 count < 25
Persistent viral loads >100,000/ml
Major AIDS-defining refractory infections or other medical conditions
Significant functional decline in ADLs
Neurologic diseases (PD, ALS, MS, MD, myasthenia gravis)
Rapid disease progression and critical nutritional state
Life threatening infections in preceding 12 months
Stage 3, 4 decubitus ulcers
Critically impaired breathing capacity, declines ventilator
Pulmonary disease
Disabling dyspnea at rest or with minimal exertion
Increasing visits to ER, hospitalizations
Hypoxemia on room air (<88 %); hypercapnia of $_pCO_2 > 50$ mmHg
FEV 1 < 30 % (helpful, not required)
Renal failure
Not seeking dialysis, not a candidate (or refusing further dialysis)
Calculated creatinine clearance < 10 (<15 for diabetics)
Creatinine >8 (>6 for diabetics)
Stroke
Coma (acute phase)
Dysphagia with insufficient intake of fluids and calories
Post stroke dementia (See dementia criteria)
LIVER DISEASE
INR >1.5 not on Warfarin
Serum albumin <2.5 g/dl
Refractory ascites
Previous spontaneous bacterial peritonitis
Hepatorenal syndrome
Recurrent variceal bleeding

Adapted from: National Hospice and Palliative Care Organization

When the *guidelines* for *disease-specific eligibility* for hospice are not met, the presence and severity of comorbid medical conditions and/or psychosocial factors may support eligibility. For example, advanced COPD or dementia may further support eligibility for hospice in a resident with late stage heart failure. Finally, there is excellent predictive value in the "surprise question":"Would you be surprised if a certain patient died in the next 12 months ?"; if so, then it would be appropriate to consider hospice care. Note that the diagnoses of failure to thrive and generalized debility are no longer accepted as a terminal diagnosis under the MHB.

Certification for hospice requires that two physicians, usually the hospice medical director and the attending or referring physician, sign a statement certifying that the patient's medical prognosis supports a life expectancy of 6 months or less if the individual's illness follows its normal course. Once on hospice a patient must be *recertified* for each benefit period. Recertification only requires a narrative statement by the hospice medical director as to continued eligibility. With the MHB, the first two hospice certification periods are each 90 days and all subsequent periods are 60 days (with no limit as to the number of 60 day periods). However, continued eligibility for hospice requires that the eligibility parameters present on admission to hospice continue to be met *and* that physical, functional and/or nutritional *decline continues* and supports that life expectancy is 6 months or less if the individual's illness follows its normal course. Note that every 60 days recertification period now requires a *face-to-face* visit by the medical director or a nurse practitioner to determine and verify continued eligibility for hospice. Every patient on hospice has the right to *revoke* their hospice benefit at any time in order to seek life-sustaining or curative treatment. In such circumstances, if the treatments are of no further benefit the discontinued patients can be readmitted to hospice if eligibility guidelines are still met.

Billing by practitioners for services rendered to patients on hospice can be confusing and dependent upon the Local Medicare Intermediary (now called Medicare Administrative Contractors). It is recommended that practitioners clarify hospice billing practices with their Medicare Administrative Contractor.

End of Life Care

As patients with advanced serious life-limiting illness enter the last months to weeks of life, practitioners need to recognize this terminal phase and inform patients and family accordingly. If not already done, goals of care need to be reviewed and modified through advanced care planning. Whether the patient and family want to continue to pursue life-prolonging treatments or are amenable to hospice care, palliative care can be integrated into either choice. Irrespective of where the patient resides, interdisciplinary management is essential to maintaining hope, dignity and the best possible quality of life until the patient dies. Eventually however, continuing life-sustaining treatments (such as IV fluids, PEG tube feeding, blood transfusions, antibiotics, pacemakers, ICDs, and hemodialysis) during the last weeks and days of life can become overly burdensome, causing more harm, pain, and suffering than benefit to the patient and the family.

The physiologic changes of dying, although complex, can be effectively managed if practitioners and the IDT understand the etiologies and underlying pathophysiology of each distressful symptom so that appropriate nonpharmacologic and pharmacologic interventions are used [15]. Given each patient's terminal illness and their comorbidities, palliative drugs, equipment, and supplies should be available in *anticipation of those symptoms* that are most likely to occur at the end of life.

As death approaches, patients and families should be advised that fatigue and weakness will increase while the desire for food and fluid intake is reduced due to the loss of both appetite and thirst. Reduced cardiac output and intravascular volume depletion result in tachycardia, hypotension, peripheral cooling, cyanosis, and mottling. Urine output will diminish with eventual anuria. Neurologic dysfunction will occur, leading to a decreased level of consciousness and eventual coma. Ten percent of patients may experience an agitated delirium during the last days of life.

Practical interventions to maintain patient comfort include periodic repositioning; decreasing food and fluid intake to prevent choking or aspiration; maintaining a moist oral mucosa; and providing moisture and lubricating agents to the conjunctiva and lips. Family members should be encouraged to participate in this care as it can often provide them with a sense of fulfillment in having helped to comfort their loved one at end of life.

Nonessential drugs (e.g., aspirin, multivitamins, calcium supplements, lipid-lowering agents) should be discontinued. Practitioners should also consider the benefits and risks of continuing any medications not needed to maintain the patients comfort such as antidepressants, antihypertensives, warfarin, and thyroid replacement. Other drugs, such as diuretics, ACE inhibitors and hypoglycemic agents (even insulin) may require a dosage reduction or even discontinuation. Reduced hepatic function and renal perfusion can precipitate an opioid-induced terminal delirium. If this occurs, consider reducing the opioid dosage while ensuring that pain is still adequately controlled.

During the last few days of life, medication reconciliation is essential to avoid polypharmacy and its potential sequelae, especially as "comfort medications" are administered to manage pain and distressful symptoms and suffering.

Remember that a peaceful death is just as important to the *family* as to the patient, perhaps even more so.

General guidelines on the use of comfort-directed pharmacologic interventions include:

- **For tachypnea or breathlessness**: use low doses of an immediate release opioid with or without a benzodiazepine, each administered sublingually or transbuccally.
- **For excessive respiratory or oral secretions**: consider an anticholinergic agent administered sublingually (e.g., hyoscyamine or an ophthalmic solution of atropine) or topically (e.g., transdermal scopolamine patch). It is beneficial to educate the family and staff to avoid suction as it will stimulate the production of even more secretions.

- **For pain**: use a concentrated oral formulation of either morphine (e.g., Roxanol® 20 mg/cc) or oxycodone (Oxyfast® 20 mg/cc). Either can be administered sublingually or transbuccally. Avoid IM or SC injections if possible as these can be painful.
- **For anxiety**: use a benzodiazepine or an opioid, possibly an antipsychotic. Remember any of these can cause paradoxical agitation.
- **For restlessness or delirium**: perform a careful medication review and rule out a rectal fecal impaction or urinal bladder retention. Ensure adequate pain control. Treat with an antipsychotic, with or without a benzodiazepine. The latter can cause paradoxical agitation.
- **For fever**: If distressing to the patient, schedule doses of acetaminophen administered orally, per rectum or per PEG (if present).
- **If excessive sweating**: Review medications, consider cooling the room or use a fan, and consider an opioid dose reduction (as opioids can cause sweating).

Compounded formulations applied topically on the skin may be effective for restlessness, though evidence is lacking. For example, ABH gel compound that comprises lorazepam, diphenhydramine, and haloperidol. Review of compounded topicals is beyond the scope of this chapter so practitioners are encouraged to contact their local compounding pharmacies and hospice agencies.

Pearls for the Practitioner

- Integrate palliative care into traditional care provided to residents and patients throughout the post-acute and long-term care continuum irrespective of whether they choose to continue disease-directed or alternative therapies.
- Support informed patient and family decision-making (i.e., advance care planning) consistent with their values and preferences for care.
- Determine, if possible, the pathophysiologic and clinical factors underlying each pain and non-pain symptom in order to choose the most appropriate interventions.
- Treat pain through the use of multiple modalities, both nonpharmacologic and pharmacologic as well as complementary and alternative therapies.
- Choose the most appropriate analgesic based on the type of pain, pain severity, potential adverse effects of the medication and the patient's individual characteristics.
- Always initiate a bowel regimen to prevent constipation when prescribing an opioid and remember to intensify the bowel regimen when the dose of the opioid is increased.
- Obtain education on Risk Evaluation and Mitigation Strategy (REMS) on the use of opioid analgesics.
- Anticipate which symptoms are most likely to occur during each patient's illness trajectory. In addition to identifying, assessing, treating, and monitoring distressful symptoms, prevent their emergence if possible.

- Consider both the general and disease specific guidelines when evaluating persons for hospice.
- Consider palliative sedation to alleviate intractable and intolerable pain or suffering that persists despite aggressive palliative care.
- Use resources in your community such as health care professionals who have expertise in palliative care and hospice.

References

1. Currow DC, Wheeler JL, Glare PA, et al. A framework for generalizeability in palliative care. J Pain Symptom Manage. 2009;37(3):373–86.
2. Young Y, Frick KD, Phelan EA. Can successful aging and chronic illness co- exist in the same individual? A multidimensional concept of successful aging. J Am Med Dir Assoc. 2009;10:87–92.
3. Aronow WS. Clinical causes of death in 2372 older persons in a nursing home during 15-year follow-up. J Am Med Dir Assoc. 2000;1:95–6.
4. Goldberg TH, Botero QA. Causes of death in elderly nursing home residents. J Am Med Dir Assoc. 2008;9:565–7.
5. Winn PA, Dentino AN. Quality palliative care in the long-term care setting. J Am Med Dir Assoc. 2005;6:589–98.
6. Winn PA, Dentino AN. Effective pain management in the long-term care setting. J Am Med Dir Assoc. 2004;5:342–52.
7. Winn PA, Salinas RC, Cook JB. End-of-life care. FP essentials, AAFP home study. 336th ed. Leawood, KS: American Academy of Family Physicians; 2007.
8. Storey CP. A resource for hospice and palliative care professionals. 4th ed. Glenview, IL: American Academy of Hospice and Palliative Medicine; 2012. UNIPAC Three. Weinstein SM, Portnenoy RK, Harrington SE. Assessing and Treating Pain; UNIPAC Four. Tucker RO, Nichols AN. Managing Nonpain Symptoms; UNIPAC Nine. Shega JW, Levine SK. Caring for Patients with Chronic Illnesses: Dementia, COPD, and CHF.
9. American Medical Directors Association. Clinical practice guideline: pain management in the long-term care setting. 4th ed. Columbia, MD: American Medical Directors Association; 2012.
10. ePOCRATES Online. End of life care. https://online.epocrates.com/u/29111020/End-of-life+care. Accessed 31 Mar 2015.
11. Brunnhuber K, Nash S, Meier D, Weissman DE, Woodcock J. Putting evidence into practice: palliative care. The BMJ Publishing Group Limited. 2008
12. Reuben DB, Herr KA, Pacala JT, et al. Geriatrics at your fingertips: 2014. 16th ed. New York: The American Geriatrics Society; 2014.
13. American Geriatrics Panel on the Pharmacologic Management of Persistent Pain in Older Persons. Pharmacologic management of persistent pain in older adults. J Am Geriatr Soc. 2009;57(8):1331–46.
14. The American Pain Society. Principles of analgesic use in the treatment of acute pain and cancer pain. 5th ed. Glenview, IL: The American Pain Society; 2003.
15. Emanuel LL, vonGunten CF, Ferris FD. Education for physicians on end-of- life care. Participant's handbook. Module 12. Last hours of living. Chicago: EPEC; 1999.
16. Teunissen SCCM, Wesker W, Kruitwagen C, et al. Symptom prevalence in patients with incurable cancer: a systematic review. J Pain Symptom Mange. 2007;34:94–104.
17. Solano JP, Gomes B, Higginson IJ. A comparison of symptom prevalence in far advanced cancer: AIDS, heart disease, chronic obstructive pulmonary disease and renal disease. J Pain Symptom Mange. 2006;31(1):58–69.

18. Cantin B, Rothuisen LE, Buclin T. Referrals of cancer versus non-cancer patients to palliative care consult team. Do they differ? J Palliative Care. 2009;25(2):92–9.

19. White C, McMullen D, Doyle J. Now that you mention it, Doctor… symptom reporting and the need for systematic questioning in a specialist palliative care unit. J Palliative Med. 2009;12(5):447–50.

Suggested Reading

20. AMDA White paper on palliative care and hospice in long term care. Accessed 31 Mar 2015.

21. AAHPM. Primer of palliative care. 6th edn. AAHPM. 2014.

22. End-of-life care overview – ePOCRATES Online. https.//online.epocrates.com/u/2911102/End-of-life + care. Accessed 31 Mar 2015.

23. Snyder L, Quill TE editors. Physician's guide to end-of-life care. American College of Physicians – American Society of Internal Medicine. 2001.

24. Matzo M, Sherman D. Palliative care nursing education: quality care to the end of life. 3rd ed. New York: Springer; 2009.

25. Flacker JM, Kiely DK. A practical approach to identifying mortality-rated factors in established long-term care residents. J Am Geriatr Soc. 1998;46(8):1012–5.

26. Center to Advance Palliative Care. Fast facts and concepts. www.capc.org. Accessed 31 Mar 2015.

27. AMDA CPG implementation series: Pain management manual. 2014.

28. McPherson ML. Demystifying opioid conversion calculations: a guide for effective dosing. American Society of Health–System Pharmacists. 2009. (now includes 2011 update section).

29. Chochinov HM. Dignity therapy: final words for final days. Oxford University Press. 2012.

30. Fishman SM. Responsible opioid prescribing. a clinician's guide. 2nd edn. FSMB Foundation. 2012.

31. Kirk TW, Mahon MM. National Hospice and Palliative Care Organization (NHPCO) position statement and commentary on the use of palliative sedation in imminently dying terminally ill patients. J Pain Symptom Manage. 2010;39(5):914–23.

32. Emanuel LL, Librach SW. Palliative care. Care skills and clinical competencies. 2nd edn. Elsevier Saunders. 2011.

Weight and Nutrition

Todd H. Goldberg and Joel A. Levien

Introduction

The nutritional needs of the geriatric patient are influenced by many factors. Changes associated with aging, individual behavior, as well as drugs and disease all increase nutritional risk. As with persons of all ages, maintaining proper nutrition and a healthy weight are important for those who reside in the community, assisted living facilities, and nursing homes. Ideally, optimal nutrition should improve health, function, quality of life, and reduce the risk of morbidity, mortality, and conditions such as osteoporosis, weakness, pressure sores, frailty, sarcopenia, and lack of resistance to infection. Weight loss is both a negative quality measure and risk factor for poor outcomes, while survival is markedly improved with adequate nutrition. Maintaining appropriate nutrition, hydration, oral intake, and weight can pose a challenge especially for those who have dementia, depression, and gastrointestinal, neurological, musculoskeletal, or psychiatric disorders. Many drugs can also affect appetite, chewing, swallowing, digestion, and bowel function that in turn can result in weight loss.

Older adults who require long-term care often reside in residential care or long nursing facilities for a variety of reasons: ranging, for example, from *temporary disability* due to a hip fracture, or *chronic disability* from COPD, CHF, or dementia. As such those with chronic illness and disability require diligent nutritional assessment. There is a strong correlation between low body mass index, low serum

T.H. Goldberg, MD, CMD, FACP (✉)
Department of Internal Medicine, WVU Health Sciences Center/Charleston Area Medical Center, 3110 MacCorkle Avenue, SE, Charleston, WV 25304, USA
e-mail: tgoldberg@hsc.wvu.edu

J.A. Levien, MD, FACG, FACP
Department of Gastroenterology, Jackson Madison County General Hospital, 27 Medical Center Drive, Jackson, TN 38301, USA
e-mail: joellevien@icloud.com

© Springer International Publishing Switzerland 2016
P.A. Fenstemacher, P. Winn (eds.), *Post-Acute and Long-Term Medicine*, Current Clinical Practice, DOI 10.1007/978-3-319-16979-8_12

albumin, and increased mortality for months to years after discharge from the hospital. Even when nutritional deficiencies are recognized, interventions are often suboptimal, leading to both poor outcomes and potential ethical and legal issues [1].

Detailed dietary guidelines and Dietary Reference Intakes are beyond the scope of this review and are available at many web sites including that of the US Dept. of Agriculture Food and Nutrition Information Center: http://fnic.nal.usda.gov/dietary-guidance/dietary-reference-intakes [2]. Table 1 summarizes the recommendations for a few key nutrients.

Table 1 Recommended intakes for some key nutrients in older adults

Nutrient	Typical recommended intake/DRI[a]	Comments for geriatrics/LTC
Calories/energy	1800+ calories	Varies by body size and activity level and desired weight loss or gain.
Protein	46 g/day Females >18 (0.36–0.66 g/kg/day) 56 g/day Males >18 10–35 % of calories	Increased protein to 1–1.2 g/kg/day suggested for geriatric LTC patients.
Fat	20–35 % of calories	
Carbohydrate	130 g/day, 45–65 % of calories	
Water	2.7–3.7 L/day	Includes total water, all beverages, in average temperate climate.
Vitamin A	700–900 mcg/day	Higher doses associated with increased toxicity and mortality.
Vitamin B$_{12}$	2.4 mcg/day. Typical oral supplement dose 100–1000 mcg.	Common deficiency in elderly; measure levels. Often malabsorbed requiring supplements.
Vitamin C Zinc	75–90 mg 11 mg	Larger doses often recommended for pressure sores but not evidence-based.
Vitamin D	800 IU (20 mcg) for adults over 70 (2011 IOM Update ref. [29]).	Older adults often deficient. Consider measuring 25 OHD levels and adding supplements ≥800 IU/day, found to reduce falls, fractures and mortality.
Vitamin E	15 mg (22.5 IU)	Supplementation >200 IU no longer recommended due to meta-analysis showing increased mortality [47].
Calcium	1200 mg/day	Calcium + Vitamin D supplements should be considered for all older adults at risk for osteoporosis.
Iron	8 mg/day	Doses >325 mg/day ineffective and cause increased constipation.

[a]Adapted from various sources, chiefly "Dietary Reference Intakes" from the Institute of Medicine, and US Department of Agriculture, Food and Nutrition Information Center (ref. [2]). What were formerly called Recommended Daily Allowances (RDA's) are now called Dietary Reference Intakes (DRI's). Not all vitamins and minerals are included; for more complete lists see the full sources cited

Risk Factors

Overall

Normal aging generally is accompanied by modest changes, if any, in appetite, metabolism, intestinal function and absorption of nutrients. Older patients will experience less hunger than younger patients after a period of underfeeding. Various physiological functions that assure appropriate nutrition; ingestion, digestion, assimilation and absorption of nutrients will be affected by the patient's medical, psychosocial, and functional status. A good bowel program and adequate fluid intake is important (see AMDA's Dehydration/Fluid Maintenance Guideline) [3]. Inadequate intake of food and fluids may lead to dehydration, constipation, slow gastric emptying, regurgitation, cognitive impairment, aspiration, infection, decubiti, and sepsis.

Every patient admitted to a LTC facility will have some *nutritional risk factors* such as:

- A history of weight loss or appetite change.
- Oral/dental problems (edentulousness).
- Reduced mobility and functional disability.
- Skin breakdown or pressure ulcers.
- Disease: depression, dementia, and chronic or terminal illness.
- Symptoms: fluid retention/edema, nausea, vomiting, or a change in bowel habits.
- Multiple medications.

Medication

Innumerable drugs can cause anorexia, GI disturbances, and weight loss. These include NSAID's, opioids, anticholinergics (which reduce salivary and gastric secretions, and GI motility); diabetic drugs such as metformin, digoxin, and cholinesterase inhibitors. Psychotropics particularly TCAs drug can cause diminished cognition, poor oral intake, and constipation. ACE inhibitors and antibiotics may distort normal smell and taste. Anti-acid drugs, especially proton pump inhibitors, may reduce absorption of nutrients such as calcium and vitamin B_{12}. Numerous drugs cause constipation, including analgesics and antihypertensives (especially calcium channel blockers). Opioids and antidiarrheals such as loperamide may decrease peristalsis and potentially result in toxic megacolon. Some drugs cause weight gain, such as the antidiabetic agents and antipsychotics. Polypharmacy can compromise appetite, weight, and nutrition. Recent surgery or trauma may result in immobility, ileus, and constipation. One of the most critical tasks of the admitting clinician is to review and verify the list of medications patients are taking, discontinue unnecessary medications, while ensuring safe transition of patients between health care settings (see AMDA's Transitions of Care Guideline) [4].

Disease

Numerous disease-related factors may cause changes in weight, appetite, swallowing and gastrointestinal function, such as: hyperthyroidism or hypothyroidism and diabetes; neurologic and psychiatric disorders such as Parkinson's, dementia, or depression; alcohol and other substance abuse; oral/dental problems; numerous GI disorders such as achalasia, malabsorption, peptic ulcers, and irritable or inflammatory bowel disease; and systemic conditions such as scleroderma, CHF, AIDS, cancer, and infection. Physiologic stress due to acute or chronic illness can increase protein and energy requirements and result in weight loss.

In community dwelling elderly the ability to obtain, prepare and eat food may be impeded by psychosocial and functional problems, sensory deficits, limited mobility, or inadequate income. Simply being admitted to a LTC facility where three good meals a day are provided may actually improve nutrition and reverse weight loss.

Assessment of Nutritional Status

Evaluation of problems with nutrition and weight entails a good medical history, physical examination, and a nutritional and laboratory assessment. The staff will often observe problems with eating or weight loss. Body weight and BMI is a basic screen of nutritional status, and subsequently serial weights are a simple tool for recognizing a change in the nutritional well-being. Obtaining accurate weights may be challenging, especially with bedridden or immobilized patients. A calibrated bed or chair scale can be used for these patients.

Monitoring for significant weight loss is required in all LTC patients and becomes part of the MDS (Minimum Data Set), and the facility's CMS Quality Measure. *According to OBRA regulations, the nursing and dietary staff must*, recognize *significant weight loss.* This is defined as 5 % weight loss over the past 30 days, or >10 % weight loss over the past 6 months [1].

General medical history questions should be asked of the patient or caregiver such as "Is there any difficulty with eating, swallowing, elimination, or maintaining weight?" No single test exists that identifies all patients at risk [5]. Brief tools for nutritional assessment that are widely used and available include the Subjective Global Assessment [6], the Mini Nutritional Assessment (MNA) [7], and the abbreviated MNA-SF (Short Form) [8]. Weight loss alone is one of the best indicators of nutritional compromise and a proven risk factor for increased morbidity and mortality [9].

An additional test to assess nutritional status is the Instant Nutritional Assessment (INA) (Table 2) [10]. The INA consists of measuring the serum albumin and total lymphocyte count, which helps identify a patients at nutritional risk.

Table 2 Instant nutritional assessment

Laboratory result	Abnormal
Serum albumin	Less than 3.5 mg/dL
Total lymphocyte count	Less than 1500/mm^3

Additional Laboratory Assessment and Monitoring

Several other laboratory parameters can also be monitored in patients who present with weight loss, fatigue, or signs and symptoms of under-nutrition or inadequate hydration. These include a CBC, comprehensive metabolic panel, lipids, and a TSH. Obtaining blood levels of vitamin B_{12} and 25-Hydroxy-vitamin D should also be considered. Low serum albumin is the single most commonly used indicator of protein malnutrition and is correlated with increased mortality in older persons [11]. These labs should be ordered not only when nutritional concerns are reported but also periodically in patients at risk for poor nutrition.

Screening for dementia and depression is an important component in the management of malnutrition in LTC [12]. Depression and dementia can impact food intake and weight, and may be the most common cause of weight loss. Medications used for these conditions (antidepressants and cholinesterase inhibitors) may further diminish appetite and cause GI upset, leading to further decrease in food intake. Mirtazapine and nortryptyline tend to increase appetite or weight more than other antidepressants, which can be of therapeutic benefit [12]. In one study of older adults depression was one of the most common causes of weight loss (30 %) followed by malignancies [13].

Weight Management

Achieving a healthy weight in LTC patients is controversial. The patient should be counseled and provided meals and nutrition in order to maintain a healthy weight. Obese patients should be put on a healthy diet with perhaps some mild caloric restriction, but dramatic weight loss should not be expected in those who cannot exercise. Giving an elderly resident a too-restrictive diet may decrease the patient's quality of life and lead to nutritional deficiencies [14]. The optimal weight range for nursing home patients has not been clearly defined but is presumably the same as the general population. A recent article reported that overall mortality rates were lowest with a "normal" BMI (body mass index) in the range of 22.5–25 kg/m^2 [16]. A longitudinal study of Canadian obese adults indicated that mortality was lowest in moderately overweight individuals (BMI 25–30) [17], indicating that older adults may benefit from extra body weight and protein stores when illness occurs; while those underweight (BMI <20) have an increased risk of illness and mortality. Therefore an optimal weight range for seniors, including LTC residents, appears to be a BMI of about 25 ± 5 (i.e., 20–30).

A more common and concerning problem in the nursing home is *underweight*. Underweight residents commonly have anorexia, leading to excessive weight loss, malnutrition and frailty, depression, low energy and activity, and associated poor skin integrity. Nursing home patients who lose at least 5 % of their body weight have been reported to be 5–10 more times likely to die [18], but even those who regain weight still have increased mortality. A workup for potentially reversible causes of weight loss should consider GI and other diseases, medication side effects, and depression. If no specific cause is found, one might then diagnose anorexia of aging, terminal stage of dementia or *failure to thrive*, and the weight loss subsequently determine the weight loss as *unavoidable*. It is often difficult to determine how aggressive interventions should be given patients' limited prognosis and decreased quality of life. The facility and family should provide residents with ample enjoyable food that includes a liberalized diet and appropriate supplements.

AMDA's Clinical Practice Guideline (CPG) on Altered Nutritional Status recommends a process of over 20 steps to evaluate and treat nutritional issues in long term care, beginning with a baseline evaluation of the patient's nutritional status, weight, height and BMI, and dietary preferences [1]. Risk factors for altered nutritional status including a history of recent weight or appetite change and impaired functional status, as well as any related medical complications such as pressure ulcers should all be documented. The presence of terminal illness, depression, or medications affecting taste or appetite should be noted. The CPG states that treatment should address the underlying issues that have been identified, tailor meals/food to individual preferences and function, limit unnecessary dietary restrictions, and add supplements when necessary. Appetite stimulants should be considered as a last resort and on an individual basis. Tube feedings should only be used in appropriate patients (see "Indications and Usage of Feeding tubes" later in this chapter as well as chapter "Ethical and Legal Issues" for further discussion). The AMDA CPG recommends that practitioners and facilities must continually monitor nutritional status.

The "feed.ME" (Medical Education) Global Study Group has recently published a Nutritional Care Pathway suggesting hospitals and LTC facilities "screen, intervene, and supervene" for the nutritional care of all patients in health care facilities [19].

Nutritional Interventions

Fluids

Recommended fluid intake for the average adult is 3.7 L/day for males and 2.7 L/day for females [2]. This assumes a typical temperate climate and includes total daily consumption of water, all beverages, and the water content derived from solid foods. Those with illness, fever, or experiencing a humid/ high ambient temperature may require additional fluids. Oral intake is preferred; IV therapy is often not available in LTC. An alternative means of hydration is *hypodermoclysis* (subcutaneous infusion of isotonic fluids) though a short term option [20]. Note that lab abnormalities of electrolytes or renal function do not necessarily indicate "dehydration" [21]. A diagnosis of dehydration may be judged as an indicator of inadequate care and is considered a *sentinel event* by regulatory agencies.

Supplements

"Food first"—nutritious food is always preferable to any artificial formula or supplement. In addition to offering and providing sufficient fruits, vegetables, starches, healthy fats, dairy products and fluids, recent position papers have suggested that increased protein intake is generally beneficial in order to maximize muscle and bone health and minimize sarcopenia and osteoporosis [22, 23]. Increasing the recommended daily intake of protein to 1–1.2 g/kg/day was recommended. Two additional studies have reported that a higher protein diet was beneficial in adults over 65 in terms of cancer incidence, function and total mortality [24, 25, 26].

Nutritional supplements such as Ensure are tasty, safe and beneficial for those who can eat and drink but cannot consume sufficient quantities of calories and nutrients via "normal" meals. One can of Ensure contains 250 calories and nutrition equal to ½ of an average modest meal. Various brands of supplements exist with different ingredients/properties, e.g., low glucose, added fiber, or higher fat for pulmonary patients. For details on ingredients and which products are available in your local facility, consult the facility dietary services supervisor or consult dietician. In order to minimize appetite suppression supplements they should be given between meals [1]. An additional option is to provide a *nutritional supplement drink* rather than water when administering medication—e.g., MedPass 2.0^R (Hormel Health Labs).

Specific vitamin and mineral supplements are generally reserved only for those noted to have specific nutritional deficiencies or medical conditions. However it is reasonable to provide a "senior" multivitamin to all LTC patients. Most women and many men should be encouraged to consume foods rich in calcium and/or receive a calcium supplement to attain a total daily intake of 1200–1500 mg. Due to hypochlorhydria commonly present in the elderly, calcium citrate is preferred due to its better absorption than calcium carbonate.

Studies have shown that even those on a multivitamin and a calcium/vitamin D supplement are often still vitamin D deficient [27]. Vitamin D deficiency is associated with numerous health problems, not only osteopenia and osteoporosis [28]. The Institute of Medicine has updated the Dietary Reference Intakes for calcium and vitamin D (to 800 IU daily) for adults over 70 [29]. Three meta-analyses have shown a benefit of vitamin D supplementation of at least 800 IU/day on falls [30], fractures [31], and total mortality [32]. Consideration should be given to supplementing all elderly LTC patients with vitamin D, or at least measuring 25-OH-vitamin D levels and *supplementing those who do not have sufficient levels (defined as ≥ 30 ng/ml)* [33].

Appetite Stimulants

All patients with problems eating should be evaluated by a dietitian and speech therapist, in order to better evaluate for the presence of swallowing problems and to provide recommendations on diet and consistency [34]. Those with oral/dental or swallowing problems may require special textures such as mechanical soft, pureed, or thickened liquids. However such diets may not be palatable and appealing to patients and can result in loss of appetite and decreased food intake. Feeding assistance should be provided when needed, and an appealing "mealtime social ambience" can be of benefit [35].

If patients are still unable to take in adequate nutrition, cautious use of an "appetite stimulant" or orexigenic medication may be considered, such as megestrol acetate, but it is expensive (up to $500 a month) and of questionable efficacy, and has safety concerns (e.g., fluid retention, edema, increased risk of DVT in up to 32 %) [36]. Orexigenic agents are officially FDA approved only for AIDS and cancer, and are of off-label use in patients with dementia, failure to thrive, etc. They have little evidence-based support for use in the elderly but are often tried. Both megestrol and cyproheptadine (another medication used off label to stimulate appetite) are on the 2012 AGS Beers list of potentially inappropriate medication use in older adults [37].

Other agents that are sometimes used to increase appetite include the antidepressant mirtazapine (Remeron[R]), which has been noted to cause weight gain (1–6 lbs) in depressed patients. There is little or no evidence that mirtazapine is effective for weight gain in the absence of depression. Dronabinol (Marinol[R]) is a cannabinoid derivative also approved for anorexia and nausea in cancer and AIDS patients. It has been used and tested in the elderly, with little evidence of efficacy, and can cause somnolence and seizures and precipitate delirium [38].

The American Geriatrics Society, in its "Choosing Wisely" campaign, stated the following: "Avoid using prescription appetite stimulants or high-calorie supplements for treatment of anorexia or cachexia in older adults; instead, optimize social supports, provide feeding assistance, and clarify patient goals and expectations" [39].

Indications and Use (or not) of Feeding Tubes

Artificial feeding with a feeding tube may be considered if a patient presents with esophageal obstruction; head and neck cancer or GI surgery; prolonged protein/calorie deprivation/depletion; moderate to severe weight loss, hyper-metabolic or hyper-catabolic state; choking or otherwise unable to swallow safety, which lead to the inability to maintain sufficient oral intake [1]. Nasoenteric or oroenteric tubes are a short term and temporary means of accessing the GI tract. A more permanent access with a gastrostomy or jejunostomy tube, may be considered if enteral support is required for more than a few weeks. A patient's advance directive or stated wishes may preclude artificial feeding.

Evidence-based literature portends that the use of feeding tubes is ethically debatable and not proven effective in preventing complications such as aspiration, pressure sores and death in elderly demented patients [40, 41]. A recent article reported that while about 5 % of demented nursing home residents had a feeding tube inserted over a 1 year period, the median survival was only 56 days with 1 year post-insertion mortality of 64 %, with many patients requiring multiple hospitalizations for complication of tube replacement [42]. Thus insertion of a feeding tube should only be considered when there is reasonable expectation or hope of recovery from a temporary condition such as an acute stroke.

Not eating can be a natural and inevitable sign of impending death, and that when considering the need for a feeding tube this should trigger recognition (and discussion with the health care proxy) that the patient is at high risk to die within the next few months, and that palliative care or hospice care would best serve the patient. Both AMDA [43] and the American Geriatrics Society [44], as part of the ABIM Foundation's *"Choosing Wisely"* initiative, have similarly stated, *"Don't insert percutaneous feeding tubes in individuals with advanced dementia. Instead, offer oral assisted feedings."* AGS has also published a position paper recommending against feeding tubes in patients with advanced dementia [45].

If tube feedings are decided upon, many different formulas are available. Standard formulas have low residue, supply 1 kcal/ml, with 13–17 % of calories as protein (*Ensure HN* and *Osmolite HN* are examples). A high fiber formula, such as *Jevity*, contains 10–14 g of fiber per liter, 1 Kcal/ml and about 14–18 % Kcal as protein. High protein formulas, such as *Replete* or *Promote* contain 20–25 % of calories as protein. Some products have added fiber, vitamins, and minerals. When patients have a problem with an increased gastric residual they may require a lower volume (i.e., higher concentrated), formula such as *Two-Cal HN* or *Magnacal*. Lower volume formulas have up to 2 kcal/ml of which 14–17 % is protein and 68–78 % water. *Vivonex Plus* and *Vital HN* are examples of some of the *hydrolyzed formulas* that are available for postpyloric or jejunal feeding. Some hydrolyzed formulas have added glutamine and arginine, which are important for bowel integrity. Medium chain triglycerides are used to replace long chain triglycerides in these postpyloric formulas. *Renal* and *hepatic formulas* are necessary in the face of renal and hepatic impairment. *Suplena* and *Nepro* are examples of renal formulas and are restricted in water and sodium, potassium, magnesium, and vitamin A. Hepatic formulas have limited aromatic amino acids and methionine, and are higher in branched chain amino acids. Immune formulas such as *Immune-Aid* are recommended in patients who suffered great physiologic stress, such as those who are on ventilators. They contain increased amounts of omega-3 and decreased omega-6 fatty acids as well as being enriched with the arginine and glutamine. A number of other additives are also available including glucose polymers, protein powder, and vegetable oil or medium chain triglycerides.

Ethical and Legal Issues Related to Feeding

The consensus of the medical and ethical literature is that withholding or withdrawing natural feedings (when unsuccessful, futile or inappropriate), is no different than initiating or not initiating tube feeding or other medical treatments based on the patient's clinical condition and patient wishes. Again, *not eating* is an expected and natural part of advanced dementia and the dying process. Tube feedings unfortunately do not reduce aspiration, pneumonia, pressure sores or infections, and *decrease rather than increase quality of life* due to tube-related complications, mobility restrictions and discomfort. Thus while the provision of food and fluids is considered basic caring and should never be withheld (unless overt aspiration or discomfort is evident), remember that artificial tube feeding is a medical intervention that has both risks and benefits and may be refused, not begun or withdrawn, when deemed not inappropriate. Under either scenario, patients and families should provide informed consent. When patients can no longer eat or swallow safely or sufficiently, careful hand feeding as tolerated should be offered. Palliative care and hospice may be most appropriate for patients nearing the end of life due to advanced illness (see chapter "Integrating Palliative Care into Practice").

Summary

It should be understood that malnutrition and weight loss, though sometimes judged as signs of poor care or neglect, in many instances is a process that is both natural and unavoidable despite the best efforts of clinicians, and attributable to the patient's advanced age, loss of functioning, and underlying medical comorbidities. To avoid claims of negligence or liability, an appropriate evaluation should be performed and interventions fully documented that are consistent with the patient's condition and wishes. The family or proxy decision maker should be duly notified. If weight loss or other nutritional conditions continue to worsen and prove to be *unavoidable*, then this fact and all its discernable causes and consequences should be clearly documented in the chart.

Pearls for the Practitioner

- All adults in LTC require careful attention to nutrition and hydration as both are a clinical, quality of life, and legal-ethical issue.
- Frequent causes of weight loss in elderly LTC patients include dementia and other neurologic disorders (e.g., Parkinson's), depression; drug effects/side effects, malignancies, and GI problems such as swallowing disorders and malabsorption syndromes.
- Optimal health and longevity are achieved with a BMI of 25 ± 5.
- Innumerable drugs and diseases affect nutritional status.
- Weight and labs should be monitored regularly in all patients.
- Most patients should receive a multivitamin, a calcium and vitamin D supplement, and a B_{12} supplement if blood levels indicate deficiency.
- Nutritional drinks such as Ensure can supplement inadequate calorie and protein intake.
- Hypodermoclysis may be used short-term to augment fluid intake and avoid dehydration.

- Restricted diets are generally not advisable or tolerated in patients and should be avoided when not necessary.
- Tube feedings are ineffective in reducing morbidity and mortality in demented patients and should be limited to carefully selected patients needing short-term nutritional support during a potentially reversible illness such as stroke.
- OBRA regulations require that the facility must ensure that a resident maintains acceptable parameters of nutritional status (*see* Fig. 1).
- Incorporate patient preferences regarding nutrition and hydration in advance directives and advance care planning.

The following OBRA regulations, state and federal requirements for nursing facilities (F-Tags 325-327; CFR 483.25, 483.35), while quite specific and strict, form a common legal and medical standard of care with which all practitioners in LTC must be familiar . [47].

CFR 483.25 (i) *Nutrition.* Based on a resident's comprehensive assessment, the facility must ensure that a resident Maintains acceptable parameters of nutritional status, such as body weight and protein levels, unless the resident's clinical condition demonstrates that this is not possible; and receives a therapeutic diet when there is a nutritional problem.

(j) *Hydration.* The facility must provide each resident with sufficient fluid intake to maintain proper hydration and health.

CFR 483.35 *Dietary services*

The facility must provide each resident with a nourishing, palatable, well-balanced diet that meets the daily nutritional and special dietary needs of each resident.... The facility must employ a qualified dietitian either full-time, part-time, or on a consultant basis.... Menus must—

Meet the nutritional needs of residents in accordance with the recommended dietary allowances of the Food and Nutrition Board of the National Research Council, National Academy of Sciences;

Be prepared in advance; and

Be followed.

(d) Food. Each resident receives and the facility provides—

Food prepared by methods that conserve nutritive value, flavor, and appearance;

Food that is palatable, attractive, and at the proper temperature;

Food prepared in a form designed to meet individual needs; and

Substitutes offered of similar nutritive valueto residents who refuse food served.

(e) Therapeutic diets. Therapeutic diets must be prescribed by the attending physician.

(f) Frequency of meals. (1) Each resident receives and the facility provides at least three meals daily, at regular times comparable to normal mealtimes in the community.

(2) There must be no more than 14 hours between a substantial evening meal and breakfast the following day.

(3) The facility must offer snacks at bedtime daily.

(4) When a nourishing snack is provided at bedtime, upto 16 hours may elapse between a substantial evening meal and breakfast the following day if a resident group agrees to this meal span, and a nourishing snack is served.

(g) Assistive devices. The facility must provide special eating equipment and utensils for residents who need them.

Fig. 1 OBRA nutrition regulations [46]

References

1. American Medical Directors Association (AMDA). Altered nutritional status in the long-term care setting. Columbia, MD: American Medical Directors Association (AMDA), Rev. 2010. Available for purhase from AMDA at www.amda.com. Accessed 24 Aug. 2014.
2. Dietary Reference Intakes. http://fnic.nal.usda.gov/dietary-guidance/dietary-reference-intakes. Accessed 1 Sept. 2015.
3. American Medical Directors Association (AMDA). Dehydration and fluid maintenance in the long-term care setting. Columbia, MD: American Medical Directors Association (AMDA), Rev. 2009. Available for purchase at www.amda.com/tools/guidelines.cfm. Accessed 1 Sept. 2015.
4. American Medical Directors Association (AMDA). Transitions of care in the long-term care continuum. Columbia, MD: American Medical Directors Association (AMDA), 2010. Guideline available free online at http://www.amda.com/tools/clinical/toccpg.pdf. Accessed 24 Aug. 2014.
5. Van Bokhorst MAE, Guaitoli PR, Jansma EP, De Vet HCW. A systematic review of malnutrition screening tools for the nursing home. J Am Med Dir Assoc. 2014;15:171–84.
6. Detsky AS, McLaughlin JR, Baker JP, et al. What is subjective global assessment of nutritional status? JPEN J Parenter Enteral Nutr. 1987;11:8–13. http://subjectiveglobalassessment.com/. Accessed 25 Aug 2014.
7. Guigoz Y. The mini-nutritional assessment (MNA). J Nutr Health Aging. 2006;10:466–87. http://mna-elderly.com/. Accessed 25 Aug 2014.
8. Messinger-Rapport BJ, Gammack JK, Little MO, Morley JE. Clinical update on nursing home medicine, 2014. J Am Med Dir Assoc. 2014;15:786–801.
9. Morley JE, Thomas DR, Kamel H. Nutritional deficiencies in long-term care. Ann Long Term Care. 1998;6(5):183–91.
10. Seltzer MH, Bastidas A, Cooper DM, et al. Instant nutritional assessment. JPEN J Parenter Enteral Nutr. 1979;3:157–9.
11. Corti MC, Guralnik JM, Salive ME, Sorkin JD. Serum albumin level and physical disability as predictors of mortality in older patients. J Am Med Dir Assoc. 1994;272:1036–42.
12. American Psychiatric Association practice guideline for the treatment of patients with major depressive disorder, 3rd edn. 2010. http://www.psychiatryonline.com/pracGuide/pracGuideTopic_7.aspx. Accessed 3 Dec 2014.
13. Wilson MM, Vaswani S, Liu D, et al. Prevalence and causes of undernutrition in medical outpatients. Am J Med. 1998;104:56.
14. Thomas DR, Ashmen W, Morley JE, et al. Nutritional management in long-term care: development of a clinical guideline. J Gerontol A Biol Sci Med Sci. 2000;55A:M725–34.
15. Bucker DA, Kelber ST, Goodwin JS. The use of dietary restrictions in malnourished nursing home patients. J Am Geriatr Soc. 1994;42:1100–2.
16. Prospective studies collaboration. Body mass index and cause specific mortality in 900000 adults: collaborative analysis of 57 prospective studies. Lancet. 2009;373:1083–96.
17. Orpana HM, Berthelot JM, Kaplan MS, Feeny DH, et al. BMI and mortality: results from a national longitudinal study of Canadian adults. Obesity. 2010;18(1):214–8.
18. Thomas DR. But is it malnutrition? J Am Med Dir Assoc. 2009;10(5):295–7.
19. Correia MI, Hegazi RA, Higashiguchi T, Michel JP, et al. Evidence-based recommendations for addressing malnutrition in health care: an updated strategy from the feed. ME Global Study Group. J Am Med Dir Assoc. 2014;15:544–50.
20. Mei A, Auerhahn C. Hypodermoclysis: maintaining hydration in the frail older adult. Ann Long Term Care. 2009;17(5):28–30.
21. Thomas DR, Tariq SH, et al. Physician misdiagnosis of dehydration in older adults. J Am Med Dir Assoc. 2003;4:251–4.
22. Bauer J, Biolo G, Cederholm T, Cesari M, et al. Evidence-based recommendations for optimal dietary protein intake in older people: a position paper from the PROT-AGE Study Group. J Am Med Dir Assoc. 2013;14(8):542–59.

23. Gaffney-Stomberg E, Insogna KL, Rodriguez NR, Kerstetter JE. Increasing dietary protein requirements for elderly people for optimal muscle and bone health. J Am Geriatr Soc. 2009;57:1073–9.

24. Levine ME, Suarez JA, Brandhorst S, Priya B, et al. Low protein intake is associated with a major reduction in IGF-1, cancer, and overall mortality in the 65 and younger but not older population. Cell Metab. 2014;19(3):407–17.

25. Imai E, Tsubota-Utsugi M, Kikuya M, Satoh M, et al. Animal protein intake is associated with higher-level functional capacity in elderly adults: The Ohasama Study. J Am Geriatr Soc. 2014;62(3):426–34.

26. Morley JE, Thomas DR. Cachexia: new advances in the management of wasting diseases. J Am Med Dir Assoc. 2008;9(4):205–10.

27. Goldberg TH, Hassan T, Grant R. High prevalence of Vitamin D deficiency in elderly nursing home patients despite vitamin supplements (abstract). J Am Med Dir Assoc. 2008;9(3):B15.

28. Holick MF. High prevalence of Vitamin D inadequacy and implications for health. Mayo Clin Proc. 2006;81(3):353–73.

29. Ross AC, Manson JE, Abrams SA, Aloia JF, et al. The 2011 report on dietary reference intakes for calcium and vitamin D from the Institute of Medicine: what clinicians need to know. J Clin Endocrinol Metab. 2011;96(1):53–8. http://fnic.nal.usda.gov/dietary-guidance/dri-reports/vitamin-d-and-calcium and http://www.ncbi.nlm.nih.gov/pmc/articles/PMC3046611/. Accessed 30 Nov 2014.

30. Bischoff-Ferrari HA, Dawson-Hughes B, Willett WC, et al. Effect of Vitamin D on falls: a meta-analysis. JAMA. 2004;291(16):1999–2006.

31. Bischoff-Ferrari HA, Willett WC, Wong JB, et al. Fracture prevention with Vitamin D supplementation: a meta-analysis of randomized controlled trials. J Am Med Dir Assoc. 2005;293(18):2257–64.

32. Autier P, Gandini S. Vitamin D supplementation and total mortality: a meta-analysis of randomized controlled trials. Arch Intern Med. 2007;167(16):1730–7.

33. Morley JE. Should all long-term care residents receive Vitamin D? J Am Med Dir Assoc. 2007;8:69–70.

34. Vitale CA, Monteleoni C, et al. Strategies for improving care for patients with advanced dementia and eating problems: optimizing care through physician and speech pathologist collaboration. Ann Long Term Care. 2009;17(5):32–9.

35. Nijs K, Graaf C, Staveren W, et al. Malnutrition and mealtime ambience in nursing homes. J Am Med Dir Assoc. 2009;10:226–9.

36. Yeh S, Lovitt S, Schuster MW. Pharmacological treatment of geriatric cachexia: evidence and safety in perspective. J Am Med Dir Assoc. 2007;8(6):363–77.

37. AGS 2012 Beers Criteria Update Expert Panel. American Geriatrics Society updated Beers Criteria for potentially inappropriate medication use in older adults. J Am Geriatr Soc. 2012;60(4):616–31. http://www.ncbi.nlm.nih.gov/pubmed/22376048 and http://www.americangeriatrics.org/health_care_professionals/clinical_practice/clinical_guidelines_recommendations/2012. Accessed 25 Aug. 2014.

38. Miller LJ, et al. Pharmacological treatment of undernutrition in the geriatric patient. Consult Pharm. 2002;17:739–47.

39. AGS Choosing Wisely Workgroup. American geriatrics society identifies another five things that healthcare providers and patient should question. J Am Geriatr Soc. 2014;62(5):950–60. http://www.americangeriatrics.org/health_care_professionals/clinical_practice/clinical_guidelines_recommendations/choosing_wisely2014. Accessed 25 Aug 2014.

40. Finucane TE, Christmas C, Travis K. Tube feeding in patients with advanced dementia: a review of the evidence. J Am Med Dir Assoc. 1999;282:1365–70.

41. Gillick M. Rethinking the role of tube feeding in patients with advanced dementia. N Engl J Med. 2000;342:206–10.

42. Kuo S, Rhodes R, Mitchell SL, et al. Natural history of feeding tube use in nursing home residents with advanced dementia. J Am Med Dir Assoc. 2009;10:264–70.

43. AMDA 5 things: Vance J. AMDA – choosing wisely. J Am Med Dir Assoc. 2013;14(9): 639–41. www.amda.com/tools/choosingwisely.cfm. Accessed 23 Aug 2014.
44. AGS Choosing Wisely Workgroup. American Geriatrics Society identifies five things that healthcare providers and patient should question. J Am Geriatr Soc. 2013;61:622–31. http://www.americangeriatrics.org/health_care_professionals/clinical_practice/clinical_guidelines_recommendations/choosingwisely. Accessed 25 Aug 2014.
45. AGS Ethics Committee and Clinical Practice and Models of Care Committee. American Geriatrics Society feeding tubes in advanced dementia position statement. J Am Geriatr Soc. 2014;62:1590–3. http://onlinelibrary.wiley.com/doi/10.1111/jgs.12924/abstract. Accessed 25 Aug 2014.
46. American Medical Directors Association. Synopsis of Federal Regulations in the nursing facility: implications for attending physicians and medical directors. Available for purchase online from AMDA at http://www.amda.com/resources/print.cfm#syn1.
47. Miller ER, Pastor-Barriuso R, Dalal D, et al. Meta-analysis: high dosage vitamin E supplementation may increase all cause mortality. Ann Intern Med. 2005;142(1):37–46.

Wound Care

Ganesh Merugu and Andrew Rosenzweig

Introduction

The medical and psychosocial complexities of wound care highlight the challenges that face practitioners in long term care (LTC). Wounds can be classified as a *medical problem*, a *geriatric syndrome*, or part of a larger *systems-based problem*. Understanding wound formation and healing is critical to the prevention and treatment of wounds. Treatment plans must not only address the wound itself but also comorbidities and medications that may hinder healing or predispose patients to acquiring wounds. The psychosocial and ethical principles of caring for patients who are no longer able to participate in their own care subsume a critical role in treatment success or failure. Though wounds may have more than one etiology, the four most common types of wounds will be reviewed: pressure, diabetic, ischemic or arterial, and venous. Pressure ulcers are emphasized due to their implications on quality of care in the LTC environment.

More than 20 % of residents who live in a nursing facility for 2 or more years will develop at least one pressure ulcer [1]. The estimated prevalence of pressure ulcers among patients residing in these facilities has been reported as between 2 and 28 % and has become an increasingly common reason for litigation [2]. The annual incidence of pressure ulceration in patients with neurologic impairment is 5–8 %, with a lifetime risk of approximately 85 % and a mortality rate of 8 % [3]. For hospitalized patients, the presence of a pressure ulcer increases nursing workload for that patient by 50 %, and adds approximately $20,000 in costs. The treatment of pressure ulcers in the USA is estimated to cost more than $1 billion annually [4].

G. Merugu, MD • A. Rosenzweig, MD, CMD, FACP (✉)
Department of Geriatric Medicine, Albert Einstein Medical Center,
5501 Old York Road, Paley 4320, Philadelphia, PA 19141, USA
e-mail: rosenzwa@einstein.edu

© Springer International Publishing Switzerland 2016
P.A. Fenstemacher, P. Winn (eds.), *Post-Acute and Long-Term Medicine*,
Current Clinical Practice, DOI 10.1007/978-3-319-16979-8_13

217

The Centers for Medicare and Medicaid Services (CMS) implemented a new payment system effective in 2008, which would cease paying hospitals for "preventable complications," including stage III and IV pressure ulcers [5]. In Medicare fiscal year 2006, pressure ulcers had the highest occurrence of preventable complications, with 322,946 cases that added an average cost of $40,381 to each admission [6]. However, in the "Guidance to Surveyors for Long Term Care Facilities," CMS acknowledges that *some* pressure ulcers are *"unavoidable"* [7]. LTC facilities are required to follow strict standards of care for evaluating pressure ulcer risk factors and implementing preventive interventions consistent with each resident's needs and goals. If a pressure ulcer develops despite the facility's best efforts to prevent it, the pressure ulcer is determined to be unavoidable. CMS has not applied this standard in other health care settings [8]. In 2010, the National Pressure Ulcer Advisory Panel held a multidisciplinary conference to address and clarify the issues of avoidable and unavoidable pressure ulcers [8]. Information from the panel's consensus report is included in this chapter.

Risk Factors for Wound Development

Wounds develop when causative factors increase a patient's susceptibility to developing a wound, or persist when factors impair the healing of an existing wound [9–12]. These risk factors are listed in Table 1. Relieving pressure on the wound

Table 1 Risk factors

Risk factor	Examples	Notes
Comorbid conditions	Diabetes, end-stage renal disease, thyroid disease	Conditions that increase risk of wounds by affecting patient's immune response, skin integrity or environment risks.
Drugs	Steroids, antimetabolites	Drugs that hinder proliferation of fibroblasts and collagen synthesis.
History of healed ulcer	History of Stage III or IV ulcer	Patient may still have the risk factors that predisposed to these ulcers
Impaired blood flow	Atherosclerosis, lower-extremity arterial insufficiency	Decrease blood flow to wounds for healing
Impaired or decreased mobility and functional ability	Bed bound, decreased lower extremity use, altered mental status (e.g., dementia)	Environmental risk of developing wounds due to increased pressure on skin, friction, or shear from transfer by others
Malnutrition and hydration deficit		Protein–calorie malnutrition and deficiencies of vitamins A, C, and zinc impair normal wound-healing mechanisms.

Adapted from American Medical Directors Association pressure ulcers in the long-term care setting clinical practice guideline 2008 (last reviewed by AMDA 2012)

area is a cornerstone of both wound prevention and treatment. Because pressure is a primary causal factor, a plan for patient repositioning needs to be tailored to the needs of each. Wounded skin has only about 80 % of the tensile properties of intact skin and thus is at increased risk of future breakdown. Patients with a history of pressure ulcers are five times more likely to develop another pressure ulcer [13]. Dermatologic conditions and limb contractures can also increase the occurrence of wounds.

The poor blood supply seen in peripheral arterial disease, hinders wound healing by depriving the injured area of oxygen and nutrients. Diabetics are at additional risk of foot wounds due to the triad of peripheral neuropathy, microvascular disease, and suboptimal glycemic control. It is estimated that among patients with diabetes, 15 % will develop a foot wound, and 12–24 % of those will eventually require amputation [2, 14]. Even with successful wound healing, the recurrence rate of diabetic foot wounds is 66 % [14].

End stage renal disease and thyroid disease are also risk factors for wound formation. Wounds may occur when medications such as steroids and anti-metabolites hinder proliferation of fibroblasts and collagen synthesis placing a patient at risk [4].

Cognitive impairment, seen in 45–67 % of assisted living residents and 69 % of nursing facility residents, creates an array of risk factors for skin breakdown [15–17]. These include functional disabilities, poor nutritional status, and a higher incidence of skin exposure to pressure, friction, or shear. Moisture-related skin breakdown is often associated with excess perspiration; heavy wound exudates, urine and/or fecal incontinence. Diarrhea is caustic and urine contains urea and ammonia, both of which damage normal skin. With prolonged exposure, these fluids soften the outer protective layer of skin and result in skin breakdown [18]. Data also suggest an association between fecal incontinence and skin ulcer development, likely related to skin exposure to bile acid and gastrointestinal enzymes [19].

The poor nutritional status frequently seen in patients with advanced dementia is another risk factor for wound development. Dehydration, deficiencies of arginine, vitamins A, C, and zinc, as well as protein–calorie malnutrition, have been implicated in wound development and impairing wound healing [20]. In dehydration, skin integrity and wound healing are impaired due to decreased tissue perfusion. Severe protein–calorie malnutrition hinders tissue regeneration, the inflammatory reaction and immune function. Albumin and prealbumin levels are indicators of protein–calorie nutritional status (see chapter "Weight and Nutrition" for further discussion) [18]. Obesity also places patients at risk for skin breakdown under the pannus or in skin folds [21]. The warm and moist environment in skin folds promote the growth of yeast and bacteria [18], that will further increase the risk for wounds to occur.

Assessment

An initial skin evaluation should be performed immediately upon admission of a resident to the LTC facility. An ulcer can develop after only a few hours of pressure. Any discovered wounds should prompt thorough patient assessment and a subsequent treatment plan that includes a timeline for wound reassessment. This assessment involves a complete medical evaluation of the patient including careful attention to conditions that may affect both wound development and healing. A comprehensive wound history should note the onset and duration of a wound, and any previous wound care. Assessment of a person's cognitive status, behavior, financial resources, and access to caregivers can impact a treatment plan.

Assessment of the patient's personal environment is also critical. Frequency of repositioning, surfaces, turning schedules, transferring techniques, and durable medical equipment (such as assistive devices, trapeze, bed rails, and padding) can all impact wound development and healing [9]. Risk assessment scales may increase awareness, but have limited predictability and effectiveness in pressure ulcer prevention [22]. A meta-analysis of 33 studies demonstrated a lack of evidence for risk assessment scales in decreasing pressure ulcer incidence, *but the scales did increase preventive interventions* [23]. The two most commonly used tools are the *Braden* and *Norton* scales. No conclusive evidence exists showing that one is superior to the other.

- *The Braden scale* evaluates six categories: sensory perception, moisture, activity, mobility, nutrition, friction and shear for predicting pressure ulcer development. Research has shown that patients with scores of 18 or less are at risk for the development of pressure sores [24].
- The *Norton Score* is another commonly used tool for assessing pressure ulcer risk that evaluates five categories: physical condition, mental condition, activity, mobility and incontinence.

Most nursing facilities use a pressure ulcer report to document identified wounds: location, stage, measurement, and description. Pressure ulcer reports fulfill standardized documentation as mandated by both state and federal (F314) regulations in the nursing facility. The clinician should document the number, location, and size (length, width, and depth in centimeters) of wounds and assess for the presence of exudates, odor, sinus tracts, necrosis or eschar formation, tunneling/undermining, infection, healing (granulation and epithelialization), and wound margins. For a pressure ulcer, the clinician should determine the stage of the ulcer according to the National Pressure Ulcer Advisory Panel (NPUAP) Staging System (see Table 2).

Risk of developing pressure ulcers is significantly high within the first 4 weeks after admission to a long-term care facility [25]. After an initial assessment, a weekly reassessment should occur for the first 4 weeks, followed by at least a quarterly assessment. Reassessments should also occur when there is a change in patient

Table 2 2007 NPUAP staging of pressure ulcers

Stage	Definition	Comment
Suspected deep tissue injury (SDTI)	Pressure-related necrosis of soft tissue with intact overlying skin	Discoloration (crimson→purple), changes in temperature, texture, tenderness. May progress rapidly
Stage I	Localized area of nonblancheable erythema. Skin is intact and sandwiched between a bony prominence and external surface.	Clinically similar to SDTI. May be harder to detect as skin pigmentation deepens
Stage II	Partial thickness destruction of dermis characterized as either a shallow open ulcer with a crimson wound bed (without slough or bruising) or as an intact or ruptured fluid-filled blister.	Do not use to describe skin tears, tape burns, dermatitis, maceration, or excoriation
Stage III	Full thickness tissue loss. Subcutaneous fat may be visible, but bone, tendon or muscle is not exposed.	Slough may be present. May include tunneling or undermining. Depth varies by anatomical location.
Stage IV	Full thickness tissue loss characterized by exposed bone, tendon or muscle. Extensive destruction, necrosis, or damage to the muscle, bone, or supporting structures.	Slough or eschar may be present on some parts of the wound bed. Often include undermining and tunneling
Unstageable	Full thickness tissue loss which cannot be staged until slough or eschar in the ulcer bed is removed	Do *not* remove eschar present on heels

Adapted from the National Pressure Ulcer Advisory Panel. Updated staging system. http://www.npuap.org/pr2.htm. Last accessed September 12, 2014

status [26]. The patient's overall clinical condition should be reassessed whenever a pressure ulcer fails to show evidence of healing within 2–4 weeks of any intervention [25]. Every nursing facility is required to develop and implement its own comprehensive wound care plan in accordance with CMS regulations.

Some patients develop pressure ulcers 2–3 days before death. These are referred to as *Kennedy terminal ulcers* and are markers of the dying process. The Kennedy ulcer often develops suddenly on the sacrum as a blister or stage 2 and rapidly progress to stage 3 or 4. These ulcers can be pear-, horseshoe-, or butterfly-shaped with irregular borders. Kennedy terminal ulcers are initially red/purple, then turn to yellow, and finally turn black. The etiology is unclear, but is thought to be part of multiorgan failure. Most of the ulcers do not heal and their treatment is the same as that for pressure ulcers [27].

Types of Wounds

A wound may not necessarily fit into one of the four general categories of wounds (pressure ulcer, diabetic, arterial and venous), but may be of *mixed etiology*. Usually the type of wound can be distinguished by its location, combined with inspection of the wound and the patient's clinical history. If the wound type remains uncertain, laboratory and/or radiographic studies may help clarify its type. For example, in lower extremity ulcers, an ankle-brachial index or Doppler arterial studies can help determine whether the ulcer is caused by vascular insufficiency, pressure or a combination of the two.

Pressure Ulcers

- 95 % develop on the lower body, 65 % over the sacrum and pelvic area, and 30 % in the lower extremities. Other common pressure ulcer sites include the coccyx, heels, ischium, iliac crest, lateral foot, lateral malleolus, and greater trochanter.
- There are three mechanical forces that, when combined, create tissue damage. These are *pressure, friction,* and *shear*. A shear injury occurs beneath the skin and cannot be seen at the skin level, but a friction injury is superficial and easily visible (e.g., an abrasion or superficial laceration). Shear and friction injuries usually occur together [28].
- A *pressure ulcer* is a localized area of damaged or necrosed tissue that develops when soft tissue is compressed between a bony prominence and an external surface for a prolonged period of time.
- In 2009, NPUAP-EPUAP *redefined pressure ulcer*, and friction was deleted from the definition. As such it defined a pressure ulcer as a compressive tissue injury that is caused by pressure alone or by pressure combined with shearing. Friction alone is not a direct cause of pressure ulcers, but it does cause shear strain in tissue, which in turn can increase the risk of tissue breakdown [28].
- Pressure ulcers can range from nonblancheable erythema of intact skin (or in dark-skinned individuals, it may have a blue or purple hue, i.e., stage I) to deep ulcers extending down to the bone (i.e., stage IV).
- The skin failure that is seen at the end of life is not considered to be a pressure ulcer [21]. In addition, skin tears, abrasions, or lacerations are not pressure ulcers [28].

Diabetic Wounds

- Commonly occur over the metatarsal heads.
- Are due to vascular complications of diabetes mellitus including decreased healing and peripheral neuropathy.

- Are typically painless; therefore the wound is usually not noticed until symptoms of infection occur such as malodor, fever or chills.
- When inspecting those ulcers, providers should probe the depth of the wound with a sterile instrument to help determine if any undermining or osteomyelitis maybe present [29].

Ischemic Wounds

- Typically occur in the lower extremities, but can also occur in the upper extremities.
- Are due to decreased arterial blood flow seen in peripheral vascular disease. Diabetes mellitus and smoking have also been implicated.
- Clinical signs of arterial insufficiency that often precede an ischemic wound include: a cold, pale or cyanotic foot, absence of digital and lower extremity hair and thin atrophic skin.
- Present either as a painful wound with discrete borders (a "punched out" appearance), or wet or dry gangrene.
- The base of the ulcer can be covered with a dry black or brown eschar or appear pale pink and fibrous.

Venous Wounds

- Commonly seen in the lower extremities.
- Are different from ischemic wounds, as these wounds are caused by peripheral edema due to venous insufficiency/stasis, medications or organ dysfunction (i.e., heart, liver, and kidney) [30].
- Are less painful than ischemic wounds.
- Have irregular borders and can be seen clustered together with hyperpigmented skin changes of surrounding skin.

Prevention

Paramount to wound care management is prevention. The Agency for Health Care Policy and Research (AHCPR) published two companion practice guidelines in 1994 with recommendations for prediction, prevention and early treatment of pressure ulcers in adults [31, 32]. The companion practice guidelines were pioneering in their scope and are still widely utilized today because they remain applicable in many settings. The first step recommended for the prevention of pressure ulcers by the Institute for Healthcare Improvement (IHI) is to identify patients at risk, and then implement prevention strategies in these patients [24]. The IHI suggests "six essential elements of pressure ulcer prevention" in its guidelines.

The six steps are [24, 33]:

- Conduct a pressure ulcer assessment of admission for all patients.
- Reassess risk for all patients daily
- Inspect skin daily
- Manage moisture
- Optimize nutrition and hydration
- Minimize pressure

The IHI recommends that prevention measures include a comprehensive treatment plan with risk factor reduction, multidisciplinary interventions, functional adaptation, environmental modifications, and a psychosocial evaluation. Evaluating and optimizing any of the residents predisposing conditions and comorbidities can help prevent the development of wounds [9]. Inspecting skin daily during bathing or personal care, as well as scheduled turning and positioning of patients, has been shown to help prevent wounds. Provide support surfaces with special mattresses and overlays to help eliminate friction, shear, and moisture [34]. Minimize pressure over bony prominences. Seats should be padded with air, foam, or gel cushioning and *avoid use of donut-shaped devices* [9]. Residents at highest risk (those who completely compress a static surface, or have pressure ulcers that fail to heal), should be placed on a dynamic surface [7, 9]. A patient should never be directly placed on the greater trochanter for more than momentary positioning. Use padding (i.e., heel or "bunny" boots, egg crates, heel lifts, suspension devices, etc.) for off-loading of heels and elbows [7, 9]. Patients should have a static support surface such as a foam overlay or gel mattress placed on their standard mattress. A supine patient should be maintained at the lowest head elevation below 30° as tolerated; head elevation ≥30° provides as much pressure as being in a seated position [35]. Repositioning every four hours has been shown to be as effective as two-hour intervals in wound healing, but this repositioning or partial turning does not always remove pressure from the sacrum or heels. Care should be taken to minimize shearing or friction during repositioning. If necessary, lift devices should be used to prevent soft tissue injury. Slow gradual turns should be used in patients with hemodynamic instability [21].

Inadequate hydration and nutrition are predisposing conditions strongly associated with pressure ulcer development [36]. *The caloric intake of 30–35 kcal/kg* and *daily protein intake of 1.2–1.5 g/kg of body weight* is recommended for nutritionally compromised patients who either have or are at risk of pressure ulcers [5]. *Adequate hydration is provided by 30–35 mL of fluid per kg body weight per day, or 1 mL of fluid per calorie for persons receiving enteral tube feeding* [9]. Enteral nutritional support can significantly reduce the risk of developing pressure ulcers in selected patients, by up to 25 % in some studies. The benefits of nutritional support in facilitating wound healing are still debated [37–39]. Use of vitamin C supplementation in wound healing is also disputed. Two well-designed randomized controlled trials compared high dose vitamin C with either low dose vitamin C or placebo, and had contradictory results [40]. (For a more in-depth discussion on nutrition please see the chapter "Weight and Nutrition.")

In clinical circumstances such as metastatic cancer, multiple organ failure, cachexia, severe vascular compromise and terminal illness, unavoidable wounds may develop [41]. The clinician should judiciously document the reasons why preventive interventions may not be appropriate or feasible, such as frequent repositioning that is causing discomfort or severe pain.

Unavoidable Pressure Ulcers

Pressure ulcers are considered to be quality of care indicator in LTC. There are many factors that are responsible for "unavoidable" pressure ulcers. According to the National Pressure Ulcer Advisory Panel (NPUAP), a pressure ulcer is considered to be *unavoidable* if it developed despite the following interventions.

1. The patient's clinical condition and risk for pressure ulcers were evaluated.
2. Interventions were consistent with the patient's needs and goals, as well as recognized standards of practice, were assessed and implemented.
3. The impact of the interventions were monitored, evaluated, and revised as necessary [21].

A pressure ulcer is considered to be *avoidable* if the facility failed to implement the above interventions. Many LTC patients are either bed or chair-bound, which significantly limits mobility and places them at risk for pressure ulcers. Patients with hemodynamic instability can make turning or repositioning difficult, as they may develop bradycardia, hypotension or hypoxemia with minimal body movement. In addition, some patients are comfortable in a particular position so they move themselves back into that same position after being turned. Vasoconstrictive medications to increase low blood pressure can predispose to ischemia and increase pressure ulcer risk. When an advanced directive for health care states that artificial nutrition and hydration are not to be used, this can put the patient at risk for malnutrition and ulcer development. Refusal of care is a common issue, especially in patients who are confused and cognitively compromised, and can significantly frustrate the staff who are attempting to offload tissue pressure. Medical *device-related* pressure ulcers can occur, if they are applied before the development of edema [21].

Staging of Pressure Ulcers

AMDA—The Society for Post-Acute and Long Term Care Medicine follows the guidelines set forth by the National Pressure Ulcer Advisory Panel (NPUAP) that define, classify and stage pressure ulcers as summarized in Table 2. Staging is based on the extent of observable tissue damage [42]. The latest version of the these guidelines describe stages I–IV along with two adjunctive terms, "*suspected deep tissue injury*" and "*unstageable*" utilized to more accurately classify these wounds (see website http://www.npuap.org). *Reverse staging should not be used*. For example, a lesion may be referred to as a, "healing stage IV" but it *cannot* be described as progressing from a stage IV to a stage III. If a Stage IV pressure ulcer reopens at the same anatomical site, it is always considered as stage IV. An ulcer covered by eschar should be categorized as a Stage IV until the eschar has been debrided. Staging cannot be used for mucosal pressure ulcers [9].

Serialized staging and pictures of wounds can be helpful for monitoring ulcer progression and healing. The Pressure Ulcer Scale for Healing (*PUSH*) tool was developed by the NPUAP in order to monitor pressure ulcer healing over time. It evaluates an ulcer with respect to surface area, exudate, and type of wound tissue. This scale has been adopted by many institutions [43]. Despite the theoretical simplicity of the PUSH tool, confusion regarding its use and interpretation still exists leading to inter-practitioner variability in staging ulcers [44]. The NPUAP guidelines have been used (at times inappropriately) as quality of care indicators or to identify suboptimal management [42].

Management

In wound care, the burden of treatment should be weighed against its benefit. Communication with the patient and family/caregivers is important and their wishes should be identified and respected. But it is also imperative to establish realistic expectations for wound healing. As with any medical treatment, if a patient with decision-making capacity declines or does not adhere to the recommended treatment,

Table 3 Wound care challenges

Wound type	Challenge to wound care	Standard medical treatment approach	Treatment
Pressure	Excess pressure and shear/friction forces	Pressure relief	Topical: packing with hydrogel or saline. Devices: Pressure reduction mattresses, padding overlying bony prominences
Ischemic	Inadequate blood flow	Revascularization or surgical removal/correction	Topical: dry or antimicrobial.
Venous	Venous insufficiency causing edema	Correct incompetent valves, reduce edema	Topical: moist environment
Diabetic	Peripheral neuropathy causing pressure points on feet	Offload pressure, careful routine evaluation of feet	Topical: pack with antimicrobial solution or hydrogel

Adapted from Takahashi et al. Wound Care Technologies: Emerging Evidence for Appropriate Use in Long-Term Care. See ref. [45]

the providers should offer alternatives and document them in the medical record. A palliative approach should always be considered when wound healing is unlikely.

Treatment

As numerous factors impede healing, an interdisciplinary approach is essential. Table 3 provides some commonly encountered challenges to optimal wound care. The team should inform the patient and/or proxy decision-maker of the treatment plan. Accepted principles of treatment for skin ulcer care include the following components [18, 34, 43]:

1. *Assess* ulcer *risk factors*, preexisting wounds, pain, and quality of life.
2. *Consider* an analgesic medication *prior to and after* wound care/dressing changes and, if needed, prescribe scheduled pain medicine for chronic wound pain.
3. *Clean* the wound surface with an isotonic solution (normal saline) to remove debris and to decrease bacterial load.
4. *Debride* necrotic tissue—sharp, autolytic, mechanical, biologic, and enzymatic debridement.
5. *Fill dead space* (undermining, tunnels) with loose absorbent wound packing.
6. *Decrease* bacterial load/infection.
7. *Keep the wound moist* to promote granulation with appropriate dressings—films, foams, alginates, hydroactives, hydrogels, and hydrocolloids.
8. *Support the wound healing process*with adjunctive treatments—vacuum-assisted closure, electric stimulation, skin grafts, and growth factor treatment.
9. *Prevent further injury* by relieving pressure and providing proper surface support to *protect the surrounding skin*.
10. Improve the patient's overall condition with *proper nutrition and hydration*.
11. *Manage risk factors and comorbidities*—diabetes, ESRD, anemia, PVD, malnutrition.
12. *Address complications*—psychosocial issues, malodor, exudates.
13. Accurately *track wound-healing* progress using tools—PUSH, Sussman Assessment Tool.

Causal factors should continue to be identified and addressed, including systemic factors and comorbidities [9]. Optimize nutritional status. Address psychosocial issues. Manage pain and infection; both are crucial for effective wound care. If necrotic tissue exists, it should be removed in order to allow viable granulation and wound healing to occur.

Wounds should be cleansed and irrigated to remove necrotic debris at each dressing change. Necrotic tissue impedes the healing process and may represent a nidus for infection. Saline should be chosen for wound irrigation over cytotoxic antiseptic agents such as Dakin's solution, iodine, acid-based and alcohol-based solutions that can retard healing [9]. Be sure to assess for pain and minimize mechanical force applied to the wound during dressing changes. Treatment can be painful, so consider administering pain medication 30 min before and after wound care or dressing change [18].

There are five *methods of debridement—sharp or surgical, autolytic, mechanical, biologic, and enzymatic debridement* [34]. Any dry black eschar on the heels should *not* be debrided unless it is tender, fluctuant, erythematous, or suppurative. Wounds with no surrounding local infection can have an occlusive hydrocolloid dressing placed over them, allowing the eschar to autodigest itself via autolytic debridement [9]. Hydrocolloids and hydrogels are used as autolytic debridement, and also help to maintain moisture in the dressing. Enzymatic debridement involves applying a topical debriding agent such as collagenase or papain-urea to devitalized tissue. This may cause some degree of pain but is more tolerable than surgical debridement. Biological debridement uses live, disinfected larvae or maggots [34]. Mechanical debridement is used when various dressings are allowed to dry and then removed, peeling off nonviable adherent tissue. This mode of debridement has fallen into disfavor as it also removes new healing tissue.

When a wound is exceptionally large, malodorous or has a large amount of necrotic tissue, more aggressive measures may be required. If all other methods of debridement have failed and/or timing is critical because of worsening infection and imminent sepsis, surgical debridement may be necessary. Obviously, the risks of an invasive procedure with sharp debridement, albeit relatively low, must be weighed against the intended benefits.

Major categories of dressings that cover wounds include films, foams, alginates, hydroactives, hydrogels, and hydrocolloids. Many products exist in combinations. A chosen dressing must be able to maintain a moist wound bed, keep surrounding skin dry, and limit contamination of the wound [9]. The ideal wound bed is not too moist or dry. The wound characteristics as well as the wound coverings' cost, ease of use, and made of action should be considered when choosing a product [9]. Wound care also includes the use of transparent, impermeable films on wounds that could be contaminated by urinary or fecal incontinence. These dressings need to be attached with waterproof tape to intact skin. Deep wounds and wounds with tunneling or undermining should be *lightly packed* with moist gauze or other filler. Packing should be changed regularly to avoid contamination with bacteria. Hydrogels are useful for deep wounds with little exudate whereas alginates help absorb tissue fluid and significant exudate. Overly dry intact skin should be protected with moisturizers. Silver impregnated dressings provide broad-spectrum antimicrobial coverage in lesions that are colonized or particularly susceptible to becoming infected based on location, mechanism or clinical context. Collagen dressings promote the development of new granulation tissue.

Several novel modalities have recently been developed with mixed results in the LTC population. These include growth factors (fibroblast growth factor, platelet-derived growth factor, and nerve growth factor); electrotherapy and negative pressure wound therapy. One type of negative pressure therapy is vacuum-assisted closure (VAC). A wound VAC is a closed system that uses negative pressure to drain wound fluid and approximate wound edges, thereby promoting wound healing. Although this therapy may improve healing, it has not been shown to be cost effective [45]. Hyperbaric oxygen therapy increases oxygen tension at the wound site and has demonstrated improved healing rates in selected patients. Its use has been limited by high cost and lack of availability. Other novel therapies that have proven successful are noncontact normothermic wound therapy, ultrasound/ultrasonic misting, as well as infrared and ultraviolet light therapy.

Complications

Pressure ulcers in LTC settings are associated with a multitude of short and long-term medical and psychosocial complications [46]. These may have a significant and damaging impact on a person's sense of well-being by worsening quality of life with isolation, increased dependence, pain, and disfigurement [47–49]. Odor, drainage, and pain from the wound are common [18]. Infection is a major complication that spans the spectrum from clinically insignificant bacterial colonization to cellulitis, deep tissue infection, osteomyelitis, and sepsis. Treating infected wounds can be difficult because they may be chronically contaminated and/or colonized and topical antibiotic agents are often caustic to cells and growth factors required for healing [50]. Osteomyelitis is more common in this population as pressure sores frequently occur over bony prominences [50].

Wound odor and heavy exudates can distress patients and result in significant feelings of embarrassment and/or depression. This then leads to decreased social interaction and poor quality of life [43]. Adequate wound cleaning, debridement, and proper disposal of used dressings can significantly control odor. Topical metronidazole can help control odor by eradicating anaerobic bacteria. Other products to decrease bacterial count and odor include cadexomer iodine, Dakin solution, medical-grade honey, and silver dressings. Excessive wound exudates can lead to maceration, breakdown, and itching. Foams and alginate dressings are good choices to reduce these exudates. However, excessive dryness in a wound causes delayed wound healing by inhibiting epithelialization. An absorptive dressing should not excessively dry out the wound [34].

Pressure ulcers in long-term care residents have been shown to increase morbidity and mortality. Osteomyelitis is associated with high levels of morbidity related to the need for several weeks of IV antibiotics, extra radiographic imaging, and surgical debridement. These things all contribute to side effects, discomfort, and immobility. Because skin breakdown can be a portal for bacteremia, nursing facility residents have been shown to be at higher risk of sepsis and death with mortality rates as high as 50 % [51]. In one study, nursing facility residents with pressure ulcers were shown to be two to three times more likely to die (as compared to their cohort who have no pressure ulcers) with a one-year mortality rate of 50 % [50]. The length of hospitalization for nursing facility residents with pressure ulcers is also approximately 2–3 times greater than those without [52]. Anyone with a large wound or large amount of drainage should be monitored for dehydration and metabolic derangements. Any non-healing wound should be evaluated for fistula formation, heterotopic calcification, and squamous cell carcinoma.

Table 4 Recommended components for documentation of wounds

Parameter	Description
Type	Pathology or disease etiology Duration of wound If applicable, what setting it occurred
Size	Measurement in centimeters: length, width, depth
Color	Define in percentage, with red indicating amount of granulation tissue, yellow indicating amount of slough present, and black indicating necrotic tissue or eschar
Exudates	Describe absence or presence of exudates If exudates present, describe if serous, serosanguinous, sanguineous, or purulent
Odor	Determine after wound is cleaned, if odor is present or absent
Peri-wound tissue	Describe if viable, macerated, inflamed, or hyperkeratotic
Undermining	Describe absence or presence of tunneling or sinus tracts

Adapted from American Medical Directors Association pressure ulcers in the long-term care setting clinical practice guideline 2008 (last reviewed by AMDA 2012)

Wound prevention and management also has financial implications. Some data estimates that the cost of care triples for a nursing home resident if a pressure ulcer is present [50]. The Centers for Medicare and Medicaid Services (CMS) periodically revises of the Interpretive Guidelines and Investigate protocol for Surveyors for use in assessing wound care in nursing homes. As of 2014 the CMS guidelines under Federal Tag 314 state that a nursing facility may be cited if they fail to prevent new pressure ulcer development; fail to promote healing of previously identified ulcers; fail to prevent ulcer progression; fail to treat an infectious complication of a pressure ulcer, or there is development of a Stage 4 ulcer, unless the wound is deemed unavoidable [25, 53].

Documentation

Accurate documentation is vital for wound care. AMDA has recently reviewed its clinical practice guideline for managing wounds in 2012 (Table 4). For optimal wound care, AMDA recommends standardized timelines for assessment, descriptions, care plans, and treatments of wounds. A timeline should include reevaluations based on the severity of the wound. As previously discussed, a thorough skin examination should occur on admission to LTC that identifies and documents any existing wounds. Scheduled 2–3 week reevaluations should be performed by trained staff members that know how to follow a consistent approach to wound care and its documentation. The Interdisciplinary team must integrate its recommendations for optimal wound care to occur in any LTC setting [9]. In community-based home care or in assisted living wound care can be accomplished when the physician and facility engage the services of a home health care agency.

Conclusion

The prevalence of wounds in LTC residents has increased due to the increasing geriatric demographic. Wounds represent a geriatric syndrome with significant medical, psychosocial and economic implications. Given the increase in morbidity, mortality, and costs related to wounds, they have become a top priority in LTC regulation at the national and state levels. LTC residents are more susceptible to developing pressure ulcers due to impaired mobility and compromised nutrition status, as well as multi-morbidities including diabetes, cardiovascular disease and dementia. If prevention through risk factor modification has failed or a resident is found to have a wound on admission, the general assessment should include a thorough and timely evaluation of the resident and their environment. In addition to documenting wound characteristics, proper staging of pressure ulcers should be completed. Management requires an interdisciplinary and multidisciplinary approach based on frequent assessment and use of wound-specific treatment modalities. The functional status of the resident, goals of care, and risk-benefit ratio of any treatment should all factor into the treatment plan. Pain should always be assessed and managed. Care should be taken to reduce pressure, friction, shearing forces, moisture, exposure to bacteria, and pain. Preventing and treating wounds can reduce medical and psychosocial complications, decrease morbidity and mortality, and improve quality of life of LTC residents.

Pearls for the Practitioner

- As the complexities of residents who reside in long-term care have increased, the prevalence of wounds has increased as well.
- An interdisciplinary and multidisciplinary team in conjunction with the patient and their family should ideally develop a *holistic wound care treatment plan* that considers available resources and incorporates all relevant resident factors into its goals of care, as well as appropriate *wound-specific care* and *adequate pain control.*
- All wounds are not pressure ulcers. Thus, the NPUAP guidelines *cannot* be applied to traumatic, ischemic, venous, or diabetic wounds.
- As pressure ulcers heal reverse staging should *not* be used.
- All ulcers covered by eschar should be categorized as a *suspected deep tissue injury.*
- Any dry, black eschar *on the heel* should *not* be debrided if it is nontender, nonfluctuant, nonerythematous, and nonsuppurative.
- Not all ulcers are preventable. Some pressure ulcers are *unavoidable* due to the overwhelming burden of risk factors, multiple diseases and advanced life limiting illness.

Websites

1. Home of the Braden Scale—http://www.bradenscale.com
2. National Pressure Ulcer Advisory Panel—http://www.npuap.org/
3. American Medical Directors Association (AMDA)—www.amda.com/http://www.amda.com/tools/library/ref-pressureulcers.cfm
4. Institute for Healthcare Improvement—http://www.ihi.org/IHI/Programs/Campaign/PressureUlcers.htm
5. Centers for Medicare & Medicaid Services. "Guidance to Surveyors for Long Term Care Facilities"—http://www.cms.hhs.gov/transmittals/Downloads/R4SOM.pdf
6. Wound, Ostomy and Continence Nurses Society—http://www.wocn.org/index.php
7. Wound Research—http://www.woundsresearch.com
8. "Push tool"—http://www.npuap.org/resources/educational-and-clinical-resources/push-tool

References

1. Brandeis GH, Morris JN, Nash DJ, Lipsitz LA. The epidemiology and natural history of pressure ulcers in elderly nursing home residents. JAMA. 1990;264(22):2905–9.
2. Bergstrom N, Horn SD, Smout RJ, et al. The national pressure ulcer long-term care study: outcomes of pressure ulcer treatments in long-term care. J Am Geriatr Soc. 2005;53(10): 1721–9.
3. Bergstrom N. Litigation or redesign: improving pressure ulcer prevention. J Am Geriatr Soc. 2005;53(9):1627–9.
4. Stillman R. Wound care. 2014. http://emedicine.medscape.com/article/194018-overview.
5. Centers for Medicare and Medicaid Services. Action plan for further improvement of nursing home quality. 2009. www.cms.hhs.gov/quality/nhqi/2009.
6. Centers for Medicare & Medicaid Services (CMS), HHS. Medicare program: changes to the hospital inpatient prospective payment systems and fiscal year 2008 rates. Fed Regist. 2007;72:47379.
7. Centers for Medicare and Medicaid Services. Guidance to surveyors for long term care facilities. CMS manual. Washington, DC: CMS; 2004.
8. WOCN Society. Wound, ostomy, and continence nurses society position statement on avoidable versus unavoidable pressure ulcers. J Wound Ostomy Continence Nurs. 2009;36(4): 378–81.
9. American Medical Directors Association. Pressure ulcers in the long-term care setting clinical practice guideline. Columbia, MD: AMDA; 2008.
10. Gosnell DJ. An assessment tool to identify pressure sores. Nurs Res. 1973;22(1):55–9.
11. Ayello EA, Braden B. How and why to do pressure ulcer risk assessment. Adv Skin Wound Care. 2002;15(3):125–31.
12. Bergstrom N, Braden B. A prospective study of pressure sore risk among institutionalized elderly. J Am Geriatr Soc. 1992;40(8):747–58.
13. Horn SD, Bender SA, Ferguson ML, et al. The national pressure ulcer long-term care study: pressure ulcer development in long-term care residents. J Am Geriatr Soc. 2004;52(3): 359–67.
14. Singh N, Armstrong DG, Lipsky BA. Preventing foot ulcers in patients with diabetes. JAMA. 2005;293(2):217–28.

15. American Health Care Association. Medical condition- mental status CMS OSCAR data current surveys; 2009.
16. US Department of Health and Human Services, Centers for Medicare and Medicaid Services. Nursing home data compendium. 2008.
17. Hyde J, Perez R, Forester B. Dementia and assisted living. Gerontologist. 2007;47(Spec 3):51–67.
18. Diane KL, Joyce B. Pressure ulcers in individuals receiving palliative care: A National Pressure Ulcer Advisory Panel White Paper. Adv Skin Wound Care. 2010;23(2):59–72.
19. Wishin J, Gallagher TJ, McCann E. Emerging options for the management of fecal incontinence in hospitalized patients. J Wound Ostomy Continence Nurs. 2008;35(1):104–10.
20. Young ME. Malnutrition and wound healing. Heart Lung. 1988;17(1):60–7.
21. Joyce MB, Laura EE, Mona M, Diane L, Margaret G, Laurie MN, Janet C, The National Pressure Ulcer Advisory Panel. Pressure ulcers: avoidable or unavoidable? Results of the National Pressure Ulcer Advisory Panel Consensus Conference. Ostomy Wound Manag. 2011;57(2):24–37.
22. Schoonhoven L, Haalboom JR, Bousema MT, et al. Prospective cohort study of routine use of risk assessment scales for prediction of pressure ulcers. BMJ. 2002;325(7368):797.
23. Pancorbo-Hidalgo PL, Garcia-Fernandez FP, Lopez-Medina IM, Alvarez-Nieto C. Risk assessment scales for pressure ulcer prevention: a systematic review. J Adv Nurs. 2006;54(1):94–110.
24. Ayello E, Lyder C. A new era of pressure ulcer accountability in acute care. Adv Skin Wound Care. 2008;21(3):134.
25. The NPUAP selected "Quality of Care Regulations" made easy: Tag F 314 Pressure ulcer, National Pressure Ulcer Advisory Panel. March 2014.
26. Ratliff CR. Wocn. WOCN's evidence-based pressure ulcer guideline. Adv Skin Wound Care. 2005;18(4):204–8.
27. Karen K-E. Understanding the Kennedy terminal ulcer. 2001. http://www.kennedyterminalulcer.com. Accessed 15 Sep 2014
28. Steven A, David B, Nancy B, Laura H, Susan L, Jeanine M, Kathy S, Maranda V, Jennifer VR, Aamir S. Friction induced skin injuries – are they pressure ulcers? A National Pressure Ulcer Advisory Panel White Paper. NPUAP WP November 2012; v1:1–3
29. Grayson ML, Gibbons GW, Balogh K, Levin E, Karchmer AW. Probing to bone in infected pedal ulcers. A clinical sign of underlying osteomyelitis in diabetic patients. JAMA. 1995;273(9):721–3.
30. Takahashi P. Chronic ischemic, venous, and neuropathic ulcers in long-term care. Ann Long Term Care. 2006;14(7):26–31.
31. Bergstrom N, Allman R, Alvaraez O. Treatment of pressure ulcers. US Department of Health Services: Rockville, MD; 1994.
32. Bergstrom N, Allman R, Carlson C. Pressure ulcers in adults: predicition and prevention. Rockville, MD: Agency for Health Care Policy and Research, Public Health Services, US Dept of Health and Human Services; 1992.
33. Ayello EA, Lyder CH. Protecting patients from harm: preventing pressure ulcers in hospital patients.[reprint in adv skin wound care. 2008 mar;21(3):134–40; quiz 140–2; PMID: 18388668]. Nursing. 2007;37(10):36–40.
34. Torrie B. Palliative care of pressure ulcers in long-term care. 2013;21(3). http://www.annalsoflongtermcare.com/article/palliative-care-pressure-ulcers-long-term-care#sthash.JD1NpjZ7.dpuf. 24 Sep 2014
35. Wound Ostomy Continence Nurses Society. Guidelines for prevention and management of pressure ulcers. Glenview, IL: Wound Ostomy Continence Nurses Society; 2003. p. 12.
36. Ayello EA, Thomas DR, Litchford MA. Nutritional aspects of wound healing. Home Healthc Nurse. 1999;17(11):719–29.
37. Stratton RJ, Ek AC, Engfer M, et al. Enteral nutritional support in prevention and treatment of pressure ulcers: a systematic review and meta-analysis. Ageing Res Rev. 2005;4(3):422–50.

38. Heyman H, Van De Looverbosch DE, Meijer EP, Schols JM. Benefits of an oral nutritional supplement on pressure ulcer healing in long-term care residents. J Wound Care. 2008;17(11):476–8.
39. Reddy M, Gill SS, Kalkar SR, Wu W, Anderson PJ, Rochon PA. Treatment of pressure ulcers: a systematic review. JAMA. 2008;300(22):2647–62.
40. Kosiak M. Etiology of decubitus ulcers. Arch Phys Med Rehabil. 1961;42:19–29.
41. Witkowshi J, Parish L. The decubitus ulcer: skin failure and destructive behavior. Int J Dermatol. 2000;39:894.
42. Black JM. National Pressure Ulcer Advisory P. Moving toward consensus on deep tissue injury and pressure ulcer staging. Adv Skin Wound Care. 2005;18(8):415–6.
43. Duncan SM. Preventing & managing pressure sores. http://www.amda.com/publications/caring/march2003/policies.cfm#refs. 24 Sep 2014.
44. Defloor T, Schoonhoven L. Inter-rater reliability of the EPUAP pressure ulcer classification system using photographs. J Clin Nurs. 2004;13(8):952–9.
45. Takahashi P, Chandra A, Kiemele L, Targonski P. Wound care technologies: Emerging evidence for appropriate use in long-term care. Ann Long Term Care. 2008;16(12). http://www.annalsoflongtermcare.com/content/wound-care-technologies-emerging-evidence-appropriate-use-long-term-care.
46. Hopkins A, Dealey C, Bale S, Defloor T, Worboys F. Patient stories of living with a pressure ulcer. J Adv Nurs. 2006;56(4):345–53.
47. Moore Z, Cowman S. Reviewing the evidence for selecting cleansing fluids for pressure ulcers. Nurs Times. 2009;105(5):22–4.
48. Bates-Jensen BM, Guihan M, Garber SL, Chin AS, Burns SP. Characteristics of recurrent pressure ulcers in veterans with spinal cord injury. J Spinal Cord Med. 2009;32(1):34–42.
49. Pieper B, Langemo D, Cuddigan J. Pressure ulcer pain: a systematic literature review and national pressure ulcer advisory panel white paper. Ostomy Wound Manag. 2009;55(2):16.
50. Smith DM. Pressure ulcers in the nursing home.[see comment]. Ann Intern Med. 1995;123(6):433–42.
51. Bryan CS, Dew CE, Reynolds KL. Bacteremia associated with decubitus ulcers. Arch Intern Med. 1983;143(11):2093–5.
52. Allman RM, Goode PS, Burst N, Bartolucci AA, Thomas DR. Pressure ulcers, hospital complications, and disease severity: impact on hospital costs and length of stay. Adv Wound Care. 1999;12(1):22–30.
53. Lyder CH. Implications of pressure ulcers and its relation to federal tag 314. Ann Long Term Care. 2006;14(4):19–24.

Dementia, Delirium, and Depression

Andrew Neal Dentino, Pamela A. Fenstemacher, and Kourtney Harrington

Introduction

Dementia, delirium, and depression will affect many residents at some point during their stay in a post-acute or long-term care (PA/LTC) facility. Cognitive disorders can either be chronic as in dementia, acute as in seen in delirium, or subacute as in depression [1]. Understanding the similarities and differences between the clinical features of dementia, delirium, and depression is paramount to evaluating the resident with a change in mentation. Assessment by the clinician is challenging when determining which of these frequently seen conditions is present as residents may be suffering with one or more of them at the same time. Careful observation by staff and providers can help the interdisciplinary team to recognize and assess any mental status changes and to initiate appropriate interventions in a timely manner. Clinical aspects of these three conditions are summarized in Table 1, while Table 2 details the clinical evaluation of depression, delirium, and dementia.

A.N. Dentino (✉) • K. Harrington, MD
Donald W. Reynolds Department of Geriatric Medicine, University of Oklahoma
Health Sciences Center, 1122 NE 13th Street, Oklahoma, OK 73117, USA
e-mail: andrew-dentino@ouhsc.edu

P.A. Fenstemacher, MD, CMD, FAAFP
Living Independently for Elders (LIFE), University of Pennsylvania School of Nursing,
Philadelphia, PA, USA

© Springer International Publishing Switzerland 2016
P.A. Fenstemacher, P. Winn (eds.), *Post-Acute and Long-Term Medicine*,
Current Clinical Practice, DOI 10.1007/978-3-319-16979-8_14

Table 1 Comparison of the clinical features of depression, delirium, and dementia

Clinical feature	Depression	Delirium	Dementia
Onset	Gradual, may be recurrent	Sudden	Gradual, progressive
Course	Chronic	Acute	Chronic
Mood	Low	Variable	Variable
Apathy	Present	May be present or absent	May be present or absent
Attention	Intact or impaired	Impaired	Intact early; impaired later
Memory	Intact or impaired	Usually impaired	Impaired
Hallucinations or delusions	Absent[a]	Present	Variable
ADL's[b]	Intact or impaired	Intact or impaired	Intact early; impaired later
IADL's[c]	Intact or impaired	Intact or impaired	Intact early; impaired before ADL's
Signs of other illness	Present	Present	Usually absent

[a]Except in depression with psychotic features
[b]Activities of daily living
[c]Instrumental activities of daily living

Table 2 Clinical evaluation of depression, delirium, and dementia*

Evaluation	Depression	Delirium	Dementia
History or interval history and physical examination	x	x	x
Screening tool	GDS, SIGECAPS Cornell Scale for Depression in Dementia	CAM	Folstein MMSE, SLUMS
CBC with differential	x	x	x
Complete metabolic panel	x	x	x
Vitamin B_{12} level	x		x
Medication review and medication level	x	x	x
Thyroid stimulating hormone	x	x	x
RPR			x
Lyme titer			x
Urinalysis with culture		x	x
Chest x-ray		x	
Arterial blood gas		x	
Electrocardiogram		x	
Brain imaging		x	x
Lumbar puncture		x	x
Electroencephalogram		x	

[a]The clinical evaluation of dementia, delirium, and depression should **always** be guided by presentation and goals of care

Dementia

Dementia is a syndrome of chronic, irreversible, progressive global decline in cognition with associated loss of memory. It is one of the most common impairments in older adults in PA/LTC and while it occurs with a clear sensorium, in its early stages it frequently complicates the evaluation of a resident with an acute change in mental status [2–4]. Dementia occurs when an abnormality in the structure and function of the brain disrupts cognition. Symptoms of dementia may be noted by the clinician, observed by the staff, or reported by the patient and/or family. Although dementia is often associated with a disrupted sleep–wake cycle, disturbances in language, recall and memory may be the most evident findings [5]. Other psychiatric disorders and medical conditions that cause cognitive dysfunction may accompany dementia making it more challenging to diagnose and treat.

Differential Diagnosis

Alzheimer's Disease (Dementia of Alzheimer's Type or DAT), vascular dementia (multi-infarct dementia or MID), Dementia with Lewy Bodies (LBD), frontotemporal dementia (FTD), and dementia due to HIV/AIDS are the most commonly seen types of dementia. Dementia can be categorized as cortical or subcortical, with DAT being a classic example of a cortical dementia. *Cortical dementias* are typically characterized by amnesia, disorientation, and relatively preserved personality. Whereas *subcortical dementias* show relatively preserved memory with difficulties in executive function, attention, and concentration. Dementia associated with Parkinson's disease is an example of subcortical dementia. It is important to remember that with increasing age persons more frequently suffer from more than one type of dementia, and this is referred to as *mixed dementia* [6].

DAT is the most common cause of dementia and is estimated to account for 55–75 % of all cases [1, 3, 7] and classified as a neurocognitive disorder (NCD) due to Alzheimer's Disease in *DSM-5* [8]. In DAT, personality and attention are preserved in the early stages of disease as opposed to other types of dementia where a more rapid deterioration of personality may occur. Executive functioning declines progressively over time in DAT, but progression of behavioral symptoms is the most common reason for admission to a memory care unit or nursing facility.

The second most common etiology for dementia is vascular disease (Vascular NCD in *DSM-5*) and accounts for 13–16 % of affected individuals [1, 3, 7]. Vascular or multi-infarct dementia (MID) is characterized by early onset of decreased attention accompanied by blunting of affect and memory disturbances. Patients usually have known risk factors for vascular disease (e.g., hypertension, diabetes mellitus, hyperlipidemia) and behavioral risk factors (e.g., smoking, obesity, sedentary lifestyle). Vascular dementia frequently progresses in a stepwise fashion as opposed to the gradual progression seen in DAT. Microcirculatory deficits accumulate over time as a result of the vasculopathic nature of the underlying disease process. On physical exam evidence of arterial vascular compromise is commonly seen as well as focal neurologic abnormalities.

Lewy Body Disease (LBD) is the third most common dementia seen and accounts for 20–25 % of all dementia, LBD NCD in *DSM-5*. LBD usually occurs at an earlier age and has a faster progression than DAT and is associated with psychiatric symptoms, fluctuations in level of alertness, and an increased sensitivity to antipsychotic medications [9]. Unfortunately psychiatric symptoms are very common and include anxiety, depression, and perceptual disturbances. Perceptual disturbances are characterized by hallucinations that are usually visual and delusions or fixed false beliefs that are frequently paranoid. LBD is closely associated with Parkinson's disease and is characterized by many of the features of the Parkinson's disease. These features include a *motor syndrome* (bradykinesia, rigidity, tremors, and gait difficulties leading to falls) and *autonomic dysfunction* (constipation and orthostatic hypotension leading to syncope). Loss of smell and sleep disturbances are frequently seen as well. Sleep disturbances include excessive daytime drowsiness and nighttime difficulty not only staying asleep but also REM sleep behavior disorder (RBD). RBD manifests as the patient acting out his or her dreams, a symptom often first recognized by a caregiver. Persons diagnosed with Lewy body dementia are also sensitive to antiparkinsonian drugs that can increase confusion and problematic behaviors. Therefore when prescribing these medications, it is important to weigh the risk of worsening cognition versus the potential benefit of improving function.

Some dementias are rapidly progressive such as *Creutzfeldt–Jakob disease* (Prion disease NCD) which is caused by a prion or infectious protein. Symptoms of this dementia develop quickly often accompanied by myoclonic jerks and eventually seizures [10]. The progression of symptoms is less obvious in frontotemporal lobe dementias (FTDs), classified as frontotemporal lobar degeneration NCD in *DSM-5*. FTD manifests as mood swings and impulsivity, with personality coarsening as well as a concomitant deterioration in functional status. Affected individuals also demonstrate inattention and affective flattening. A more unusual cause of dementia is Huntington's disease, which is inherited and begins at a very young age (e.g., 35–45). Huntington's disease causes subtle mood changes and cognitive problems that progress fairly rapidly to dementia with behavioral disturbances, which are accompanied by a lack of coordination and chorea (i.e., involuntary writhing movements).

Other etiologies of dementia to consider in the differential diagnosis include HIV disease, Parkinson's disease (where the Parkinson's motor symptoms will *precede* cognitive decline by several years), Wilson's disease, traumatic brain injury (i.e., from falling in older adults), or other neurological conditions (e.g., ALS, multiple sclerosis, Korsakoff's syndrome/alcoholic encephalopathy). Medical conditions that can cause cognitive dysfunction include obstructive sleep apnea, metastatic disease, neurosyphilis, and substance abuse. The possibility of substance abuse or prescription medications influencing cognition should always be considered in anyone presenting with memory complaints, even if the medication had been taken for many years [8]. *Remember to look for the more common potentially reversible causes of dementia*: B_{12} deficiency, thyroid disease, subdural hematoma, normal pressure hydrocephalus, and primary tumors of the brain.

Diagnosing Dementia

When the staff in the PA/LTC facility is trained and experienced in caring for persons with dementia, those residents who develop early symptoms of dementia are more readily recognized. In nursing facilities (NFs) MDS evaluations can be compared to determine changes in resident cognition, memory, and other manifestations such as:

- Inability to perform activities or tasks of daily living.
- Changes in hygiene.
- Altered interactions with staff and other residents.

The diagnosis of dementia starts with a patient history, often obtained from a family member and/or staff in PA/LTC. It is important to determine if the onset of the condition was insidious and difficult to pinpoint in time or if the progression was gradual or stepwise (i.e., DAT vs. MID). Any specific neurologic and psychiatric symptoms that have occurred also need to be considered [3]. The diagnosis can then be refined on the basis of the neurologic signs and symptoms, mental status, physical examination and the results of neuropsychologic testing (though often not needed), brain imaging, and laboratory studies.

The Importance of Screening

It is important to thoroughly evaluate a resident with suspected dementia, as many medical conditions can cause or worsen dementia, some of which can be reversed (See Table 3). In particular, a patient presenting with new symptoms of memory or cognitive impairment should be evaluated for depression as well. Depression can cause a form of cognitive impairment referred to as *pseudodementia* (for further discussion see section on depression).

Evaluation of the Resident with Cognitive Impairment

The *"gold standard"* for the diagnosis of dementia is **clinical**, based upon the patient history and physical assessment, with ancillary information such as formal neuropsychologic testing [11] and brain imaging performed as needed. A basic evaluation of the resident with new cognitive impairment includes laboratory tests such as a complete blood count with differential, comprehensive metabolic panel,

Table 3 Medical conditions that can cause or worsen dementia

Delirium
Developmental disability
HIV/AIDs
Hyperglycemia or hypoglycemia
Hypothyroidism
Mental retardation (i.e., neuropsychologic impairment)
Normal pressure hydrocephalus
Sequelae of traumatic brain injury
Subdural hematoma
Tertiary syphilis
Vasculitides
Vitamin B_{12} deficiency

vitamin B_{12} level, thyroid function panel including a TSH, and possibly blood levels of medication such as digoxin, lithium, theophylline, anticonvulsants (e.g., phenytoin, valproic acid), and tricyclic antidepressants (e.g., amitriptyline). Other tests to consider are: HIV, RPR or perhaps a test for Lyme disease (depending on local prevalence and other risk factors) as possible causes for a change in cognition [3, 4].

It is also necessary to evaluate underlying medical conditions and to optimize their management. Medical conditions commonly implicated in cognitive dysfunction include: recent coronary artery bypass grafting, hypertension, nutritional deficiencies including B vitamins, diabetes mellitus, stroke, Parkinson's disease, and diseases that cause hypoxia such as COPD and obstructive sleep apnea [4].

Quantifiable scales that may be used as benchmarks for diagnosing and monitoring dementia progression include the Montreal Cognitive Assessment (MOCA), the Folstein Mini Mental Status Exam (MMSE), the St. Louis University Mental Status Exam (SLUMS) or other commercially available instruments [11, 12]. The MMSE is a simple 30-point screening tool frequently used to evaluate for cognitive impairment. Recently, the official form has been copyrighted and must be purchased (www.minimental.com.) Because of this expense, some practitioners have chosen instead to use the SLUMS available at http://medschool.slu.edu/agingsuccessfully/pdfsurveys/slumsexam_05.pdf. More tools can be found in "Other Resources" at the end of this chapter. Keep in mind that the MDS in skilled nursing facilities will also provide an evaluation of the resident's cognitive status (Brief Interview for Mental Status or BIMS) and functional status.

Finally, neuro-imaging of the brain may be performed to rule out structural lesions such as a neoplasm or other potentially reversible conditions such as normal pressure hydrocephalus or a subdural hematoma. A neuro-imaging study should be considered especially when the onset of the dementia has occurred within the past 6–12 months, is rapidly progressive, or is following an unpredictable course.

If there is a question of diagnosis, or if the resident or their family has difficulty accepting the diagnosis of dementia, neuropsychologic testing may be done to more definitively diagnose the resident's cognitive status. Not only may neuropsychologic testing help determine the type of dementia, but it can also help to delineate the patient's strengths and weaknesses; to identify particular areas of cognitive dysfunction in order to suggest compensation strategies, and to aid in behavioral management [5]. The diagnosis of dementia can aid in the care of the resident. Its diagnosis will provide a framework for prognostication and will aid in health care decision-making by both resident and family. Although dementia is a chronic, progressive, and ultimately terminal illness, it is often unrecognized in its early stages. The goals of care in the management of dementia are to provide a safe environment, educate caregivers and family, and provide emotional support for the healthcare team, patient, and family.

Prognosis

Different types of dementia have varied manifestations at onset, with the common pathway being one of progressive loss of ability to perform daily tasks of living (i.e., ADLs and IADLs). Residents eventually become unable to care for themselves, incontinent of bowel and bladder, and unable to safely swallow and to maintain sufficient nutrition to sustain life. Even when carefully hand fed, the resident with end stage dementia will eventually develop progressive weight loss and be at high risk for developing pressure ulcers. The demented resident may also develop urinary retention, constipation, and repeated urinary or respiratory infections (the latter due to aspiration of food and secretions) [5]. It is imperative that the family be educated on the disease process of dementia and its course. This may be difficult for families to accept, as many do not understand that dementia is a terminal illness (see Chaps. "Integrating Palliative Care into Practice" and "Weight and Nutrition" for further reading).

Pharmacologic Treatment

Pharmacologic treatment of dementia should focus on the underlying medical and psychological condition(s) affecting the individual, with the goal being maximization of his or her functional well-being. For example, in those with coexistent depression, the use of antidepressants with serotoninergic activity may improve both depressive symptoms and cognition [3].

Alzheimer's Disease (DAT)

In Alzheimer's disease, the mainstay of treatment is neurotransmitter modulation to lessen the symptoms of the disease. Although it is an area being avidly researched, no medication has yet been found that slows the progression of DAT.

Specific treatment for DAT includes the use of two major classes of medications, *cholinesterase inhibitors* and the *NMDA receptor antagonists* [13, 14]. The most widely used cholinesterase inhibitor is donepezil (Aricept) but other medications include rivastigmine (Exelon) and galantamine (Razadyne). Cholinesterase inhibitors are currently indicated for mild (MMSE >19), moderate (MMSE 19–10), or severe (MMSE < 10) DAT. The only currently available NMDA receptor antagonist is memantine (Namenda). Memantine is currently indicated for moderate to severe AD either in conjunction with a cholinesterase inhibitor or as monotherapy [3, 4]. Monitoring for and management of potential common side effects of these two classes of medications should be as much a part of patient care as their prescribing. Because *these medications are not curative but palliative* decisions about whether to continue them must be individualized as the benefits and risks are weighed on an ongoing basis.

Other medications and treatments have not been shown effective in treating or preventing AD. These include anti-inflammatory medications such as NSAIDs, hormone replacement therapy such as estrogen, gingko biloba, and antioxidants such as vitamin E. Research in this area continues predominantly investigating the prevention of CNS inflammation and the formation of beta-amyloid plaques, both hallmarks of DAT [3].

Non-DAT Dementias

The mainstay of treatment for non-DAT dementias is preventing progression of the underlying disease process (as in the case of vascular dementia) and treating the symptoms that arise in the course of the disease (as in the case of hallucinations in LBD.) Donepezil has been tested (off label) in other cognitive disorders, including LBD and MID, but it is not currently FDA approved for these diagnoses.

Challenging Behaviors in Dementia

Pacing, wandering, hoarding, agitation, insomnia, aggression, hypersexuality, perseveration, hallucinations, paranoia, and emotional lability are challenging behaviors seen in dementia [4, 15]. Agitation frequently is seen with "sundowning," which is a syndrome of disorientation, confusion, and agitation that often starts in the middle to late afternoon and progressively worsens through the evening into the night. An environment and medical evaluation often gives insight into ways in which these behaviors can be mitigated or prevented. Frequently, these behaviors are a natural manifestation of the dementing process, but they may be exacerbated by stimuli in the environment or a medical illness. On one hand, commonly seen environmental causes of disruptive behavior include a new caregiver, an absent family member or another disruptive resident. On the other hand, commonly seen medical causes of disruptive or changed behaviors include pain, constipation, urinary retention, drug effect(s), dehydration, or infection. It is important to first evaluate any reversible environmental and/or physical stimuli that may be implicated in precipitating the behavior before initiating any treatment interventions for the behavior [4]. Communication becomes increasingly difficult for patients as their dementia progresses. Often what may be deemed as "agitation" or other abnormal behavior might be reformulated to questions of, "What is this behavior attempting to communicate?" "What are their unmet needs, if any?" "What is this behavior attempting to convey?" Whether it is pain or discomfort due to constipation or inability to urinate, boredom or hunger, attempting to identify and address the antecedents to these underlying behaviors should be a first-line intervention rather than prescribing a pharmacologic agent for "agitation."

Psychosocial interventions constitute a mainstay for the creation and promotion of a sense of well-being for those with progressive dementia. Learning about and acknowledging individual resident preferences and personhood, as well as providing care with dignity can help establish a fulfilling and meaningful activity program. Physical activity, even if limited to the upper extremity for wheelchair-bound residents, may be a welcomed and enjoyable part of the day. Social activities such as listening to reading, singing, or reminiscing and reality orientating may bring solace and peace to patients, families, and staff. Respect for privacy, sleep and meal preferences, and effective verbal, visual, and tactile cueing may further benefit the resident with dementia and others at the end of life [16].

Treatment of Behaviors in Dementia

Behaviors in dementia may be addressed using non-pharmacologic and/or pharmacologic treatment.

Non-pharmacologic Treatment

An adjustment of environmental factors (both physical and human) may lesson or resolve distressing behaviors. For example, although providing areas in the facility with more home-like furnishings and wall decorations did not reduce wandering and pacing, residents were kept safe and were easier to monitor because they preferred to remain in the home-like areas [15].

Suggested interventions include:

- Establish a daily routine for personal care and meals while maintaining some flexibility to accommodate the resident's needs and preferences. If the resident is resistant, re-approach the resident a short time later and they may then be more willing to allow care or eat.
- Reduce isolation; segregate noisier or disruptive residents from quieter ones.
- Maintain adequate and appropriate lighting at all times.
- Provide pleasant experiences, such as ethnic foods and other culturally oriented activities, pet therapy, or stuffed animals [4].

Interventions for disruptive or challenging behavior:

- For inappropriate sexual behavior: use clothing that reduces access to genitalia, provide care from same-sex caregivers, seat away from residents of the opposite sex [15].
- Redirect with individual and group activities.
- Know the resident's social history and preferences, which will often give insight into behaviors and preferred activities. For example, the resident who continuously moves tables and chairs in the dining room may be repeating his former motor activity of returning grocery carts from the parking lot to the supermarket. When staff observed him moving furniture safely, he was allowed to continue this activity with supervision and his agitation was reduced.

Pharmacologic Treatment

If modifying the environment cannot alleviate distressing behaviors, medication management may need to be considered. As with other changes to a resident's plan of care, the risks and benefits of any medical treatment need to be carefully considered. The staff and family should be advised of the issues and interventions that have been tried before instituting medical therapy. There has not been a great deal of consensus on which medications to treat challenging behaviors in dementia, or research to prove efficacy [15]. *One must also take into consideration State regulations and facility policies regarding medications that are considered chemical restraints.* The following may be considered:

- Residents who exhibit agitation with psychotic features such as hallucinations, delusions, or preservative behaviors such as pacing or hoarding may respond to treatment with antipsychotic medication.
- Residents with sundowning or insomnia may improve with a medication that promotes sleep (trazodone) or reduces confusion (antipsychotic).
- Residents who exhibit behaviors with an anxiety component may benefit from a serotonergic reuptake inhibitor or trazodone.
- Residents with hypersexual behaviors may respond to antipsychotic medication or to antiandrogenic hormone therapy such as estrogen (in male residents).
- Residents with anger or aggression may respond to the use of serotonergic agents, mood stabilizing agents such as divalproex, carbamazepine, gabapentin, or antipsychotic medication such as risperidone and olanzapine [15].

Medication regimens must be reviewed on a regular basis to evaluate their effectiveness. This includes periodic attempts to reduce dosing or discontinue medications. For example, 3–6 months after admission to a facility, it is not uncommon that a resident is able to have medications that were necessary at the time of admission be reduced or even discontinued. *Beware that antipsychotics and benzodiazepines can cause paradoxical agitation and/or worsen confusion.*

Medication Management in Cognitive Impairment

The average nursing facility resident takes seven medications, and nearly a third of residents take nine or more medications [16]. Therefore, when evaluating cognitive impairment it is crucial to consider medications and medication interactions that can alter cognitive function. Medications that are commonly implicated include antiarrhythmics, hypnotics, psychotropics, sedatives, analgesics, and medications with significant anticholinergic properties such as those used for urinary urge incontinence. Toxicity from certain medications such as digoxin can also cause changes in cognition. In 1991, Dr. Mark Beers created a list of *potentially inappropriate* medications used in the geriatric population. The Beers list continues to be updated and is used for guidance by practitioners in PA/LTC and by state surveyors (See Chap. "Medication Management in Long-term Care for further discussion") [13].

Delirium

Delirium is a medical emergency. Its differential is vast and maintaining patient safety is paramount. Because undiagnosed or untreated delirium can result in increased morbidity and mortality, a timely and prudent workup is essential. In contrast to dementia and depression, delirium is a medical condition that can be either *acute* or *subacute with its onset frequently unrecognized*. It is caused by an imbalance in brain acetylcholine that occurs either because of changes in the body's homeostatic internal environmental (e.g., fever) or changes in the metabolic milieu (e.g., ischemia, hypoxia), which then disrupt normal neuronal circuitry [17, 18]. *It is so common that it should be anticipated* whenever an older adult undergoes surgery, is hospitalized, or suffers an acute medical illness.

Nevertheless, regardless of its pathophysiology, the behavioral manifestations of delirium include symptoms of abnormal attention, arousal and awareness [19]. Most striking is the patient's inability to maintain attention for all but extremely short periods of time, frequently changing topics mid-sentence. The patient will also experience a change in cognition including perceptual impairments such as illusions, delusions, or hallucinations [20]. Delirium can be described according to the level of psychomotor activity manifested by the patient, either *hyperactive* or *hypoactive*, or *mixed*. A patient with *hyperactive delirium* experiences increased psychomotor activity and may appear anxious or agitated. In contrast, *hypoactive delirium* causes reduced psychomotor activity and is often under-recognized due to the "absence of a complaint" or the attribution of the apathy to another illness such as depression. The staff will describe patients with a hypoactive delirium as, "quiet and requiring little or no attention". This may lead to the delirium being overlooked and therefore untreated. The third type of delirium is a *mixed delirium*, the resident exhibits fluctuating levels of psychomotor activity ranging from immobility to extreme agitation [4, 21].

Table 4 Delirium risk factors

Dementia
Older age
Functional impairment
Multiple comorbidities
Dehydration
Malnutrition
Sensory impairment
History of depression
History of substance abuse

Any resident who has an acute change in sensorium or behavior (i.e., suspected delirium) warrants an immediate review as to the antecedents and consequences of the behavior with consideration as to its possible etiology. Delirium is likely to occur in a vulnerable resident who develops an acute illness, affecting at least one third of hospitalized elders [22]. It may last for weeks to months and has been associated with poor health outcomes including increased in-hospital mortality, longer length of stay, functional decline and risk of institutionalization. As pressure increases to discharge individuals sooner from acute inpatient facilities, many of these acutely confused elderly transition from hospital to a post-acute facility, where they remain delirious and can experience potentially life-threatening complications [21, 23]. Many of the residents in PA/LTC facilities are at particular risk of developing delirium due to multiple risk factors (See Table 4). In PA/LTC, the identification, assessment, and management of delirium are urgent as delirium may signify an underlying medical emergency and delirium is frequently the presenting symptom of a resident's change in condition. If hospital admission or readmission is going to be prevented, quickly addressing any acute change in mental status is essential (see chapter 9 Preventing Hospital Admissions and Readmissions for further discussion). Consider how frequently delirium occurs when a NF resident develops an infection or dehydration that has underlying dementia, multi-morbidities, and a complicated medication regimen.

Identification

Each resident with delirium should be evaluated for the multiple risk factors of delirium, especially those that are reversible. When investigating the cause of delirium it is important to review the medical history and medication list for all chronic medical illnesses and medications that increase the risk for delirium. Dementia is a leading risk factor for delirium as are anticholinergic and analgesic medications. *An unfamiliar environment or change in staff, such as experienced during a hospital stay, can by itself precipitate delirium.* In the hospital setting up to one third of the cases of delirium are thought to be either preventable or iatrogenic. For other risk factors for delirium, see Table 4 [24].

Assessment of Delirium

One of the simplest ways to evaluate a resident for delirium is the Confusion Assessment Method (CAM) [25]. It is a four-item evaluation that was developed by Inouye et al. and entails the following characteristics:

1. Acute onset and fluctuating course.
2. Inattention.
3. Disorganized thinking.
4. Altered level of consciousness.

The diagnosis of delirium is made by the presence of *both* (1) and (2), with *either* (3) or (4). The CAM has been shown to have excellent sensitivity and specificity and has been validated in a number of care settings [26].

As with any change in mental status, an evaluation of the resident/patient must investigate all potentially reversible causes. This should include a complete interval history to determine not only when there was a change in mental status but also the time course of the resident's mental status. Another essential part of the history is medication review. Medications that were recently prescribed, had a dosage change, or were recently discontinued should be noted. All prescription medications, over-the-counter medications, supplements, and substances with potential for abuse (alcohol, illicit and prescription drugs as well) should be reviewed carefully. It is also important to include any topical medications, such as eye drops, nasal sprays, or suppositories. A *withdrawal syndrome* from prescription drugs (e.g., analgesics, benzodiazepines, or antidepressants), alcohol or illicit drugs should be considered as a possible cause of the delirium. These medications may have been prescribed at the facility or discretely brought into the facility by the resident, a family member, or a friend.

Medication interactions, changes in metabolism with aging (such as decreased renal or liver function), or recently acquired or progressing disease (such as dementia or diabetes) all increase the likelihood that a medication will cause or contribute to delirium. Medications that were previously necessary or recommended may now be causing unwanted effects and thus may need to be discontinued.

A physical exam should include vital signs: temperature, pulse, and blood pressure, as well as pulse oximetry, and blood sugar. A careful mental status and neurologic examination should be performed. The remainder of the physical exam should focus on signs and symptoms that may indicate either an acute underlying disease process, or a chronic condition that has worsened.

Diagnostic tests should be guided by findings from the history and physical examination. Laboratory tests should include a complete blood count, electrolytes, renal function, and a urinalysis. Other lab tests to consider are: thyroid function tests, B_{12} level, and serum levels of prescribed medications (such as digoxin, lithium, and valproic acid). If indicated, an arterial blood gas or chest X-ray should be done. Other diagnostic testing to consider are neuroimaging and an EKG. Neuroimaging may reveal a subdural hematoma, stroke, brain tumor or normal pressure hydrocephalus. An acute coronary syndrome and/or arrhythmia may be seen on EKG. On rare occasion there may be an indication for either a lumbar puncture to evaluate for infectious or neoplastic processes or an EEG to look for seizure activity [4, 20–22]. *In most cases of delirium the EEG will show nondiagnostic generalized showing that does not contribute to establishing the cause of delirium nor helpful in its treatment.*

Prevention

Most of all, it is important to strive to prevent delirium. As noted studies in the hospital setting have shown that up to one third of cases of delirium are either potentially preventable or iatrogenic. Interventions used in the hospital that may also help prevent delirium in the PA/LTC setting are listed in Table 5.

Treatment

A safe and calming environment needs to be established for the patient with delirium, while adequate nutrition and hydration are maintained. Patient reassurance, redirection, reality orientation, with involvement of family and caregivers can assist in alleviating the delirium. On occasion treatment of the underlying medical condition causing the delirium will not be sufficient to lessen symptoms in a timely manner to prevent harm to the patient, other patients, staff, and/or the caregiver. In such cases, short-term use of an antipsychotic may be necessary. Use of haloperidol is the most clinically established, with only limited studies on the use of the atypical antipsychotics. Benzodiazepines have not shown efficacy except in acute withdrawal from sedatives, hypnotics, or alcohol. *Be aware that antipsychotics and benzodiazepines can cause a paradoxical worsening of anxiety, agitation and confusion.*

Table 5 Interventions to prevent or ameliorate delirium

Problem	Intervention
Cognitive impairment	Reorientation to time, location, care team Provision of cognitively stimulation activities Caffeine-free warm beverages Music Back massage
Dehydration	Volume repletion (encouragement of oral intake)
Hearing impairment	Disimpaction of cerumen, use of hearing aids and portable amplifiers
Immobility	Encourage early ambulation or active range of motion
Sleep deprivation	Noise reduction measures in patient care areas Minimize sleep deprivation by staff or medication aide
Vision impairment	Use of eyeglasses, magnifying lenses, and adaptive equipment

From: Aging in the Know: www.americangeriatrics.org

Depression

Depression is a major illness affecting many elderly who reside in PA/LTC, frequently having an impact on every aspect of their life from mental to physical health. A recent review of the literature showed the prevalence of major depressive disorder in nursing facility residents was 10 %, with 29 % of residents having depressive symptoms [27]. Depression is more likely to occur in patients because of *comorbid medical* (e.g., dementia, stroke, cancer, coronary artery disease or Parkinson's disease) *and psychiatric conditions* that are frequent in this population. Although depression is very common, it can remain undiagnosed when its symptoms are confused with those of another illness. When depression is untreated, it can worsen any coexisting medical illness and lead to poorer outcomes and increased risk of suicide [1, 4, 28]. In 2004 the World Health Organization reported that unipolar depressive disorders ranked as a leading cause of the global disease burden and that by 2030 it would be ranked first [29]. Depression is associated with increased disability, greater medical burden, and patients perceiving they have poor health [30, 31].

It is important to be able to differentiate the symptoms of depression from those of delirium and dementia. These disorders often coexist making the diagnosis difficult. Depressive symptoms can be vague, atypical, and non-diagnostic in and of themselves, thus challenging to establish a diagnosis. Both long-term care residents and community-dwelling elders often have undiagnosed and untreated (or undertreated) depression [32].

Symptoms and Risk Factors

The symptoms of depression can be typical or atypical in nature and are commonly overlooked or under recognized. The elderly tend to report less symptoms of depression due to fear of being stigmatized. When they do complain, their somatic symptoms of depression may be incorrectly attributed to physical illness. Finally, even when symptoms of depression are recognized, the false belief that depression is a normal part of aging can keep the depression from being treated [19].

The classic symptoms of depression include [10]:

- Depressed mood.
- Loss of interest or pleasure (i.e., anhedonia).
- Weight loss or gain, with change in appetite (decreased or increased).
- Change in sleep pattern.
- Psychomotor disturbance.
- Lack of energy or fatigue.
- Guilt.
- Inability to concentrate.
- Suicidal thoughts.

Multiple illnesses can mimic or mask symptoms making it even more difficult for the clinician to recognize depression. Studies have demonstrated a need for *late-life depression* to have a separate classification and diagnostic criteria as it presents differently than depression in younger people [33]. A depressive syndrome that is prevalent in the elderly is *"depression without sadness"* where patients present with lack of vigor, social withdrawal, and apathy [10]. *"Depression-executive dysfunction syndrome"* has also been described in the elderly. It includes psychomotor retardation, loss of interest and task initiation as well as a language dysfunction characterized by difficulties with visual naming and verbal fluency [33]. When the elderly are depressed they are also more likely to experience anergia, anhedonia, appetite changes, and sleep dysfunction [34]. Rather than self-report depression or sadness the elderly are more likely to report somatic complaints (i.e., anxiety or hypochondriasis). It is critical to have a low threshold for screening for depression when the organic causes of symptoms are ruled out or when no physical cause of symptoms can be established.

There are several risk factors for late-life depression that encompass social, demographic, psychological, and health domains. One study showed that low economic status, psychosocial stressors, chronic illness, disability, and disrupted relationships all are associated with late-life depression [35]. Another study showed that poor self-rated health, comorbidities, frequent hospitalizations, and lack of friends at the NF are associated with depressive symptoms [12]. Other risk factors included in the health domain that have been found associated with depression are delirium, dementia, or mild cognitive impairment at a younger age, a myocardial infarction or coronary artery disease, and pain or diabetes. Physical disability and hearing loss are other risk factors associated with depression [11, 28].

Differentiating Depression from Dementia

Many patients in long-term care facilities have dementia or some degree of cognitive impairment. It can be difficult to differentiate between cognitive impairment and depression, but it is important to do so as their treatments and potential outcomes are different. *Pseudodementia* is an entity in which cognitive impairment is actually due to a depressive disorder and not dementia [1]. The symptoms of depression and dementia frequently overlap, which can make it difficult for clinicians to differentiate between the two. The Cornell Scale for Depression in Dementia is a tool that uses an interview with the patient and the caregiver (see diagnosis/screening tools below). *Any resident with newly recognized memory or cognitive impairment should also be evaluated for depression,* as they may actually be suffering from pseudodementia rather than dementia. Aggressive treatment of depression in the resident with suspected pseudodementia will lead to a gradual improvement or resolution of the cognitive impairment associated with their depression [36]. Dementia is a known risk factor for depression and there is also evidence that depression may be a precursor to dementia. So when depression or dementia is present, the other should be considered [37].

In summary depression is frequently undiagnosed or under-diagnosed in the geriatric patient population. It is postulated that this occurs for many different reasons. The reasons include an overlap between symptoms of depression and those of dementia, a lack of a biologic gold standard test that would diagnose geriatric psychiatric disorders, and preconceptions that depression is a natural part of aging. There is also concern that clinicians have inadequate diagnostic skills and are unable to recognize subtle clinical features of depression in geriatric patients [4, 36].

Diagnosis

It is important to note that a resident may experience a depressed or sad mood and yet not meet the criteria for depression. The key to the diagnosis and treatment of depression is determining whether or not the mood has a significant negative impact on the resident's quality of life. The diagnosis of depression may be guided by the American Psychiatric Association Diagnostic and Statistical Manual of Mental Disorders–version V [10]. *If a resident has significant psychiatric disease, comorbid substance abuse, or depression with psychotic features, it may be helpful to consult a psychiatrist for help with a resident's diagnosis and treatment.*

The DSM-V criteria are currently used to diagnose a major depressive disorder (MDD). In order to make this diagnosis the patient must have *five or more symptoms present for a continuous 2-week period* in which at least one of the symptoms is either *depressed mood or lack of interest or pleasure* [10]. Other symptoms are:

- Significant weight loss or gain.
- Increase or decrease in appetite nearly every day.
- Insomnia or hypersomnia.
- Psychomotor agitation or retardation.
- Fatigue or anergia.
- Feelings of excessive or inappropriate guilt or worthlessness.
- Lack of concentration.
- Recurrent thoughts of death, suicidal ideation, or a suicide attempt.

When using symptoms to diagnose depression, the symptoms should be different from the patient's previous level of functioning and not due to a general medical condition. Two other depressive disorders may occur in long term care: *depressive disorder due to a medical condition* or *other specified depressive disorder.* Other specified depressive disorders include *recurrent brief depression, short duration depressive episode* (lasts 4–13 days), and *depressive episode with insufficient symptoms* to meet criteria for major depressive disorder [10]. These depressive disorders should be considered when a patient is not thought to be suffering from a major depressive episode. It is necessary to ensure that neither a medical condition nor a medication is the cause of the patient's depressive symptoms as treatment would be aimed at the underlying disease (e.g., hypothyroidism).

The evaluation of depression, as with the evaluation of delirium and dementia, should begin with a history, physical exam and testing guided by the patient's presentation to determine any causative or contributing factors. The investigation should be guided by the goals of care and life expectancy of each patient. For example, in the case of a patient whose life expectancy can be measured in weeks, it may be less important to determine the cause of the depression than it is to treat the depression with therapy that will help relieve symptoms. Careful attention should be given to medication reconciliation and investigating whether the patient recently received any new medications as many medications and some drug–drug interactions may cause or worsen depression. If so, then medication and dose reductions could lessen these effects. Commonly used medications that may cause symptoms of depression include [28]:

- Cardiac medications such as antiarrhythmic or antihypertensive drugs.
- Psychotropic medications such as benzodiazepines or barbiturates.
- Antiseizure medications.
- Steroids.
- GI drugs such as H2 blockers and metoclopramide.
- Opioid analgesics.
- Carbidopa/levodopa.

Laboratory tests that should be considered include: electrolytes, a complete blood count, thyroid function studies, B_{12} and folate levels. If indicated consider medication levels (including, but not limited to antiepileptic drugs, digoxin, lithium, and tricyclic antidepressants). Other investigations may include evaluation for infection (e.g., urinalysis and culture, blood cultures) and an EKG to evaluate for a cardiac ischemia or arrhythmia [4].

Screening Tools

Many different diagnostic and screening tools for depression have been developed and studied. In PA/LTC facilities the Beck Depression Index (BDI), Geriatric Depression Scale (GDS), and the Cornell Scale for Depression in Dementia (CSDD) have been proven useful [38]. A simple screening tool for evaluating depression is SIGECAPS, it is a mnemonic reminder with eight questions (a version of this tool shown in Table 6), which only requires a patient interview. *Five or more positive answers* (indicated in bold) *on SIGECAPS **may** indicate depression.* The GDS-30 is favored by many, consisting of a 30-question interview that evaluates feelings and behaviors of the resident using a "yes/no" format. Scores of 0–10 are considered in the normal range, 11–20 indicates mild depression, and 21–30 severe depression. Use of the GDS-30 is limited because it has a poor predictive value in patients with a MMSE score of 15 or lower. The GDS-15 (see Table 7) is a short form of the GDS-30 that has been reported to be valid in the elderly, but it is thought to still have the same limitation as the GDS-30 in patients with severe cognitive impairment [39].

Table 6 SIGECAPS
mnemonic

S	Are you **S**ad? (**YES**/NO)
I	Do you suffer from **I**nsomnia (**YES**/NO)
G	Do you have feelings of **G**uilt (**YES**/NO)
E	Do you have a lack of **E**nergy (**YES**/NO)
C	Do you have difficulty **C**oncentrating (**YES**/NO)
A	Have you had changes in your **A**ppetite (**YES**/NO)
P	Do you receive **P**leasure from anything in your life (YES/**NO**)
S	Have you had thoughts of **S**uicide (**YES**/NO)

Table 7 Geriatric depression
scale—short form

Choose the best answer for how you have felt over the past week:
1. Are you basically satisfied with your life? YES/**NO**
2. Have you dropped many of your activities and interests? **YES**/NO
3. Do you feel that your life is empty? **YES**/NO
4. Do you often get bored? **YES**/NO
5. Are you in good spirits most of the time? YES/**NO**
6. Are you afraid that something bad is going to happen to you? **YES**/NO
7. Do you feel happy most of the time? YES/**NO**
8. Do you often feel helpless? **YES**/NO
9. Do you prefer to stay at home, rather than going out and doing new things? **YES**/NO
10. Do you feel you have more problems with memory than most? **YES**/NO
11. Do you think it is wonderful to be alive now? YES/**NO**
12. Do you feel pretty worthless the way you are now? **YES**/NO
13. Do you feel full of energy? YES/**NO**
14. Do you feel that your situation is hopeless? **YES**/NO
15. Do you think that most people are better off than you are? **YES**/NO

Answers in **bold** indicate depression. Although differing sensitivities and specificities have been obtained across studies, for clinical purposes a score > 5 points is suggestive of depression and should warrant a follow-up interview. If the patient has a score > 10, they almost always have a depression

The CSDD is a 19-item tool used to assess a wide variety of depressive symptoms in patients with cognitive impairment. Its use has been validated in patients with a wide range of cognition, from intact to severely impaired. The CCDD shortcomings are that information needs to be gathered from interviewing the patient *and* interviewer observations, causing it to not only require more time but also a trained clinician to conduct the assessment [39]. The Mood Questionnaire is a modified version of the PHQ-9 and can be completed in a short amount of time, and can either be answered or conducted by patient interview. The scale of the Mood Questionnaire ranges from 0 to 27 with increasing scores indicating more severe depression. The Mood Questionnaire is easy to use, has a simple format, and good validity in patients with varying degrees of severity in cognitive function [39]. These tools can be selected on a case-by-case basis according to each patient's characteristics and symptoms. SIGECAPS and the GDS include questions that are asked *only of the resident* as opposed to the Cornell Scale that is comprised of questions asked of *both the caregiver and the resident.* SIGECAPS and the GDS are in the public domain and therefore available for use by anyone.

Once a patient has been diagnosed with depression it is important to assess suicide risk. All patients should be questioned about suicidal ideation, a suicide plan, and previous attempts. Caucasian males and elderly men older than 80 have been shown to have the highest risk for completed suicide, followed by males 65–80 years of age. The most important risk factors for suicide are [4]:

- History of a suicide attempt.
- Poor social support.
- Severe depression.
- Psychotic depression.
- Alcoholism.
- Recent loss or bereavement.
- Abuse of sedatives/hypnotics.
- Development of disability.
- Analgesic abuse.

Treatment

Treatment of depression should be aimed at symptom reduction, addressing suicidal thoughts, improving quality of life and function, and preventing relapse with the ultimate goal of remission. However, accomplishing remission can be difficult with one study showing a sustained remission rate of only 30 % after treatment with citalopram [40].

The mainstay of therapy remains psychotherapy and pharmacotherapy. It is important to consider patient characteristics. Psychotherapy may not be helpful in those who have severe cognitive impairment. For patients who have the cognitive ability, cognitive behavioral therapy and learning based therapy have been shown to be useful. Therapy can be provided by a primary care practitioner, social worker, or psychologist [28]. Other non-pharmacologic measures include lessening the institutional appearance of the facility, especially the resident's own space; providing opportunities for meaningful interaction; as well as social, physical, spiritual, and religious activities.

Pharmacotherapy

There are several variables to consider prior to prescribing an antidepressant. These include:

- Characteristics and symptoms of the patient's depression.
- Mode of action of the antidepressant.
- Potential medication side effects.
- Potential drug–disease interactions.
- Concomitant medical and psychiatric illness.

For example, patients with bipolar disorder are at risk for developing manic episodes when placed on *selective serotonin-reuptake inhibitors* (SSRI).

The classes of medications used to treat depression include SSRIs, serotonin-norepinephrine reuptake inhibitors (SNRIs), tricyclic antidepressants, monoamine oxidase inhibitors (MAOIs), bupropion, and mirtazapine. *SSRIs are typically used as first-line therapy* due to ease of use and low side effect profile. In the elderly the most tolerated SSRIs are sertraline, citalopram, and escitalopram with fluoxetine being least desirable due to its long half-life. *Paroxetine is not preferred in the elderly because it is anticholinergic and sedating* [41]. *The side effects of SSRIs* include nausea, dyspepsia, hyponatremia (due to SIADH), and anorexia. *Serotonin syndrome* is not infrequent and typically occurs when a SSRI is used with other medications that increase serotonin levels in the brain (e.g., SNRIs, buspirone, oxycodone, St. John's wort, linezolid). Serotonin syndrome is characterized by fever, confusion, muscle rigidity, tachycardia, hyperreflexia, and agitation. Muscle rigidity and hyperpyrexia can lead to rhabdomyolysis, which can then cause renal failure. Not only does paroxetine have more side effects, but because of its short half-life, when stopped it can precipitate a *discontinuation syndrome* characterized by increased anxiety, agitation, and tachycardia.

SNRIs (e.g., duloxetine) are useful in patients who have coexistent pain, in particular neuropathic pain. Nausea, agitation, insomnia and an increase in diastolic blood pressure are side effects often seen with SNRIs. TCAs are useful for treating depression, but are no longer considered first line due to their higher side effect profile and the cardiac risk for arrhythmias or cardiac arrest in the event of overdose and possibly even at therapeutic blood levels. *The most concerning side effects of*

TCAs are their anticholinergic effects and hypotension. TCAs are contraindicated in patients with cognitive impairment, recent history (<2 weeks) of myocardial infarction, cardiac conduction abnormalities, orthostatic hypotension, narrow angle glaucoma, urinary retention, and benign prostatic hypertrophy. Nortriptyline and desipramine are more desirable TCAs due to less anticholinergic effects [41].

MAOIs are *typically not used in the elderly* due to possible *drug–drug interactions and dietary modifications that make them difficult to use.* Mirtazapine has both serotonergic and noradrenergic properties and may be useful in patients with insomnia and weight loss owing to its side effects of improved appetite and weight gain and nighttime sedation. Bupropion has noradrenergic effects and its benefits include stimulant properties and low risk for sexual side effects. However, *bupropion lowers the seizure threshold and thus should not be used in patients with a seizure disorder* [41].

Attention should be given to the duration of antidepressant treatment as it has implications in the long-term management of depressive episodes. Recurrence is common in the elderly so it is important to consider a longer duration of treatment. The PROSPECT trial demonstrated that geriatric patients benefit from longer treatment. However, it is also important to assure compliance and follow-up with the patient to assess tolerance to the antidepressant. Other studies have found that geriatric patients had a lower mortality rate after more than 4 years of treatment for depression with antidepressants and psychotherapy as compared to those receiving usual care [42]. *Maintenance therapy* should be *considered for patients with one or more episodes of depression and for those at deemed high risk for recurrence.* For a first episode of depression between 6 and 12 months of antidepressant therapy should be given before reassessment that evaluates continued benefit and potential for relapse. *Patients with three or more lifetime episodes of depression should be considered for lifelong antidepressant therapy* [41].

Summary

Dementia, delirium, and depression comprise a diagnostic challenge for the clinician as one, two or all three conditions may occur in the same individual at the same time or separately over time. An understanding of each of these three conditions will assist the practitioner in providing appropriate clinical evaluation, intervention and treatment. Evaluation and treatment should be tailored to the goals of care of each resident, guided by the resident's prognosis, level of functioning, comorbidities, and life expectancy. It is essential that monitoring of response to diagnostic and therapeutic interventions be continued, and to consider consultation with specialists or hospitalization if needed. The patient and family should be involved in decision-making in order to accommodate choice, preferences, and goals of care that evolve or change over time.

Pearls for the Practitioner

Dementia

- Dementia is a chronic, irreversible, progressive condition often with insidious onset.
- There is a high prevalence of dementia as a primary diagnosis in the PA/LTC setting.
- Residents with dementia can exhibit challenging or disruptive behavior, as a natural part of their disease process or unmet needs.
- Remember the potentially reversible causes of dementia and the frequent occurrence of a mixed dementia.

Delirium

- Delirium is a potentially life-threatening condition.
- Hyperactive delirium is more easily recognizable than hypoactive delirium.
- Interventions to prevent delirium have been shown to be effective.
- Be aware that many medications and acute medical conditions can precipitate delirium in frail older adults.

Depression

- The prevalence of a depressive disorder or depressive symptoms in the long-term care population has been estimated to be as high as 70 %.
- Depression is not an inevitable consequence of aging.
- Depression frequently occurs in the setting of the other medical conditions.
- Several commonly used medications can cause symptoms of depression, even antidepressants.

Websites

1. Alzheimer's Association, www.alz.org.
2. American Geriatrics Society, www.americangeriatrics.org.
3. American Medical Directors Association for their Clinical Practice Guidelines, www.amda.com.
4. Hospitalized Elder Life Program for information on delirium, www.elderlife. med.yale.edu.
5. Folstein Mini Mental Status Exam (MMSE), the official form has been copyrighted and must be purchased from www.minimental.com.
6. St. Louis University Mental Status Exam (SLUMS) is available at: http://med-school.slu.edu/agingsuccessfully/pdfsurveys/slumsexam_05.pdf.
7. St. Louis University Geriatrics www.aging/SLU.edu.

References

1. Gagliardi JP. Differentiating among depression, delirium, and dementia in elderly patients. Virtual Mentor. 2008;10(6):383–8.
2. National Nursing Home Survey 2004. Centers for Disease Control. 2009. http://www.cdc.gov/nchs/data/series/sr_13/sr13_167.pdf. Accessed 9 Jan 2010.
3. Rosenblatt A. The art of managing dementia in the elderly. Cleve Clin J Med. 2005;72 Suppl 3:S3–13.
4. Hazzard WR, Blass JP, Halter JB, Ouslander JG, Tinetti ME. Principles of geriatric medicine & gerontology. 5th ed. New York: McGraw-Hill; 2003.
5. Blackwell T, Yaffe K, Laffan A, et al. Associations between sleep-disordered breathing, nocturnal hypoxemia, and subsequent cognitive decline in older community-dwelling men: the osteoporotic fractures in men sleep study. J Am Geriatr Soc. 2015;63(3):453–61.
6. Turner M, Moran N, Kopelman M. Subcortical dementia. Br J Psychiatry. 2002;180:148–51.
7. American Medical Directors Association. Dementia in the long term care setting clinical practice guideline. Columbia, MD: AMDA; 2009.
8. American Psychiatric Association. Diagnostic and statistical manual of mental disorders. 5th ed. Arlington, VA: American Psychiatric Association; 2013.
9. Donaghy PC, McKeith IG. The clinical characteristics of dementia with Lewy bodies and a consideration of prodromal diagnosis. Alzheimer's Res Ther. 2014;6(4):46.
10. Kim MO, Geschwind MD. Clinical update of Jakob-Creutzfeldt disease. Curr Opin Neurol. 2015;28(3):302–10.
11. Carney RM, Freedland KE. Depression, mortality, and medical morbidity in patients with coronary heart disease. Biol Psychiatry. 2003;54:241–7.
12. Santiago LM, Mattos IE. Depressive symptoms in institutionalized older adults. Rev Saude Publica. 2014;48(2):216–24.
13. Hogan DB. Long-term efficacy and toxicity of cholinesterase inhibitors in the treatment of Alzheimer's disease. Can J Psychiatry. 2014;59(12):618–23.
14. Kurz A, Grimmer T. Efficacy of menantine hydrochloride once-daily in Alzheimer's disease. Expert Opin Pharmacother. 2014;15(13):1955–60.
15. Buhr GW, White HK. Difficult behaviors in long-term care patients with dementia. J Am Med Dir Assoc. 2007;8:E.101–13.
16. Doshi JA, Shaffer T, Briesacher BA. National estimates of medication use in nursing homes: findings from the 1997 Medicare beneficiary survey and the 1996 medical expenditure survey. J Am Geriatr Soc. 2005;53:438–43.
17. Zhang QH, Sheng ZY, Yao YM. Septic encephalopathy: when cytokines interact with acetylcholine in the brain. Mil Med Res. 2014;1:20.
18. Choi SH, Lee H, Chung TS, et al. Neural network functional connectivity during and after an episode of delirium. Am J Psychiatr. 2012;169(5):498–507.
19. Conner KQ, Copeland VC, Grote NK, et al. Mental health treatment seeking among older adults with depression: the impact of stigma and race. Am J Geriatr Psychiatry. 2010;18(6):531–43.
20. American Medical Directors Association. Delirium and acute problematic behavior in the long-term care setting clinical practice guideline. Columbia, MD: AMDA; 2008.
21. Inouye SK. Delirium in older persons. N Engl J Med. 2006;354:1157–65.
22. Fick DM, Agostini JV, Inouye SK. Delirium superimposed on dementia: a systematic review. J Am Geriatr Soc. 2002;50:1723–32.
23. Ozbolt LB, Paniagua MA, Kaiser RM. Atypical antipsychotics for the treatment of delirious elders. J Am Med Dir Assoc. 2008;9:18–28.
24. Elie M, Cole MG, Primeau FJ, Bellavance F. Delirium risk factors in elderly hospitalized patients. J Gen Intern Med. 1998;13:204–12.
25. Fong TG, Tulebaev SR, Inouye SK. Delirium in elderly adults: diagnosis; prevention and treatment. Nat Rev Neurol. 2009;5:210–20.

26. Marcantonio ER, Ngo LH, O'Connor M, et al. 3D-CAM: derivation and validation of a 3-minute diagnostic interview for CAM-defined delirium: a cross-sectional diagnostic test study. Ann Intern Med. 2014;161(8):354–61.
27. Seitz D, Purandare N, Conn D. Prevalence of psychiatric disorders among older adults in long-term care homes: a systematic review. Int Psychogeriatr. 2010;22(7):1025–39.
28. American Medical Directors Association. Depression clinical practice guideline. Columbia, MD: AMDA; 2003.
29. World Health Organization. Depression. http://www.who.int/mental_health/management/depression/wfmh_paper_depression_wmhd_2012.pdf?ua=1.
30. Barry LC, Murphy TE, Gill TM. Depressive symptoms and functional transitions over time in older persons. Am J Geriatr Psychiatry. 2011;19:789–91.
31. Alexopoulos GS, Buckwalter K, Olin J, et al. Comorbidity of late life depression: an opportunity for research on mechanisms and treatment. Biol Psychiatry. 2002;52:543–8.
32. Cepoiu M, McCusker J, Cole MG, et al. Recognition of depression in older inpatients. J Gen Intern Med. 2007;22:559–64.
33. Jeste DV, Blazer DG, First M. Aging-related diagnostic variations: need for diagnostic criteria appropriate for elderly psychiatric patients. Biol Psychiatry. 2005;58:265–71.
34. Rothschild AJ. The diagnosis and treatment of late-life depression. J Clin Psychiatry. 1996; 57(Suppl5):5–11.
35. Alexopoulos GS. Depression in the elderly. Lancet. 2005;365(9475):1961–70.
36. Peskind ER. Management of depression in long-term care of patients with Alzheimer's disease. J Am Med Dir Assoc. 2003;1(Supp Nov/Dec):S141–5.
37. Vilalta-Franch J, Lopez-Pousa S, Llinas-Regla J, Calvo-Perxas L, Merino-Aguado J. Depression subtypes and 5-year risk of dementia and Alzheimer disease in patients aged 70 years. Int J Geriatr Psychiatry. 2013;28(4):341–50.
38. Koopmans RTCM, Zuidema SU, Leontjevas R, Gerritsen DL. Review: comprehensive assessment of depression and behavioral problems in long-term care. Int Psychogeriatr. 2010;22(7): 1054–62.
39. Anna Azulai, Christine A Walsh. Screening for geriatric depression in residential care facilities: a systematic narrative review. J Gerontol Social Work. 2014.
40. Zisook S, Ganadijan K, Moutier C, et al. Sequenced Treatment Alternatives to Relieve Depression (STAR*D): lessons learned. J Clin Psychiatry. 2008;69:1184–5.
41. Rojas-Fernandez C, Mikhail M. Contemporary concepts in the pharmacotherapy of depression in older people. Can Pharm J (Ott). 2012;145(3):128–35.
42. Gallo JJ, Bogner HR, Morales KH, et al. The effect of primary care practice-based depression intervention on mortality in older adults: a randomized trial. Ann Intern Med. 2007;146: 689–98.

Ethical and Legal Issues

David A. Smith and Randall D. Huss

Introduction

Ethical and legal issues are common in long-term care and are separate, but closely interrelated. Health care ethics is the application of *values* (patient, caregiver and societal) to the process of clinical decision-making. This process requires the intellectual and empathetic weighing of values, facts and prognostications in order to produce a supportable decision. Clinicians often encounter competing values, e.g., *the right of self-determination of an individual versus the interests of society as a whole, and must take into consideration the facts, as well as the likelihood and consequences of various outcomes.*

The *law* is a society's compilation of rules, which are intended to be uniformly applied (equal protection under the law), mandatory (ignorance of the law is no excuse), and modifiable only through the legislative process. Fortunately, the tenants of health care ethics have not been ignored in the process of evolution of the law as it interfaces with clinical medicine.

There is no shortage of challenges for the long-term care practitioner in applying health care ethics within the tenets of existing state and federal law. It should be noted that all state and federal survey long-term care facility regulations are dictated by law. Clinicians are admonished to know the laws of their jurisdiction and to seek legal counsel when needed. The contents of this chapter are educational only and not formal legal advice.

D.A. Smith, MD, FAAFP, CMD (✉)
Geriatric Consultants of Central Texas, Brownwood, TX 76801, USA
e-mail: geriatricconsult@aol.com

R.D. Huss, MD, CMD
Department of Family Medicine and Geriatrics, Mercy Clinic,
1605 Martin Springs Drive, Suite 360b, Rolla, MO 65401, USA
e-mail: randall.huss@mercy.net

© Springer International Publishing Switzerland 2016
P.A. Fenstemacher, P. Winn (eds.), *Post-Acute and Long-Term Medicine*,
Current Clinical Practice, DOI 10.1007/978-3-319-16979-8_15

Principles of Health Care Ethics

The principles of health care ethics include *autonomy, beneficence, justice, non-maleficence*, and *fidelity*. These principles do not stand alone or in a hierarchy, but must be considered in the context of each other. Frequently, different aspects of each ethical principle compete. Within the framework of the law an ethical judgment must be made by considering one of the ethical principles more strongly.

Autonomy is the principle attesting to an individual's right to sovereignty over oneself. It encompasses the right to self-determination and privacy. The law recognizes the right to privacy in statutes that codify the privacy of medical records such as the Health Insurance Portability and Accountability Act (HIPAA), informed consent, and the individual's right to decline life-sustaining treatment. Competency and mental capacity issues may alter the principle of autonomy.

Beneficence is the principle that holds a caregiver responsible to do good for others. Good Samaritan laws are designed to protect individuals when they act by this principle. Similarly, laws that require health care professionals to report suspected elder abuse is an example of this principle. Laws related to guardianship and other forms of surrogate decision-making for those adjudicated incompetent by a judge in a court of law or clinically determined not to have mental capacity derive from the principle of beneficence.

Non-maleficence, a corollary to beneficence, holds that it is the responsibility of the caregiver to do no harm. Avoiding unnecessary surgery and optimizing patient safety are examples. Laws regarding medical malpractice are based on this principle and claims for punitive damages stem from what plaintiffs perceive as breaches of this principle.

Justice is the principle espousing the responsibility of the medical professional to treat a patient fairly, to treat all patients equally and to consider not only one's patient but also the good of society in medical decision-making. This principle is applied when a physician assists with terminating the driving privileges of an unsafe driver.

Finally, *fidelity, a corollary to the principle of justice*, involves the medical professional's responsibility to keep the terms of the "doctor/patient contract." Truthfulness and substantial compliance with informed consent are components of fidelity as is *non-abandonment*. A medical professional should not summarily cease to act for the benefit of one's patient even when that patient has not lived up to their side of the doctor/patient contract (e.g., noncompliance) or exerted their autonomy and chosen a course of medical action with which the physician disagrees. The physician should attempt to provide the best possible outcome in the context of the patient's noncompliance and their treatment choices. Alternatively, the medical professional may exit the doctor/patient contract by providing emergency care as needed, while affording the patient sufficient time to become established with another health care professional.

Historically, until the middle of the twentieth century, physicians often made such decisions for their patients as they exercised the principle of beneficence without an appreciation of patient autonomy, which is paternalism. Society's response was a consumerism movement, including a Patient's Bill of Rights. While this was needed, it potentially elevated autonomy above other ethical principles. Today we must recognize that the principles of autonomy, beneficence and justice all be considered with equal weight as we formulate an ethical decision. For example, autonomy and the right to privacy would be subordinate to the principles of beneficence and justice in the case of an individual with chronic active hepatitis B who willingly refuses to follow guidelines to prevent the transmission of the disease to others. Conversely, beneficence and justice (the state's interest in protecting life) would be subordinate to autonomy when a capacitated adult Jehovah's Witness declines a life saving blood transfusion. However, if a patient were a child below the age of consent, the state's interest in protecting life would prevail.

The vast majority of applications of these principles are not played out in the legal arena, but in everyday medical decision-making. The practice of medicine within the long-term care continuum commonly involves issues related to diminished mental capacity and mental illness, treatments with narrow risk/benefit ratios, end-of-life care, potential for elder abuse and exploitation, and high utilization of limited and expensive medical resources. Practicing in long-term care challenges every practitioner to hold these principles dear and competently apply them with skill and confidence. Input from others on the interdisciplinary team and from the family is essential when applying these principles and choosing the most appropriate course of action. Finally, every practitioner must be able to communicate and balance these principles as they apply to the specifics of the clinical scenario at hand and to succinctly record his/her reasoning in the medical record.

Common Areas of Concern

Resident Rights

When an individual enters into any facility or program within the long-term care continuum they do not lose their fundamental rights. Providers have an obligation to inform residents of their rights and to encourage or assist them in exercising those rights. It is illegal for a facility, program or any employee to infringe upon an elder's human rights by threatening, coercing, intimidating or retaliating against an elder who is exercising their rights. A facility or program should educate elders on how to use their complaint process if they ever feel their human rights are violated. Specific responsibilities of long-term care institutions are described in the Abuse, Neglect, and Exploitation section of this chapter. Resident rights are delineated in state and federal regulations for nursing facilities as detailed in Table 1 [1].

A resident's rights may only be restricted when it is necessary to protect the resident or another individual from potential harm, or to protect the rights of another resident, e.g., infringements on another's privacy. Facility rules that have been fully disclosed before admission, such as scheduled smoking breaks or a nonsmoking policy, can only be enforced if the resident or their legally recognized surrogate has agreed to these rules as a condition of admission. Furthermore, problem behaviors may be addressed by providers through behavior modification programming or behavioral contracting with the resident, or even as a condition of continued residence in the facility if done as part of a therapeutic plan of care and in keeping with nursing facility regulations. A resident with mental incapacity still retains all of the human rights outlined in Table 1. However if an individual lacks capacity, their rights are both advocated for and managed by the legally designated surrogate decision-maker. For instance, a mentally incapacitated resident with diabetes mellitus who wants to spend all of their money on candy and soda may be care planned to receive budgeted amounts of spending money from their facility account and be supervised in spending this on diabetic snacks and sugar-free soft drinks, if the care plan is agreed upon by their surrogate decision-maker. Providers and practitioners should note that litigation alleging infringement on human rights might not be covered by medical malpractice insurance.

Elder Abuse, Neglect, and Exploitation

Residents within the long-term care continuum represent a population vulnerable to abuse, neglect, and exploitation by a family member, another person, a member of the health care team or even an institution. Abuse, neglect, and exploitation may be purposeful or due to inadequate knowledge and/or training.

Abuse is an act of commission intended to do harm. Abuse can be physical, sexual, or emotional in nature. Many episodes of physical and emotional abuse are sporadic and occur as an unguarded response to an elderly, demented, or mentally ill person's behavior toward the caregiver. Resistive, combative, and assaultive behaviors by the resident may trigger retaliation if the caregiver fails to understand the behavior as part of the disease process. Caregivers are more likely to be abusive if they lack knowledge of alternative behavioral approaches or become overly obsessed with completion of care giving tasks (feeding, bathing, etc.). Unresolved stress, depression, and cultural acceptance of violent punishment increase the chance that a caregiver will be abusive. Abusive caregivers are also more likely to have been abused by their now elderly parent.

Neglect is an act of omission, the failure to meet one's obligation to anticipate and meet the needs of a vulnerable elderly person. Elders who have not yet been recognized as mentally incapacitated may be neglectful of themselves, refusing assistance, living in squalor, and not attending to their health, hygiene, or safety (a common situation in Adult Protective Services). Neglect may be purposeful or retaliatory. When the elder shows no gratitude or is critical of the care they receive neglect is more frequently seen. But more often, neglect is the result of inadequate understanding and anticipation of a vulnerable elder's needs. Poor knowledge and training on the specifics of care giving of a vulnerable elder, inadequate care planning to delineate anticipated needs, lack of "job ownership," unprofessional

Table 1 Statement of resident rights

You have a right to:
1. All care necessary for you to have the highest possible level of health;
2. Safe, decent and clean conditions;
3. Be free of abuse and exploitation;
4. Be treated with courtesy, consideration, and respect;
5. Be free from discrimination based on age, race, religion, sex, nationality, or disability and to practice your own religious beliefs;
6. Privacy, including privacy during visits and telephone calls;
7. Complain about the facility and to organize or participate in any program that presents residents' concerns to the administrator of the facility;
8. Have facility information about you maintained as confidential;
9. Retain the services of a physician of your choice, at your own expense or through a health care plan, and to have a physician explain to you, in language you understand, your complete medical condition, the recommended treatment, and the expected results of the treatment, including reasonably expected effects, side effects, and risks associated with psychoactive medications;
10. Participate in developing a plan of care, to refuse treatment, and to refuse to participate in experimental research;
11. A written statement or admission agreement describing the services provided by the facility and the related charges;
12. Manage your own finances or to delegate the responsibility to another person;
13. Access money and property you have deposited with the facility and to an accounting of your money and property that are deposited with the facility and of all financial transactions made with or on behalf of you;
14. Keep and use personal property, secure from theft or loss;
15. Not be relocated within the facility, except in accordance with nursing facility regulations;
16. Receive visitors;
17. Receive unopened mail and to receive assistance in reading or writing correspondence;
18. Participate in activities inside and outside the facility;
19. Wear your own clothes;
20. Discharge yourself from the facility unless you have been adjudicated mentally incompetent;
21. Not be discharged from the facility, except as provided in the nursing facility regulations;
22. Be free from any physical or chemical restraints imposed for the purposes of discipline or convenience and not required to treat your medical symptoms;
23. Receive information about prescribed psychoactive medication from the person who prescribed the medication or that person's designee, to have any psychoactive medications prescribed and administered in a responsible manner, as mandated by the Health and Safety Code, § 242.505, and to refuse to consent to the prescription of psychoactive medications; and
24. Place an electronic monitoring device in your room that is owned and operated by you or provided by your guardian or legal representative

attitudes, and low motivation of caregivers are all potential risk factors for neglect. Elders with burdensome needs due to morbid obesity or elders who are slow assisted feeders have been shown to be at increased risk for neglect as well. Neglect often occurs when caregivers fail to recognize that an elderly individual's disability is progressing and they now have increased care needs. Changes in the plan of care should not wait for a quarterly facility care plan update, but should occur when a change of resident condition is recognized.

Neglect may also occur at the institutional level due to understaffing, or as a result of inadequate supervision, orientation, or training. Poor work group cohesion, excessive staff turnover, and inadequate resources may also lead to institutional neglect.

Exploitation refers to acts of misappropriation of a vulnerable elder's money or property. This is not necessarily for the purpose of enriching the perpetrator. For example, two daughters have their mother's best interest in mind as they hurriedly sell their mentally capacitated mother's home and furnishing while she is in a nursing facility recuperating from a surgery. They sell the house to prevent their mother from returning home to live alone, because they feel she will be unsafe. More often, however, exploitation is overt fraud or theft. Misappropriating an elder's pension and Social Security checks for their own use, and illegal transfers of property without proper consent are the types of exploitation most commonly perpetrated by families. Nursing home staff taking a resident's property or medications is the type of exploitation commonly perpetrated by facility staff. Occasionally, guardians and those designated as Power of Attorney may exploit the elderly they are supposed to protect. Although Courts require yearly reports from guardians in order to discourage exploitation, no such oversight is required for persons with other forms of surrogate decision-making. The practitioner in long-term care should be alert to evidence of exploitation and report concerns to the appropriate authority. Consider the situation of an aged and non-ambulatory resident with schizophrenia who wanted to buy a thermos to keep coffee in his room. When the facility's social worker was asked if the resident could purchase the thermos, they indicated that the resident would have a small amount of spending money left over from his Social Security check after the nursing home payment. When, 1 month later, the resident did not have a thermos, the physician discovered the resident's family routinely pocketed all his spending money. The state government agency for nursing home surveys is typically the authority to investigate abuse of a nursing home resident by facility staff or a family member. Adult Protective Services is the appropriate authority to investigate abuse, neglect, or exploitation of an individual who lives in the community.

Abuse, neglect, and exploitation perpetrated by a family member, unpaid caregiver, or other private individual are usually resolved without bringing criminal charges. In contrast, abuse, neglect, and exploitation by an institution or a certified or licensed caregiver within the long-term care continuum, are handled by the formal survey process, and increasingly by licensure procedures and even criminalization. The Centers for Medicare and Medicaid Services State Operations Manual requires nursing facilities to make efforts at abuse prevention by:

- Having abuse prevention policies and procedures.
- Screening potential employees to be hired.
- Providing initial and ongoing training on elder abuse.

- Making an effort to identify potential abuse events including setting expectations among staff for reporting.
- Investigating alleged abuse events and incidents that might constitute abuse.
- Protecting residents from retaliation or distress during investigations.
- Reporting incidents, alleged abuse events, investigations, and facility actions in response to investigations as required by state and federal authority.

Mental Capacity, Competence, and Options for Surrogate Decision-Making

All adults are considered mentally competent by law unless adjudicated otherwise. A court makes a competency or incompetency designation. Physicians and other providers, as recognized by individual state law, may make a determination of an individual's mental *capacity* or *incapacity*. This may be partial or complete and it may be specific to a particular circumstance. Capacity, then, is somewhat decision related. Similarly, incapacity may be permanent as in dementia, or temporary as in delirium or intoxication. While often used interchangeably, *competency is a legal determination and mental capacity is a clinical one.*

There are several distinct types of competency under the law. A person is competent to stand trial for a crime if they know the difference between right and wrong and are able to participate in their own defense. Different criteria exist for competency to make or change a will; this is referred to as *testamentary capacity*. When changing a will, a person is considered competent if they know the nature/extent of their property; know the natural objects of their bounty (heirs); the disposition that their will is making; and the implications of this plan of distribution. Additionally, they must be free of undue influence or coercion.

Practitioners are rarely asked to opine on mental capacity as it relates to competence to stand trial, though in cases of resident-to-resident physical or sexual assault this may occur. More often practitioners are asked to evaluate mental capacity as it relates to testamentary capacity. When this is likely to be contested, the practitioner may wish to perform the capacity evaluation on videotape with the appropriate consents, or in a lawyer's office with full transcription. Asking questions that relate to criteria for testamentary capacity as well as performing a standard test of cognition, are both helpful when determining capacity.

Mental capacity assessment is often needed in long-term care practice to determine an elder's ability to make decisions in their own best interest of a personal, medical and financial nature. Often an adult child is listed as the "*Responsible Party*" on the nursing facility demographic face sheet and delegated to make decisions without any formal authority, and no attempt is made to determine whether the resident is partially or fully able to make their own decisions. This practice runs contrary to the ethical principle of autonomy and exemplifies ageism. Indeed, cases have occurred where a mentally capacitated individual has been kept in nursing home care against their will through the combined efforts of the facility, attending physician, and family.

Conversely, there are nursing or assisted living facilities, which list the resident as the "Responsible Party" even though the resident is moderately or severely demented, psychotic, or neuropsychiatrically impaired, and clearly do not have decisional capacity. This usually occurs when the resident has no close family or proxy legal representative.

When an elder is found to be mentally incapacitated and is facing a situation requiring an informed decision, the practitioner must consider all the surrogate decision-making options. In all situations of surrogate decision-making, look for documents such as living wills or advance care directives, or any individuals that can provide a "substituted judgment" for what the individual would have decided if he or she were able to express an informed decision. Any surrogate decision-maker is always expected to act in that individual's best interest.

In many states, statutes exist listing a hierarchy of family decision-making usually beginning with the spouse, then the oldest adult child and so forth, who assume the decision-making role without need for a more involved legal process. Clinicians simply make a determination of temporary or permanent mental incapacity in the medical record, and then contact the family member highest on the list who is both capable and willing to undertake surrogate decision-making. Should a clinician initially or subsequently believe that this individual is not acting in the best interest of the patient, then the clinician should challenge their surrogate decision-making status by submitting a report to Adult Protective Services or perhaps to the court as appropriate to that jurisdiction and circumstance.

Other forms of surrogate decision-making include *Power of Attorney* and *conservatorships*. The latter typically deals only with financial matters while Powers of Attorney may be designated as to decision-making related to "person" or "estate" or both.

- A **General Power of Attorney** is a legal instrument by which a mentally capacitated (presumed competent) person chooses another to make decisions on their behalf commencing from the time the instrument is executed and *endures until either death or a future time of mental incapacity*. These instruments may convey broad powers or may be very specific, e.g., to complete a real estate transaction.
- A **Springing Power of Attorney** may be made by a mentally capacitated person to give their chosen surrogate decision-making powers *at some future time when the person may become mentally incapacitated*.
- A **Durable Power of Attorney** *goes into effect at execution* (if agreed to by the capacitated person) and continues to grant surrogate decision-making power to the chosen person *beyond the occurrence of mental incapacity* of the person who established the power of attorney.

Long-term care providers should remain alert to the circumstance under which a family and lawyer draw up a Power of Attorney and encourage a mentally incapacitated person to sign it. Only *a person who has mental capacity can execute a Power of Attorney*. Once a person is mentally incapacitated a Power of Attorney cannot be created and another form of surrogate decision-making must be established, such as a *guardianship*.

Guardianship. This may be temporary or permanent. A physician will often be asked to provide an opinion on an elder's mental incapacity (in part or total) stating the reason for incapacity and elaborating on any medical condition and medications that might affect the elder's mental status. This is typically done on a standardized legal form and submitted to the court. Upon making a ruling of incompetence, the court will name a guardian for surrogate decision-making. The guardianship for surrogate decision-making has limitations. For example, in some jurisdictions a guardian may not sign consent for admission to inpatient psychiatric care, sign a DNR, or authorize withdrawal of life sustaining treatment. Such medical decisions may require separate court action, which differs from state to state. In most states a surrogate decision-maker cannot give permission for the nursing facility to hide antipsychotic medication in food, give it by force, or by injection on a routine basis. Even a severely demented or mentally ill person who has objected to taking the medication cannot be forced or tricked into taking the medication. This usually does not apply to the treatment of a psychiatric emergency in which the behavior puts the patient at imminent danger to self or others. In some states, the need for psychiatric treatment is sufficient to seek a forced medication order but in others the standard of danger or imminent danger to self or others must be met.

In decision-making, the guardian should attempt to represent resident/patient choices that follow existing advanced directives. If no such directives exist then the guardian should make a best effort to make choices on behalf of their ward, which are consistent with the historical value system, culture, and life history of the ward. When partial capacity exists, the wishes of the ward should be respected for those decisions for which they have the capacity to make. When totally incapacitated, the guardian and caregivers should still attempt to ascertain the resident/patient opinions on different choices, especially when the probable outcomes of various choices are likely inconsequential. Wherever possible *assent* should be solicited even when *consent* cannot.

Evaluation of Capacity

When undertaking a capacity evaluation the practitioner must maintain a high level of intellectual honesty. An elder's capacity is challenged when they make a decision that others do not agree. Obviously, this cannot be a stand-alone criterion. Similarly, neither can the level of cognitive impairment be a sole criterion. Capacity is less an issue when various choices differ little in their risk and benefit. Of note, *lifelong poor judgment does not necessarily indicate mental incapacity. People have a right to make mistakes, and some exercise this right again and again. However, poor judgment resulting from disease of the central nervous system and representing a decline from prior intellectual functioning is noteworthy evidence of mental incapacity.*

A capacity evaluation should include a formal mental status examination (Table 2). This includes testing of judgment, orientation (time, person, place), memory (recent and remote), and the ability to think in the abstract, as well as do calculations. Formal mental status testing such as with the *Mini Mental Status Examination* (MMSE) or the *Saint Louis University Mental Status Exam* (SLUMS) evaluates memory and orientation as well as other domains of cognition.

Judgment can be tested with hypothetical scenarios such as requesting a solution to the problem, "What would you do if you were the first person in a crowded movie theater to discover that it was on fire?" Answers not recognizing the need to avoid causing a panic would indicate faulty judgment. If the need for a specific and important decision has induced the evaluation, the clinician may specifically explore the individual's ability to explain the nature of the decision at hand, the individual's thoughts on the personal ramifications of various choices and their assessment of the risks and benefits. An individual with capacity should also be able to articulate how they have come to a decision, what factors were important to them, and what values or principles they applied to come to the decision. The clinician must make allowances if hearing or eyesight interfere with the individual's grasp of the issues at hand.

Adequate *judgment* also involves the *ability to negotiate*. A capacitated individual should be able to negotiate in their best interest, unless the issue at hand is related to one of their fundamental human or religious values. Thus, an individual who declines a blood transfusion because they are a Jehovah's Witness can be capacitated but still unwilling to negotiate on this issue in any way. An elder with a compelling need to be admitted to long-term care who absolutely refuses to discuss the matter and insists that her daughter will meet her needs (housekeeping, medical care and personal assistance), even though the daughter has categorically stated she cannot, would fail to meet this test of mental capacity. Sometimes, if the potential medical consequences are not too high a dilemma may best be handled by allowing the elder to experience the consequences of their decision. *Self-neglect* by the elder should be recognized and would support a determination of mental incapacity.

The *ability to think in the abstract* can be evaluated by asking the individual to explain the "underlying or poetic" meaning of a proverb. The proverb should be one with which the individual is likely familiar. A concrete (non-abstract) answer may indicate low IQ, low educational level or an organic impairment of the brain.

Ability to calculate can be tested by requesting the individual to subtract 7 serially from 100. When specific to decisions at hand, a value comparison of certain assets may be helpful, e.g., "Which is worth more-your farm or your antique car?"

A dysfunctional family such as an "enmeshed" family is at increased risk for placing undue influence or coercion on an elder family member. However, practitioners should also be aware that in certain cultures the opinion of a family leader or a family consensus is the accepted norm for decision-making and would not be considered undue influence or coercion.

Mental illness, e.g., depression and psychosis, often are the basis of a finding of mental incapacity. However, decisions that conform to the individual's historical

Table 2 Elements of a
mental capacity evaluation

• Mental Status Testing (JOMAC)
– Judgment
– Orientation (time, person, place)
– Memory (recent, remote)
– Ability to think in the abstract
– Ability to calculate
• Ability to explain the nature of the needed decision at hand
• Ability to explain personal implications of choices, understand risks/benefits
• Ability to explain the rationale for choices
• Ability to explain how their decision best matches their personal goals
• Ability to persist in a decision unless new facts or circumstances arise
• Ability to negotiate (unless the issue at hand is a core value)
• Evaluate for undue influence or coercion
• Consider the effect of mental illness on decision-making

value system, culture and life history prior to the onset of mental illness may well be capacitated decisions. Additionally, the reasoning underlying a decision should be examined such that choices made as a result of the individual's mental illness may be incapacitated while others may be capacitated. A patient with paranoid schizophrenia who while scowling at the examiner refuses evaluation and treatment of a breast mass "because it's probably nothing," probably lacks capacity. Or a patient with suicidal depression who declines electroconvulsive therapy because "it won't do any good" or because "I don't deserve to feel better" is likely incapacitated, while a similar patient who declines because "I'm scared I'll have memory loss, you told me ECT can cause that" is likely capacitated.

Dementia does not automatically imply mental incapacity. Determination of mental capacity depends on the severity of cognitive loss, the domains affected by cognitive loss, the kind and complexity of the issues at hand, and the potential consequences of the decision. The level of cognition is important to the determination of capacity. Marson, Ingram, and Cody showed that most participants with Alzheimer's disease had capacity to make and communicate choices, consequences of choices and their rationale for choices if they had a MMSE score of 19 or greater [2]. The clinician should not use a MMSE score as a sole criterion when determining capacity. Standardized, structured capacity evaluations such as the *MacArthur Capacity Assessment Test* are available, but they are not designed to determine if an elder is capacitated at a certain score [3].

End-of-Life Issues

Residents of long-term care facilities often have a limited life expectancy. Thus end-of-life issues are common for clinicians working in post-acute and long-term care. It has become a federal mandate upon admission to a hospital or a long-term care facility to inquire whether a patient has made an *advance directive*, though the law does not require the patient to have one. Persons without a known advance directive in emergencies are presumed to have elected to pursue life-saving and life-sustaining treatment. In some states, persons with an advance directive that includes a decision of "Do Not Resuscitate" (DNR) are presumed to have verbally withdrawn their DNR if they call for an ambulance. Should a person wish to have such an advance directive for DNR continue to be respected, they may need to exercise a second advance directive such as an *Out-of-Hospital DNR*.

Any advance directives should be routinely and compassionately reviewed on admission to the hospital or a long-term care facility. Crisis driven prerogatives by caregivers for a patient to create an advance directive, should be viewed with apprehension that there may be other motives than the caregiver's desire to follow the wishes of the patient.

An Advance Directive for health care may take the form of a *Living Will*. Springing and Durable Powers of Attorney are also forms of advance directives, but these involve use of a proxy decision-maker. The Living Will is a document outlining the general and/or specific wishes of a capacitated individual (or previously capacitated person) for various health care procedures and strategies to be (or not be) carried out irrespective of their future mental capacity. If a capacitated person has a known, potentially fatal medical condition it is wise to construct a Living Will that mentions the person's wishes concerning any clinical circumstances that are likely to occur given the natural history of their terminal disease. As most Living Wills lack sufficient detail to speak directly to a specific disease or an actual clinical circumstance, Living Wills often leave room for doubt and controversy. However, they can provide a general framework that is useful to family as a guideline for that person's substituted judgment in the specific situation. This may lessen discord among family members and relieve potential guilt.

Note that a Living Will may state a person's wishes to receive aggressive treatment such as cardiopulmonary resuscitation (CPR), use a respirator or feeding tube, etc. though this is seldom seen.

Areas of concern not usually addressed by Living Wills but that should be considered by the individual completing a Living Will include:

- Whether the individual wishes or declines to give a Power of Attorney the prerogative to consent for them to enter into research.
- Whether they wish to be an organ donor.
- Whether they wish to accept or decline psychotropic drug treatments by class and accept/decline electroconvulsive treatment.
- Whether they wish to be allowed to enter into an emotional, physical, or sexual relationship with another person when they demonstrate assent.

- Whether they wish to continue to have a physical relationship with their spouse when they demonstrate assent. The practitioner should be aware that some state surveyors and caregivers (both formal and informal) believe that once mentally incapacitated, an individual can no longer consent to be intimate with their spouse.

The wishes expressed by an individual in their Living Will or by their surrogate, however, *do not* oblige the practitioner to perform *futile care*. The American Medical Association defines futile care as medical treatment that has very little or no potential for benefit. Practitioners may not recognize this obligation to avoid futile medical care. Offering futile care (e.g., CPR in an unwitnessed cardiopulmonary arrest in the nursing home or feeding tube placement in a patient with end stage dementia), as if it were a reasonable treatment option breaches the ethical principles of beneficence, non-maleficence, and fidelity. Offering futile care can make the family that declines care feel guilty that they are not doing enough. It may be prudent to educate families about futile medical treatments and discuss them as such.

There is no ethical difference between withholding a treatment and withdrawing it at such time as it becomes apparent that it is futile. For instance, placing a person on a respirator when in acute respiratory failure does not oblige one to continue artificial ventilation when it is evident that the patient has intractable adult respiratory distress syndrome.

End-of-life issues include controversial subjects such as *active euthanasia* and *physician-assisted suicide*. The AMA and AMDA have both spoken about these and other end-of-life issues. The reader is referred to policy statements and white papers stating the collective wisdom of these professional organizations [4, 5].

Ethical and Legal Aspects of Research in Long-Term Care

Given the unresolved issues in long-term care, the value of research cannot be understated. Studies rarely focus on the long-term care population because the potential research subjects have many confounding diseases and conditions, and are at risk to drop out of a study due to unexpected death or intervening multimorbidities. They are also considered a "vulnerable population" with a higher than usual ethical and legal standard for informed consent before participating in research.

The high prevalence of cognitive impairment in the long-term care population makes this population vulnerable to abuse in recruitment for research. The protections and processes required for the ethical and legal recruitment of incapacitated persons does allow for a legally recognized surrogate decision-maker to consent on behalf of the incapacitated person to be a research subject. However, an elder who in any way demonstrates lack of assent to the research should be either not enrolled or withdrawn. Further information on the ethical and legal aspects of research in vulnerable populations is reviewed in ref. 6.

Liability in Long-Term Care

A discussion of liability issues is crucial to practitioners and also germane to patient access, delivery of care, and care transitions. An American Medical Directors Association survey in 2005 on attitudes and responses to the risk of litigation indicated that more than half of the respondents had in some way limited their work as a medical director to avoid risk. Some 38 % had limited their long-term care patient numbers as an attending physician. Almost the same number increased their use of consultations. Seven percent of respondents reported they had left long-term care practice due to risks of liability [7].

Most practitioners agree that when medical errors occur as a result of either negligence or purposeful misdeeds that the injured party should be reasonably compensated. Common liability issues in long-term care are listed in Table 3 [8]. Many long-term care providers feel that inevitable bad medical outcomes, inevitable decline in function or cognition and unavoidable accidents are frequently litigated irrationally or unfairly. A negatively held view of long-term care by the public, which is frequently validated by the press, may predispose the facility and practitioners to criticism and liability.

In order for a *medical malpractice* action to have merit, plaintiffs must show:

- Defendant(s) had a *duty* to the patient.
- A *breach of* an existing *standard of care* occurred.
- The breach was a *proximate cause* of harm suffered by the plaintiff.
- Harm, injuries, (e.g., *damages*) and their value.

Given that many nursing facility residents have a limited remaining life expectancy and are not employable, actual damages in these cases are often not of great magnitude. But, *non-economic damages*, e.g., pain and suffering or family/spouse loss of counsel and consortium may increase damage claims. Additionally, *punitive damages* can be sought that are designed as a financial punishment for outrageously bad practices by the defendant(s).

Duty exists when a long-term care practitioner or facility has an existing relationship with the patient, e.g., the patient is a resident of the nursing facility or is attended by a certain physician. Practitioners are duty bound to act in accordance with their *professional standards*. Facilities, likewise, are duty bound and also must act within existing state and federal regulations. Institutional policies and procedures that exceed professional standards or regulations can appear to raise the standard. *A practitioner is expected to exercise the degree of care and skill that would be expected of a reasonably prudent practitioner of that same kind under the same or similar circumstances.*

Standards of care once thought to be unique to a local geographic area are now viewed as national. *Regulations, clinical practice guidelines* and *evidence-based practice*, as well as the testimony of expert witnesses, are often used to establish standard of care. *A breach of a standard of care may be either a matter*

Table 3 Common liability
issues in long-term care

• Dehydration
• Elopement
• Emotional distress
• Falls/fractures
• Improper use of restraints
• Medication errors
• Pressure ulcers
• Sexual assault
• Single event injuries
• Weight loss

of omission or commission. Collectively, medical professionals create standard of care, while state and federal regulations should reflect standards of care, the state and federal regulations should not be viewed as the origin of any professional standards of care.

Not all breaches of a standard of care will connect to causation of harm. For example, failing to chart one meal intake as ordered by the physician is a breach of a nursing standard of care but could not reasonably be the cause of weight loss. A *proximate cause* is an event or act that results in an injury that would not have occurred were it not for that event or act. It should be recognized that there could be more than one reason for an injury. Breaches of standard of care that do not connect to causation are of great interest and concern to quality improvement processes, but may only be relevant to medical malpractice as evidence of a defendant's inadequate training, experience, or professional conduct.

Practitioners should be aware of several pitfalls that place them at risk for nursing facility litigation. Risk is created by:

- Inadequate documentation, criticisms or bickering in the medical record.
- Failure to follow policies and procedures without documentation of a clinically supportable reason.
- Routine documentation of care in a manner not concurrent with that care.
- Failure to notify the physician and family of changes in condition.
- Outdated and unnecessary policies and procedures.
- Care plans not updated to reflect the current condition of the resident and the care being delivered,
- Failure to follow the care plan.
- Unrealistic goals documented in the care plan.

These pitfalls predispose the facility, staff, and physician to litigation. Once a malpractice action is initiated, failure to protect the integrity of the medical record and *alterations of the medical record* (*whether these relate to the cause of action or not*) *can be severely damaging to the defense.*

Summary

Ethical and legal issues abound in the everyday practice of post-acute and long-term care medicine. The clinician must have a thorough understanding of medical ethics and the law in one's jurisdiction and be able to communicate these issues to other members of the interdisciplinary team, the family, and patients in a way that will foster collaboration and consensus within an ethical and legal framework. A clinician skilled and confident in these areas can do much to guide patients, families and other caregivers through the process of medical decision-making. This guidance will provide clarity, comfort, and consistency to the plan of care within the goals and personal values of the person receiving that care. Our adherence to the principles of medical ethics defines our professionalism and creates the matrix within which all clinical care must be delivered.

Pearls for the Practitioner

1. The principles of health care ethics include *autonomy*, *beneficence*, *justice*, *non-maleficence*, and *fidelity*. For ethical decision-making, these must each be considered in the context of the others.
2. No individual should lose his/her human rights upon entering the long-term care continuum.
3. Federal and state regulations require nursing facilities to proactively prevent abuse, neglect, and exploitation.
4. Practitioners in long term care need to have the skills to assess mental capacity in order to determine an elder's ability to make decisions in their own best interest of a personal, medical, and financial nature.
5. End of life issues are common in post-acute and long-term care, and the practitioner must be well versed in tools for surrogate decision-making and applicable laws in their jurisdiction.
6. While litigation is common in long term care, for a malpractice action to be successfully pursued, all of the 4 elements of duty, breach of the standard of care, causation, and harm (damages) must be proven.

References

1. www.dads.state.tx.us.
2. Marson DC, Ingram KK, Cody HA, et al. Assessing the competency of patients with Alzheimer's disease under different legal standards. Arch Neurol. 1995;52:949–54.
3. Grisso T, Applebaum PS, Hill-Fotouhi C. The MacCat-T:Clinical tool to assess patient's capacity to make treatment decisions. Psychiatr Serv. 1997;48:1415–9.
4. www.ama-assn.org/ama/pub/physician-resources/medical-ethics.

5. www.amda.com/governance/papers.cfm.
6. www.amda.com/governance/resolutions/m03.cfm.
7. AMDA Health Policy Advisor. AMDA liability survey shows more than half work as a medical director. 2005;9(2).
8. Huss R, Smith DA. Nursing facility litigation and liability: a case-based tutorial. American Medical directors Association 32nd Annual Symposium, Charlotte N.C., March 2009.

Caring for Families

David Brechtelsbauer

Introduction

Too often physicians and other members of the interdisciplinary team (IDT) shudder when the note, "Please call Mrs. Jones' daughter" appears on the chart. The goal of this chapter is to examine attitudes, review and apply knowledge, and illustrate skills that will improve the performance of all practitioners who must work with families in the Post-Acute and Long-Term Care (PA/LTC) setting.

Family caregivers, usually adult children, face many challenges. Family members vary widely in their level of knowledge of their loved ones condition and of how to work effectively with the health care system. Poorly implemented hospital–nursing facility transitions can leave family caregivers frustrated and confused [1]. Adult children are often uncomfortable with the role-reversal experienced when caring and advocating for an elderly parent. The realities of being separated by long distances and having employment and nuclear family obligations can limit an adult child's opportunities to assess the situation firsthand, or to actively participate in care giving. Family members are often unprepared when thrust into the new role of caring for a parent, and need education and support [2].

The 2008 Institute of Medicine report, Retooling for An Aging America [3], recommends an even greater role for family and other informal caregivers as part of the response to workforce challenges created by the baby boomer generation's entry into old age and the resulting stresses on the health care system, especially long-term care. This demographic reality will require PA/LTC professionals to become even more efficient and effective when working with families.

D. Brechtelsbauer (✉)
Department of Family Medicine, University of South Dakota Sanford School of Medicine,
1115 East 20th Street, Sioux Falls, SD 57105, USA
e-mail: David.Brechtelsbauer@usd.edu

© Springer International Publishing Switzerland 2016
P.A. Fenstemacher, P. Winn (eds.), *Post-Acute and Long-Term Medicine*,
Current Clinical Practice, DOI 10.1007/978-3-319-16979-8_16

This chapter provides guidance and a concise reference for physicians and other PA/LTC professionals who wish to improve their performance when working with families.

Attitudes

It is useful to examine one's attitudes towards families and the issues that commonly arise when working with families. Prejudicial assessments, blind spots in problem solving, and ineffective interventions can result when the professional is unaware of his or her own beliefs and values relative to how families are defined and how they (should) function.

Some of the discomfort in dealing with family issues probably relates to the lack of attention to communication, particularly communication with persons other than the patient, in many professional training programs. The emphasis placed on the doctor–patient relationship and confidentiality is often the first attitudinal barrier that must be negotiated before one can work effectively with families. Practitioners who feel they are exclusively responsible to the designated patient may respond by trying to avoid dealing with families, a response that only worsens most issues.

Overcoming an exclusive focus on the patient will allow the professional to consider the family system, as well as the patient, to be a focus of care. Many times this can result in a collaborative relationship between the IDT and the family, to the benefit of the resident and the facility. Other families, due to personal preferences or the barriers created by living far away or holding down two jobs, will want to be kept informed, but will not be able to share in the care of the resident. Finally, a few families (the vast minority in the experience of the author) have no desire to be involved. It is useful to determine the level of involvement desired by each family, and periodically check to determine if the desired level of involvement has changed.

It is important to recognize the influence of one's family of origin on attitudes toward family issues. While professionals are encouraged to set aside personal biases when engaged in a professional relationship, *feelings* about traditional verses nontraditional family structures, gender roles, locus of decision-making, and filial obligation all can impact a professional's attitudes, and therefore effectiveness, when dealing with families.

A major attitudinal issue is reflected in the use of the word "*dysfunctional*" when describing families. Too often the word signals a professional caregiver's feeling hopeless or powerless to intervene in a difficult family situation. Whenever a care team member utters this word, that person needs to be encouraged to examine exactly what he/she understands the word to mean and why use of "dysfunctional" seems necessary or appropriate in the situation at hand. At times dysfunctional may be an accurate description, but dwelling on that aspect of the problem will interfere with problem solving.

Cross-cultural issues can also raise attitudinal issues and create blind spots in one's thinking. Increasing diversity in the population is a second demographic trend that requires reexamination of systems of care and communication skills. Cultural issues will be discussed later in this chapter.

Knowledge

The physician's knowledge of the resident *and* of the health care system, particularly the post-acute and long-term care system, are important prerequisites to success when working with families. It is important for the PA/LTC professional to remember that families are generally not expert in how the health care system works, and much of the knowledge families do have was gained through experience obtained in the acute care setting. For example, it is useful to discuss restraints preemptively as the family has probably seen their loved one "protected" by side rails in the hospital and will be at best confused, and at worst angry, that such a simple and common sense safety device is not available in the nursing home.

Displaying and sharing knowledge of the health care system in a non-condescending manner is an important first step in building credibility and rapport with the resident and family. Studies have shown that the move to a long-term care setting, which for many PA/LTC professionals is routine and straightforward, is a major stressor for residents and families [4]. Compassionately and effectively guiding the family through the initial transition from acute care to post-acute or long-term care will get the physician–patient and physician–family relationship off to a positive start, and in turn help create a collaborative and positive tone for the ongoing relationship between the *professional (formal)* and *family (informal) caregivers*.

Subsequent situations that are likely to be new to the family and that will benefit from proactive efforts by the physician and IDT to meaningfully engage the family include: the response to the first incident, the first acute illness or exacerbation of a chronic illness, the need to explicitly address goals of care and possible limitation of treatment options, formal code status discussions, and end of life care issues [4].

Beyond knowledge of the resident's medical condition and the functioning of the medical system, some knowledge of *clinical psychology* and *family systems* medicine is useful to provide a foundation for effective work with families. Full discussion of this knowledge base is beyond the scope of this chapter. Excellent texts [5] and review articles [6, 7] discussing this aspect of care with particular reference to long-term care are available.

Chronic illness in general, and particularly moving from the family home, creates stress for residents and their families. Most families cope well most of the time. Explicitly asking, "What stressful events have you (your family) dealt with in the past" and "How did you cope?" is helpful. The best predictor of future behavior is past behavior. Knowledge of past coping skills can inform plans being made to deal with a new crisis. Responses to the above questions can raise "red flags" for ineffective coping and dissatisfaction with care. Communication difficulty is more likely to occur if family members bring with them a pattern of chronic financial stress, active substance abuse, chronic psychiatric problems, or criminal behavior [8].

Prudence requires that the physician and other members of the care team proactively engage family members when red flags are noted. Make extra and persistent efforts to communicate. Seek agreement or at least acknowledgement of realistic goals of care, and monitor the resident's progress and the family's progress in managing their stress. Give family members permission to take time for themselves as a way to manage stress and preserve caregiver health. If things are not going well with the family, consider referral to a family therapist, religious counselor, or a community resource (Alzheimer's Association, Adult Day Care Program, etc.).

Skills

Skills in dealing with families are learned and improve with practice. If one finds him/herself struggling when returning phone calls from family members, avoiding family contact, or unable to participate in family meetings, it is helpful to find someone who is skilled and effective in this area. Practicing these skills under the watchful eye of a mentor, and being open to feedback and the use of new or refined approaches will lead to improvement.

In an encounter likely to be emotionally charged it is important to choose one's words very carefully [9]. The phrase "there is nothing more to do" often is spoken when dealing with frail elderly residents and their families. A more complete, accurate, and less provocative phrase would be, "There is nothing more to do *to cure the illness.*" This statement opens the door to discussion of symptom management, psychosocial and spiritual support, and other measures that promote comfort and dignity for the resident and caring and support for the family.

A similar problematic question posed to residents or their families is, "Would you like us to do everything?" Clinicians often equate this with the use of high tech interventions and need for acute hospital level of care. For families, it is a question that often precipitates a "yes" answer when they are thinking about everything to relieve pain and suffering, not about transferring their loved one back to the hospital. A better phrase is, "I recognize your mother is in distress, and that in turn is distressing to you. I don't think sending her to the hospital for more tests would help her distress, but let me explain what we can do here in the nursing home to get her pain (or any distressing symptom) under better control."

There are times a resident may need to be admitted for symptom control, but many symptoms can be managed by a skilled nursing facility IDT without hospitalization. The physician's awareness of the nursing facility team's level of skill and confidence will also influence the recommendation to treat in the nursing facility or in the hospital [10].

Selection of a Family Spokesperson

In most circumstances communication efficiency is enhanced when the physician and other IDT members communicate with the family through a family spokesperson. This person's contact information needs to be conveniently available. While the physician or IDT may have a preference as to which family member should be the spokesperson, the choice rests with the family. The family's choice is often revealing as it typically reflects how the family has functioned in the past.

The team needs to inquire as to the spokesperson's preferred method of communication—telephone (home, work, cell), email, face-to-face, and the alternative plan if the designated spokesperson is not available. It is also useful to let the spokesperson know the best times and locations for contacting team members, generally which team members are most knowledgeable in which areas, and who to contact when it is not obvious to the spokesperson. Typically, the administrator is ultimately the point person for facility issues, and the attending physician or medical director for medical issues.

Responding to a Phone Call from an Unhappy Family Member

A useful phrase to use when returning phone calls is, "Hello Mrs. Jones. This is Dr. Smith. *I understand you are concerned about your mother.*" Use of this phrase communicates to the family member that you have some level of awareness about the concern. If you don't have an idea about what is going on, call the nurse, social worker, or other staff member to get basic information about what might be going on before returning the call. If it's a particularly dicey situation, making a face-to-face visit to the resident and more thorough data collection is important if it can be accomplished without causing too much delay in returning the call. The need for prompt communication needs to be balanced with the need for preparation.

Mrs. Jones is likely to have to agree with your opening statement, which gets the conversation off on the right foot. Next, *very briefly* state your understanding of the issue—"I think at least some of your concerns relates to your mother's bruises, but please explain to me what you are noticing." Then, with the chart open in order to record what you are about to hear, do what too many professionals find difficult: listen to the whole story before attempting to explain. On one level, families often are as concerned that they are not being heard as they are about the problem itself. Important things to listen for are family perceptions and interpretations that you did not expect, and if the caller is an eager or reluctant family spokesperson. Sometimes the caller has been put up to calling by another family member and the caller's own feelings and perceptions are not congruent with the feelings and perceptions of the family member with the concern. While working through a family spokesperson is generally recommended, in this case the professional might want to ask the spokesperson if it would be better to speak directly to the person with the concern.

After listening, and with review of your notes, reflect back what you heard with enough detail for the family member to be convinced that you have heard and understood what was said. Depending on the issues involved, you may be able to provide education, reassurance, or an action plan that will satisfy the caller. If you are not able to do so, in the absence of a true emergency, the best response is, "I'm going to have to look into your concerns in order to better understand what is going on. I will visit the nursing facility tomorrow and get back to you later in the day. What is the best way to reach you tomorrow afternoon after three?"

Effective communication by phone, including keeping a succinct record of what was said, is an extremely important skill.

Consider the following example of a phone call from a family member who's loved one had been transferred from the nursing facility to the hospital the prior afternoon. The phone call was transcribed verbatim (names have been changed) in order to enter it into the medical record.

> This is Donna Smith. I am Richard Jones' daughter. Richard was taken yesterday from Sunset Manor to the hospital, at first with thoughts of a stroke or whatever. I guess we are just really, really frustrated. Nobody, Dr. B or I know he has students or whatever that come in and are under him [the caller is referring to resident physicians], my mom has not heard anything from him as far as treatment, what is the plan, what are they going to do? If it was a stroke, what the blood test results were? We need to know. He has been laying up there for a full day with nothing to eat, we don't know if he can eat. He can't speak. It is pretty frustrating and I believe probably somebody needs to get on the ball and find out what is going on and let the family know. My number is xxx-xxxx, and my mother's number is xxx-xxxx. Her name is Darla Jones and she is retired. She is on her way up to the hospital right now. Again, we do want some answers and we want to know what is going on. Thank you.

Obviously the ball was dropped in this situation. When this call is returned, an apology needs to be promptly stated. What is really informative in this example is the concerned tone of the message when it was reviewed by *listening to the voice mail*, in contrast to the hostile character one quickly picks up when reading the transcription. A major lesson here is not to read too much into a transcribed message. In situations where there seems to be hostility (and, in contrast to the example, there may be hostility), it's best to respond by phone in order to hear the tone of voice and inflection, or even face-to-face so the clinician can observe and respond to nonverbal cues.

It is becoming more common for families to communicate by email. Email allows the convenience of asynchronous communication and convenient record keeping. Like the above example however, email messages generally cannot accurately convey the emotional state of the family member sending the message or the empathy of the responding professional. When the content of the email message is not routine it is generally better to pick up the phone than to hit the reply button. It is also very important to carefully proofread your email before sending it, and be extremely careful if you are sending it to the correct person; inadvertently striking the "reply all" key can create problems.

Emerging technology will allow virtual face-to-face encounters. These hold promise to overcome some of the disadvantages of current technology, but their use and role are still in evolution [11].

Convening and Conducting a Family Meeting

Effective phone communication and face-to-face meetings with the family spokesperson can sometimes resolve family concerns. Other situations, either because of complex family dynamics, or because of the complex medical or ethical issues that are causing the concern, require a much more formal process to achieve resolution. The "rules" for family meetings are a product of the "Family Systems" literature and are summarized here. A more detailed description is referenced at the end of this chapter [12].

Preparation for a family meeting needs to be even more thorough and thoughtful than preparation for a phone call. The practitioner needs to learn as much as possible about the resident, be as familiar as possible with the facility environment and culture, and understand the medical issues as completely as possible. This often involves an examination of the resident and review of the chart for the purpose of clarifying the current status of the medical issue(s), obtaining as much knowledge as possible about the family, and discussing the concern with relevant staff members including the floor nurse and certified nursing assistant, the social worker, and chaplain. If the issue involves a conflict about nursing facility regulations or internal polices, the administrator should also be consulted. Once the above preparation is complete, set a date, time, and place for the meeting. Professionals need to, as much as possible, clear schedules to allow for uninterrupted participation. All *relevant* professionals should attend, but avoid having too many staff members attend in order not to appear to be ganging up on the family. By the same token, all family members should attend. Out of town family members should be encouraged to participate via conference call or speakerphone.

The person moderating the meeting should begin with introductions and state the "rules" for the meeting. Many physicians, with training and experience, are comfortable in the moderator role, but the moderator can be anyone on the professional team. Many social workers have formal training and are skilled moderators of family meetings.

The first rule is that everyone will be invited to state his or her perception of the problems. This is to be done without interruption, if another person at the table wants to make a comment, the comment should be written down and reported during that person's time to speak. Generally speaking, the resident, if present, or the least empowered person should speak first. The person who is least empowered may be the person who is present only by speakerphone, or the person with the least familiarity with the problem or the least formal education. In an effort to put family members at ease, assure everyone that all comments are useful to help understand the concerns that precipitated the need for the meeting. If you are aware that a particular family member might be intimidating to other family members, or has very strong feelings about the issue at hand, call on that person last.

This may seem like a time consuming process, especially with large families. Often however, family members begin to report that they agree with a previous speaker and have nothing to add.

After the family has spoken, the moderator should summarize what has been said and secure assent that the summary is basically correct. Then each professional is called upon to state his/her perception of the issue. Avoid offering solutions at this point. Once again, after the professional team has spoken, the moderator should offer a brief summary of what was said.

Next the person with the most credibility (this is often, but not always, the physician) can provide education and suggest realistic goals and expectations. Discussion, problem solving, and hopefully agreement on next steps follow. It is useful to explicitly define what will be measured to monitor the results of the intervention(s). Ask, "If this plan works, how will we know?" Also, agree on how the results of the monitoring will be communicated to both the family and the IDT, particularly the front line caregivers.

Most of the time this process will lead to a plan that is acceptable to the family and the IDT. If things go poorly it may be possible only to state that the outcome, for now at least is "we can only agree we disagree."

The team and family at this point can be *assigned tasks* (obtaining a second opinion, obtaining a copy of the advance directive, searching the Internet for references) that may impact the situation and provide useful information for a future meeting. ,It is sometimes helpful to have the next meeting moderated by a skilled and disinterested family therapist. Other options are to refer the situation to an ethics committee or formal arbitration.

While in the long run formal family meetings often save time (and improve outcomes and satisfaction) and can sometimes be quite efficient, there are barriers to equitable reimbursement for the time involved in preparation and participation in a family-IDT meeting. If the resident is present the physician can bill and be reimbursed for education, counseling, and coordination of care using appropriate nursing facility subsequent visit codes. Some facilities will recognize the value of family meetings, both in terms of resident/family satisfaction and risk management, and be willing to pay the moderator a reasonable consultation fee.

Writing a Progress Note for Families

The *degree of involvement families' desire* in the care of their loved ones varies dramatically. For the family who has frequent questions it can be useful to, with the consent of the resident, send a copy of the physician's progress note after each routine nursing facility visit. It is of course necessary to write a less technical note, or provide a brief cover letter, to make this a useful intervention. Sending a copy of progress notes routinely can sometimes dramatically decrease the number of phone calls to the physician or facility.

Families quickly learn that, generally speaking, no news from the nursing facility is good news. Ongoing communication about routine and nonurgent matters can build rapport and a common understanding of the resident's situation. This in turn can make communication at critical times more efficient and productive. An example of a cover letter to the family spokesperson is as follows:

Dear Mrs. White

A copy of my note from your sister's most recent nursing home checkup is enclosed. Tilly was pleasant and cooperative during my visit. I did not find any major changes.

If you have any questions or comments please feel free to call the office (XXX–XXXX) and leave a message with my office nurse, Sandy H.

Sincerely,
Dr. Good Apple

Creating and Using a Genogram

Creation of genograms, a diagrammatic representation of a family, is taught in many social work and nursing training programs, but is less familiar to most medical professionals. The ability to create *a genogram is a useful skill, providing an efficient way to document and recall the "anatomy" of the family.*

By convention, male family members are represented as squares and females as circles. An arrow indicates the resident. A horizontal line connecting the two individuals involved indicates a marriage, a slash though the line indicates a divorce. Each generation occupies a separate "layer" on the genogram. Notations can be added indicating supportive or problematic relationships [13]. An example of the Brown family, whose matriarch is unhappy with being placed in a nursing facility, is shown in Fig. 1.

A review of the genogram illustrates Grandma Ethel's likely belief that "in our family we take care of people at home" and the likely pressure this family story creates for daughter Beth and daughter-in-law Heidi. The genogram also provides a "snapshot" of potential family resources and likely sources of conflict.

Families change over time and the genogram that has been placed in the chart needs to periodically be updated. Reference to the genogram before returning a phone call or participating a family meeting can quickly refresh one's memory of family structure and dynamics, making the call or meeting more productive and efficient.

When There Are Cultural Barriers

Like unexamined attitudinal issues, *cultural barriers can also create blind spots and interfere with success when working with families.* In an age where political correctness sometimes trumps confronting a problem directly, examining possible cultural issues can be intimidating.

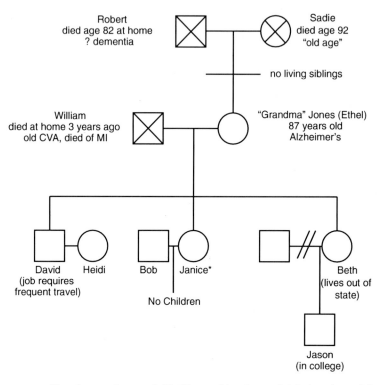

*lives in same town as Bob's 87 year old mother and visits her almost daily

Fig. 1 Genogram of the extended Jones Family

Begin by examining your personal and professional cultures. What assumptions might others make based on knowing you are an African-American physician, or a Filipino nurse? If things often thought about a cultural or professional group were true, how much would they apply to you?

Next, consider the cultural background of the resident and his/her family. What do you know, or think you know, about the culture in question? No one expects a health care professional to have an intimate knowledge of each resident's culture, but some basic knowledge is useful. Professional colleagues from the culture of the resident may be helpful. Other resources include, "CultureGrams" (www.culturegrams. com) ©2007 ProQuest-SCA and Brigham Young University [14], which provide concise, reliable and up-to-date reports on more than 200 countries, and your local librarian. Just as you may recognize yourself as being an American physician, but meet none of the stereotypes, you cannot assume the resident and the resident's family will be well characterized by generalizations made about their culture. A useful way to begin to address this is to ask; "I have heard that it is common in Bulgaria for adult children to care for their elderly parents. How true is that for your family?"

Sometimes, despite being knowledgeable and respectful of the family and the family's cultural background, communication still seems ineffective. In this case it is *usually helpful to find a mutually acceptable mediator*. This person selected is often a community or religious leader from the cultural group involved. This person can often "bridge the gap" between the prevailing and/or professional culture and the minority and/or lay culture.

Effective communication when a translator is necessary requires behaviors that may not be intuitive. When a translator is being used it is important to talk directly to the resident and not to the translator. "How are you feeling today?" is more likely to engender engagement and a meaningful response than "Ask her how she is feeling today." Talking directly to the resident also makes the translator's job easier.

Professional translators are preferred over use of family members, although financial and logistical barriers often force the use of untrained family members. Companies offering telephone and computer-based translators can be found by searching "language line" on the Internet. Prices and available languages vary.

Summary

A practitioner seeking to achieve excellence in working with families in the post-acute or long-term care setting needs to critically examine his or her attitudes towards families, and display detailed knowledge of PA/LTC medicine, the resident, the family system, facility, and IDT function. Excellence can only be achieved through the development of nonintuitive communication skills, including communication in the setting of a family meeting. The ability to create and utilize a genogram is a powerful asset that will enhance communication with families.

Cultural issues can make communication more difficult. Successful communication can be assured by a obtaining a basic knowledge of the family culture, and when necessary make use of a skilled professional translator.

Pearls for the Practitioner

- Recognize and acknowledge that chronic illness and PA/LTC placement are major stressors for residents and their families.
- In almost every situation it is important to listen before offering solutions.
- Determine the level of involvement the family desires, whenever possible support that involvement.
- Practice until you can comfortably and skillfully.

  - Return a phone call from a family member.
  - Respond to an email communication from a family member.
  - Participate effectively in a family meeting.
  - Create and utilize a genogram.
  - Communicate with a resident/family when using a translator.

- Develop resources that can efficiently provide background information when dealing with residents/families from cultures different from the dominant culture.

Websites

- Culture Grams: http://www.culturegrams.com
- AMDA: http://www.amda.com
- Center to Advance Palliative Care: www.capc.org
- Center to Advance Palliative Care hosts "Fast Facts" which provide succinct and practical information about palliative care—select "Communication" for information most relevant to this chapter, including particularly Fast Fact 222 Preparing for the Family Meeting, and Fast Fact 223 The Family Meeting: Starting the Conversation.

References

1. Marziali E, Shulman K, Damianakis T. Persistent family concerns in long-term care settings: meaning and management. J Am Med Dir Assoc. 2006;7:154–62.
2. Henry SM. The eldercare handbook: difficult choices, compassionates solutions. New York: Harper-Collins; 2006.
3. Institute of Medicine. Retooling for an aging America: building the health care workforce. Washington: National Academies Press; 2008.
4. Bern-Klug M. The emotional context facing nursing home residents' families: a call for role reinforcement strategies from nursing homes and the community. J Am Med Dir Assoc. 2008;9:36–44.
5. Conn DK, Herrmann N, Kaye A, et al., editors. Practical psychiatry in the long-term care home: a handbook for staff. 3rd ed. Cambridge: Hogrefe & Huber; 2007.
6. Winn P, Cook JB, Bonnel W. Improving communication among attending physicians, long-term care facilities, residents, and residents' families. J Am Med Dir Assoc. 2004;5:114–22.
7. Bluestein D, Bach PL. Working with families in long-term care. J Am Med Dir Assoc. 2007;8:265–70.
8. Kidder SW, Smith DA. Is there a conflicted surrogate syndrome affecting quality of care in nursing homes? J Am Med Dir Assoc. 2006;7:168–72.
9. Pantilat SZ. Communicating with seriously ill patients: better words to say. JAMA. 2009;301:1279–81.
10. Cheng HY, Tonorezos E, Zorowitz R, et al. Inpatient care for nursing home patients: an opportunity to improve transitional care. J Am Med Dir Assoc. 2006;7:383–7.
11. Hensel BK, Parker-Oliver D, Demiris G, Rantz M. A comparison of video-based resident-family communication in a nursing home and a congregate living facility. J Am Med Dir Assoc. 2009;10:342–7.
12. Bloom MV, Smith DA. Brief mental health interventions for the family physician. New York: Springer; 2001. p. 262–3.
13. McGoldrick M, Gerson R, Petry S. Genograms: assessment and intervention. 3rd ed. New York: Norton; 2008.
14. CultureGrams. www.culturegrams.com. Accessed 4 May 2015.

Documentation and Coding

Alva S. Baker and Leonard Gelman

Introduction

The provision of care to residents of long-term care facilities presents different complexities in documentation and coding for both physician and practitioner services than those provided in the office or hospital setting. Proper documentation of the care provided and use of the appropriate billing code is essential to receiving appropriate reimbursement for rendered services. Practitioner familiarity with a glossary of common terms (see Fig. 1) is critical to ensure accurate documentation, coding, and billing.

Documenting the Visit

The AMA is responsible for establishing and maintaining the CPT codes. The AMA defined documentation guidelines for Evaluation and Management (E/M) codes in 1995 and these were revised in 1997. These are available on the CMS website. Either set can be used but one cannot mix the guidelines for any one encounter, except that, starting September 10, 2013, physician's using the 1995 guidelines may use the 1997 definition of Extended History along with the other elements of the 1995 guidelines. AMDA has issued a *Guide to Long Term Care Coding, Reimbursement and Documentation* based upon the AMA's CPT guide (available for ordering at www.amda.com).

There are seven components that define provider encounters. In most cases the first three are called the Key components and are used to define the level of E/M service.

A.S. Baker, MD, CMD (✉)
CMDR, HMDC, 747 Northern Avenue, Hagerstown, MD 21742, USA
e-mail: dr.alva.baker@grnmd.com

L. Gelman, MD, CMD
Capital Care Family Medicine, 20 Prospect St., Ballston Spa, NY 12020-1367, USA
e-mail: gelmanl@msn.com

© Springer International Publishing Switzerland 2016   291
P.A. Fenstemacher, P. Winn (eds.), *Post-Acute and Long-Term Medicine*,
Current Clinical Practice, DOI 10.1007/978-3-319-16979-8_17

Admission – when a patient enters a NF or SNF and there are no open clinical or financial records pertaining to the current stay

Re-Admission – there is no clarity from CMS concerning the definition of this term, and it may be used in two ways, the more logical of which, based on the CMS wording in the Medicare Carrier Manual, is number two below

1. When a patient returns to a NF or SNF after leaving with a bed hold status; the clinical and financial records have remained open and the patient is considered to be continuing the current stay that began prior to leaving with the bed hold status; all services are billed using the subsequent care codes (99307-99310)
2. When a patient returns to a NF or SNF after leaving with a discharged status; the clinical and financial records from the prior stay have been closed and the patient is considered to be starting a new stay; an initial visit is again required and this is billed using the initial care codes (99304-99306)

Discharge – when a patient leaves a NF or SNF to go to another venue of care (home, hospital, assisted living, group home, etc.) and the clinical and financial records pertaining to the current stay are closed, even if there is a possibility or probability that the patient will return to the same NF or SNF

Bed Hold – when a patient leaves a NF or SNF to go to another venue of care (usually, hospital) and the clinical and financial records pertaining to the current stay remain open in expectation of the patient's return

MDS – acronym for Minimum Data Set, the comprehensive multidisciplinary evaluation performed for a patient on admission and periodically thereafter as long as the patient remains a resident in the NF or SNF; the MDS is submitted electronically to State and Federal agencies

Initial Visit – "the initial comprehensive assessment visit during which the physician completes a thorough assessment, develops a plan of care and writes or verifies admitting orders for the nursing facility resident."

CMS – acronym for The Centers for Medicare and Medicaid Services

Nursing Facility (NF) – an institution (or a distinct part of an institution),which is primarily engaged in providing nursing care and related services for residents who require medical or nursing care. *Residents in a NF do not receive Medicare Part A benefits.*

Skilled Nursing Facility (SNF) – an institution (or a distinct part of an institution) which is primarily engaged in providing skilled nursing care and related services for patients who require medical or nursing care, or rehabilitation services for the rehabilitation of injured, disabled, or sick persons. *Patients in a SNF are receiving skilled services that are being paid for by the their Medicare Part A benefits.*

Fig. 1 Glossary of terms

- *History*
- *Physical examination*
- *Medical decision making*
- **Patient counseling**
- **Coordination of care**
- **Severity of the presenting problem and**
- **Time or duration needed to render the service**

The three Key Components each has four levels of extensiveness or complexity.

History

The four types of history and their definitions are as follows:

- *Problem focused*: <u>brief</u> history of present illness or problem
- *Expanded problem focused*: <u>brief</u> history of present illness: <u>problem pertinent</u> system review
- *Detailed*: <u>extended</u> history of present illness; <u>problem pertinent</u> review of systems; pertinent past, family and/or social history directly related to patient's problems
- *Comprehensive*: <u>extended</u> history of present illness; review of systems that is directly related to the problem(s) indentified in the history of the present illness plus a review of all additional body systems; <u>complete</u> past, family and social history.

   A Chief complaint is needed for each encounter.

Examination

The four types of physical examination are defined as follows:

- *Problem focused*: A <u>limited</u> examination of the affected body area or organ system.
- *Expanded problem focused*: A <u>limited</u> examination of the affected body area or organ system and other symptomatic or related body area(s) or organ system(s).
- *Detailed*: An <u>extended</u> examination of the affected body area(s) and other symptomatic or related body area(s) or organ system(s).
- *Comprehensive*: A general multisystem examination or a complete examination of a single organ system and other symptomatic or related body area(s) or organ system(s).

Medical Decision Making

The four types of medical decision-making are based on:

- The number of possible diagnoses
- The number of management options that are considered
- The amount and complexity of medical records and other information that must be reviewed
- The risk of significant complications, i.e., morbidity and/or mortality, in addition to comorbidities and their respective severity and how all these can impact management options

The four levels of complexity of medical decision-making are as follows:

- *Straightforward*: <u>minimal</u> number of diagnoses or management options; <u>minimal</u> or no data to be reviewed; <u>minimal</u> risk of complications, morbidity, and mortality.
- *Low complexity*: <u>limited</u> number of diagnoses or management options; <u>limited</u> amount or complexity of data to be reviewed: <u>low</u> risk of complications, morbidity, and mortality.
- *Moderate complexity*: <u>multiple</u> diagnoses or management options: <u>moderate</u> amount of complexity of data to be reviewed: <u>moderate</u> risk of complication, morbidity, and mortality.
- *High complexity*: <u>extensive</u> diagnoses or management options; <u>extensive</u> amount or complexity of data to be reviewed; <u>high</u> risk of complication, morbidity, and mortality.

Time

Time can be used to define a level of E/M service if counseling and coordination of care predominates the encounter (>50 % of time spent). Time is also used for prolonged service codes (see below). Otherwise the times associated with the E/M codes are not used to define the level of service provided and are to be only used as estimates. Document time spent with the patient in conjunction with the medical decision-making involved and a description of the coordination of care or counseling provided. Documentation must be in sufficient detail to support the claim.

Coding and Billing for Nursing Facilities

The E&M service code selection is based upon fulfilling the requirements of the individual CPT codes as well as fulfilling medical necessity requirements. Having provided the service and properly documented the care, the selection of the most accurate CPT code is relatively straightforward.

Skilled Nursing and Nursing Facility Visits

For attending physician services, there are four groups of service codes:

- *Initial Nursing Facility Care* (services provided on admission to the SNF or NF for the initial comprehensive assessment): 99304, 99305, 99306. The patient's attending physician of record must append the modifier "AI" to the bill when performing initial visits.

- *Subsequent Nursing Facility Care* (services provided subsequent to or prior to the initial comprehensive assessment): 99307, 99308, 99309, 99310.
- *Services provided for discharge*: 99315 or 99316.
- *Services provided for annual health evaluation*: 99318.

   Note that all codes apply to either new or established patients.

   The appropriate *Initial Nursing Facility Care* code is determined by the extensiveness and complexity of the components of the E/M service provided: with the most comprehensive service being billed at level 99306 (see Fig. 2). *All the initial codes require that all three E/M components be performed (history, physical, medical decision making)*. These codes are used for the initial admission (or readmission, if the patient has previously resided in the nursing facility and had been discharged, i.e., no bed hold). The *Subsequent Nursing Facility* care codes are reviewed in Fig. 3. Again, the appropriate subsequent care code is determined by the complexity of the components of the E/M service provided, with the most complex and comprehensive services being coded at the 99310 level.

   Note that when billing for subsequent care, only two of the three E/M components need to be performed, though optimal medical care is likely best provided if all 3 components are performed.

   The codes for services provided upon discharge from a SNF or NF include 99315 and 99316 (see Fig. 4). For these discharge services, the differentiation of the appropriate code is determined by the time spent performing all of the tasks and services required for the patient's discharge (final exam, instructions for continuing care, preparation of discharge records, prescriptions, referral forms and communications with providers of care for the patient following discharge). *It is important to remember that these discharge visit codes, as do all the other visit codes, require a face-to-face visit*, and that if the visit is performed on a day different than the actual day of discharge, the date of service for the billing should be the actual date of the visit. These same codes can be used for a visit when a patient has died, but are only billable if the physician fulfills the requirement of a face-to-face visit and actually pronounces the death.

   The code for services provided for the annual (or periodic) health evaluation is 99318 (see Fig. 5). The visit for this health evaluation and the billing with this code are to be used in place of, not in addition to, a routine or regulatory visit code.

   CMS requires that any E/M code for a SNF visit be noted with the Place of Service Code "31" and that for a NF visit with the Place of Service Code "32".

Other Coding Issues in Nursing Facilities

Consultations

A specialist consultant or a primary care physician may perform consultations in the nursing or skilled nursing facility. A billable consultation requires a request from the physician caring for the patient. As of January 1 2010, (see below for CMS

99304

- REQUIRES THREE OF THREE E&M COMPONENTS

    - DETAILED OR COMPREHENSIVE HX

    - DETAILED OR COMPREHENSIVE EXAM

    - MEDICAL DECISION MAKING:

        · STRAIGHTFORWARD LOW

    - 25 minutes

- USED FOR:

    - INITIAL ADMISSION / READMISSION

    - Usually, the problem(s) requiring admission are of low severity

---

99305

- REQUIRES THREE OF THREE E&M COMPONENTS

    - COMPREHENSIVE HX

    - COMPREHENSIVE EXAM

    - MEDICAL DECISION MAKING:

        · MODERATE

    - 35 minutes

- USED FOR

    - INITIAL ADMISSION / READMISSION

    - Usually, the problem(s) requiring admission are of moderate severity.

99306

- REQUIRES THREE OF THREE E&M COMPONENTS)

- COMPREHENSIVE HX

    - COMPREHENSIVE EXAM

    - MEDICAL DECISION MAKING:

        · HIGH

    - 45 minutes

- USED FOR:

    - INITIAL ADMISSION / READMISSION

    - Usually, the problem(s) requiring admission are of high severity.

Fig. 2 Initial SNF or NF visit codes: 99304–99306

```
99307

•    REQUIRES TWO OF THREE E&M COMPONENTS

        –   PROBLEM FOCUSED HX

        –   PROBLEM FOCUSED EXAM

        –   MEDICAL DECISION MAKING:

                •   STRAIGHTFORWARD

        –   10 minutes

   •    USED FOR

        –   PATIENT STABLE, RECOVERING, OR IMPROVING

        –   "ROUTINE / REGULATORY" VISIT
```

```
99308

•    REQUIRES TWO OF THREE E&M COMPONENTS

        –   EXPANDED PROBLEM FOCUSED HX

        –   EXPANDED PROBLEM FOCUSED EXAM

        –   MEDICAL DECISION MAKING:

                •   LOW

        –   15 minutes

•    USED FOR

        –   PATIENT RESPONDING INADEQUATELY TO RX OR DEVELOPED

            MINOR COMPLICATION

        –   "ROUTINE / REGULATORY" VISIT
```

Fig. 3 Subsequent SNF or NF visit codes: 99307–99310

99309

- REQUIRES TWO OF THREE E&M COMPONENTS
    - DETAILED HX
    - DETAILED EXAM
    - MEDICAL DECISION MAKING:
        - MODERATE
    - 25 minutes
- USED FOR
    - PATIENT DEVELOPED SIGNIFICANT COMPLICATION OR SIGNIFICANT NEW PROBLEM
    - "ROUTINE / REGULATORY" VISIT

99310

- REQUIRES TWO OF THREE E&M COMPONENTS
    - COMPREHENSIVE HX
    - COMPREHENSIVE EXAM
    - MEDICAL DECISION MAKING:
        - HIGH
    - 35 minutes
- USED FOR
    - The patient may be unstable or may have developed a significant new problem requiring immediate physician attention.

Fig. 3 (continued)

99315 - 30 MINUTES OR LESS DURATION OF TIME

99316 - MORE THAN 30 MINUTES DURATION OF TIME

- USED FOR:
    - FINAL EXAM
    - INSTRUCTIONS FOR CONTINUING CARE
    - PREPARATION OF DISCHARGE RECORDS
    - PRESCRIPTIONS
    - REFERRAL FORMS
    - COMMUNICATIONS WITH AFTER-DISCHARGE PROVIDERS

Fig. 4 SNF or NF discharge visit codes: 99315 or 99316

99318

- REQUIRES THREE OF THREE E&M COMPONENTS

    – DETAILED INTERVAL HX

    – COMPREHENSIVE EXAM

    – MEDICAL DECISION MAKING:

        . LOW TO MODERATE

    – 30 minutes

- USED FOR

    – Annual exam

    – Usually, the patient is stable, recovering, or improving.

Fig. 5 Annual (periodic) nursing facility health evaluation code: 99318

informational website) the initial consultation evaluation is billed using the nursing facility initial assessment E/M codes (99304–99306). The patient's principal physician of record must append the modifier "AI" to the bill when performing initial visits to differentiate the attending initial visit from a consultant performing an initial visit as a consultation at which time no modifier is needed. The principal physician of record is identified in Medicare as the physician who oversees the patient's care, which differs from other physicians who may be furnishing specialty care.

Any follow-up visits for consultation are billed using the subsequent nursing facility visit codes (99307–99310).

Hospice Care

If the patient is receiving care under the Medicare Hospice Benefit, there are additional guidelines for billing for provided services that depends on whether the provider has any relationship with the hospice and whether care is related to the terminal illness or not (see Fig. 6). However, physicians should ask their Medicare Administrative Contractor (formerly called Medicare Fiscal Intermediary or Carrier) to verify whom to bill for physician services related to the terminal diagnosis (i.e., whether the hospice or Medicare Part B).

Physicians in Group Practice

In certain circumstances, provider members of a group practice of the same specialty may bill for services provided to a patient on the same day as indicated in Fig. 7.

For care **not** related to terminal illness:

- Bill Medicare Part B – modifier GW

For care **related** to terminal illness:

- Check with your Medicare Administrative Contractor
  - If the physician is *not associated* with the hospice
    - Bill Medicare Part B– modifier GV
  - If the physician is *associated* with/employed by the hospice
    - Bill Hospice unless services are covered by the contract or agreement with hospice

Fig. 6 Billing for patients receiving the Medicare hospice benefit

Same Group - *Same* Specialty
- Bill and be paid as though they were single physician
- One E/M code per day per problem
- Can combine same day visits and submit appropriate code
- Unrelated problems: can submit different bills; documentation critical

Same group – *Different* Specialty
- Bill and be paid without regard to membership in group

Fig. 7 Group practice

Multi-site Same Day Visits

The only case in which Medicare will pay for two different services provided by the same physician to the same patient on the same day at different sites of service is for hospital discharge management (99328, 99329) and the nursing facility admission (99304, 99305, 33906). Documentation must be adequate at each site of service to demonstrate that each service with all the appropriate E/M components was actually provided.

Split or Shared Visits

Medicare does *not* recognize split or shared E/M visits in the nursing facility and thus these may not be billed.

"Incident To" Services

"Incident To" services provided in the nursing facility are not recognized by Medicare and will not be reimbursed. However, if the physician establishes an office in the nursing facility (a discrete space that the physician rents and controls the use of for patient care visits), "incident to" services provided in that discrete office space are billable to and reimbursable. In this case, the "incident to" services are billed utilizing the office service codes.

Visits by Qualified Non-physician Practitioners

Non-physician practitioners (NPP) include Nurse Practitioners (NP), Physician Assistants (PA) and Clinical Nurse Specialists (CNS). All E/M visits must be within their State scope of practice and licensure requirements where the visit is performed. All the federal and state requirements for physician collaboration and physician supervision must also be met. Refer to Table 1 for the Federal regulations related to which services may be provided by the various NPPs in differing employment and care settings.

Prolonged Services

Medicare does pay for prolonged care services in the nursing facility. These are billed along with the visit charge for a standard E/M visit. The prolonged care timing starts at the completion of the typical time for the E/M visit being billed plus additional time as summarized in Fig. 8. The service must be face-to-face. For further guidance on this complex issue go to http://www.cms.hhs.gov/transmittals/downloads/R1490CP.pdf.

Services Provided in the NF or SNF that are not Reimbursable by Medicare

Care plan oversight, telephone calls, medical team conferences (Interdisciplinary team meetings), and prolonged services without face-to-face service are not reimbursable.

Table 1 Non-physician practitioner services

	Order to admit	Admission treatment orders	Initial comprehensive visit	Other required visits	Other medically necessary visits	Other medically necessary orders	Certification, recertification
SNF							
PA, NP, and CNS employed by facility	N	N	N	Y (alternate)	Y	Y	N
PA, NP, and CNS not a facility employee	N	N	N	Y (alternate)	Y	Y	Y
NF							
NP, CNS, and PA employed by facility	N	N	N	N	Y	Y	N/A
NP, CNS, and PA not a facility employee	Y	Y	Y	Y	Y	Y	N/A

99356 – First hour of prolonged service	
99357 – Each additional 30 minutes beyond the first hour	
• Including both SNF or NF	
• Time of prolonged service included in these codes is face to face, continuous or not, beyond the typical time for the E/M visit code plus 30 minutes	
• Documentation not required to be sent with the bill, but is required in record as to duration and content of the service provided	

Fig. 8 Prolonged care services: 99356–99357

Initial		Subsequent	
Code	Time	Code	Time
99324	20 minutes	99334	15 minutes
99325	30 minutes	99335	25 minutes
99326	45 minutes	99336	40 minutes
99327	60 minutes	99337	60 minutes
99328	75 minutes		
Note: These Visit Codes with typical service duration for Assisted Living Facilities, Group Homes, Custodial Care Facilities, and Residential Substance Abuse Facilities			

Fig. 9 Assisted living visit codes

Coding and Billing for Assisted Living Facilities

Levels of E/M services are defined by the same components. See Fig. 9 for the billing codes used for assisted living facilities, group homes, custodial care facilities and residential substance abuse facilities. It is important to use the correct place of service code for each of these venues (13, 14, 33, and 55, respectively).

Coding and Billing for Home Visits

Visit services provided in the patient's home are billed using still a different set of codes. These nevertheless follow the same pattern of E/M service intensity and also linked to typical duration of service. These codes are used for services provided in the patient's private residence (place of service code 12) and may not be used for services provided to persons residing in any type of congregate/shared facility living arrangement, including assisted living facilities and group homes. See Fig. 10 for a listing of these codes.

Initial		Subsequent	
Code	Time	Code	Time
99341	20 minutes	99347	15 minutes
99342	30 minutes	99348	25 minutes
99343	45 minutes	99349	40 minutes
99344	60 minutes	99350	60 minutes
99345	75 minutes		
Note: Visit Codes with typical service duration for E/M services provided in the patient's home.			

Fig. 10 Home visit codes

Pearls for the Practitioner

- Appropriate medical necessity along with fulfilling the requirements of the individual CPT codes are necessary for choosing the level of E&M code.
- Appropriate and thorough documentation in the medical record must support the level of service E/M code chosen.
- The extensiveness of the history and physical examination and the complexity of medical decision-making must be appropriate to the presenting complaint(s) or clinical situation.
- The three Key components of any E/M code are history, physical examination, and medical decision-making.
- For billing purposes, it is essential to use the appropriate place of service and modifier codes.
- Contact your Medicare Administrative Contractor for information on billing and coding in your locale.
- The home visit codes are <u>NOT</u> to be used for practitioner visits performed at assisted living facilities, residential care facilities, group homes, custodial care facilities, and residential substance abuse facilities.
- Be cognizant that the E/M code numbers and documentation requirements do change over time and the responsibility rests with practitioners to keep informed of these changes.

Websites

1. Centers for Medicare and Medicaid Services Manual Update on Prolonged Service Codes from April 2008. http://www.cms.hhs.gov/transmittals/downloads/R1490CP.pdf.
2. AMA Website CPT Code/Relative Value Search Engine based on Current CPT codes and Medicare payment information. https://catalog.ama-assn.org/Catalog/cpt/cpt_search.jsp

3. Find-A-Code, a commercially available website that helps find ICD and CPT codes. http://www.findacode.com.
4. CMS Revisions to Consultation Services Payment Policy, information for physicians. http://www.cms.hhs.gov/MLNMattersArticles/downloads/MM6740.pdf
5. AMDA's Website where a *Guide to Long Term Care Coding, Reimbursement and Documentation* can be obtained. http://www.amda.com.

References

1. Current procedural terminology CPT, professional edition. 2015. American Medical Association. All rights reserved.
2. Guide to long term care coding, reimbursement and documentation. AMDA, 2015.

Medication Management in Long-Term Care

Susan T. Marcolina and Peter Winn

Introduction

Two-thirds of Americans over the age of 65 have multiple chronic conditions (i.e., multi-morbidities) that affect both quality of life and longevity. The most common chronic diseases and the leading causes of death in this population are heart disease, cancer, stroke, chronic lower respiratory disease, and diabetes mellitus. Census projections estimate that by 2030, 20 % of the US population will be 65 years of age and older. As pharmacotherapy is an essential component of care in older adults, optimization of their drug regimen (where benefit will outweigh risk) is an important public health issue [1]. Multiple chronic diseases, limited physiologic reserves, changes in drug metabolism, and impaired immune and inflammatory mechanisms all result in frail elders being susceptible to serious adverse drug events (ADEs) such as falls, hip fractures, weight loss, cognitive and functional decline.

Since 27 % of patients who reside in a long-term care facility (LTC) routinely take nine or more medications a day, it is not surprising that over 65 % will have an ADE occur during a 4-year period, with one in seven of these ADEs resulting in a hospital transfer [2]. Therefore the prevention and recognition of medication-related events is a principal *health care quality* and *safety* issue for LTC facilities, hospitals, and community settings. Understanding the basics of drug pharmacokinetics and pharmacodynamics is essential to quality and safe prescribing.

S.T. Marcolina, MD, FACP (✉)
Public Health Seattle and King County, 401 Fifth Avenue, Seattle, WA 98104, USA

Eastgate Public Health Center, 14350 SE Eastgate Way, Bellevue, WA 98007, USA
e-mail: dr_marcolina@me.com

P. Winn, MD, CMD
Department of Family and Preventive Medicine, Geriatric Assessment Clinic,
OUHSC Family Medicine Center, University of Oklahoma,
Oklahoma, OK, USA
e-mail: Peter-Winn@ouhsc.edu

© Springer International Publishing Switzerland 2016   307
P.A. Fenstemacher, P. Winn (eds.), *Post-Acute and Long-Term Medicine*,
Current Clinical Practice, DOI 10.1007/978-3-319-16979-8_18

Pharmacokinetics

Physiologic changes that occur with normal aging can have an important influence on the pharmacokinetics or disposition of a specific drug within the body that includes its absorption, distribution, metabolism, and elimination. Significant physiologic changes that occur in these four parameters must be considered when prescribing medications.

Absorption

Medications enter the systemic circulation via oral, rectal, inhalation, percutaneous, subcutaneous, intravenous, and intramuscular routes. The effect of aging on decreased gastric and intestinal motility and permeability has not shown to have consistent effects on drug absorption. Gastric hypochlorhydria seen with normal aging can affect the absorption of some medications such as ketoconazole. The widespread use of acid suppressive therapies (proton pump inhibitors (PPIs) and H2 antagonists) has made hypochlorhydria and its consequences on drug and vitamin B-12 absorption more prevalent [3, 4].

Comorbid conditions can further alter the oral absorption of some medications. Congestive heart failure causing bowel wall edema can interfere with absorption of diuretics such as furosemide, thus diminishing its clinical efficacy. With regard to the transdermal or intramuscular absorption of medications, several changes occur in the aging integumentary system that can result in a significant decrease in a drug's absorption [5]. These are summarized in Fig. 1.

Distribution

After absorption, how a drug is distributed within the body compartments depends upon its lipid and water solubility and the extent to which it is bound to plasma proteins. The volume of distribution (Vd) is the pharmacokinetic variable that relates the drug dose administered to its resulting concentration in body fluids.

- Diminished peripheral blood flow with impaired microcirculation (especially in patients with cardiovascular and peripheral vascular disease)
- Increased keratinization
- Decreased hydration and surface lipid content which affect both water-soluble and fat-soluble topical medications
- Decreased permeability with increased percentage of intramuscular connective tissue

Fig. 1 Factors that affect drug absorption in aging integument (Adapted from [5])

Aging decreases the body's lean-to-fat ratio and total body water 10–15 % by age 80 [6]. Subsequently, this results in a reduced Vd for water-soluble drugs and those drugs distributed to lean body tissues. Therefore a reduced loading dose is recommended for water-soluble medications such as digoxin, lithium, and theophylline. Conversely, the age-related increase in body fat content increases the Vd for lipid-soluble medications such as benzodiazepines, amiodarone, and hormones (thyroid), thereby resulting in reduced clearance and elimination time from the body.

Albumin and alpha-1-acid glycoprotein are the most common plasma proteins to which many drugs are bound. Although the concentrations of these plasma proteins do not normally decline significantly with normal aging, reduced nutritional status or catabolic states may cause a clinically important decline. Medications that are highly protein-bound, such as the warfarin and phenytoin, will have *higher free serum concentrations* in the elderly who have reduced plasma proteins [7]. For example, a patient may have a low total phenytoin blood level in the presence of hypoalbuminemia, yet a normal therapeutic free phenytoin level. So in order to avoid phenytoin toxicity, dose adjustments may need to be based on *free* dilantin level, not on the total blood level.

Metabolism

Liver mass and blood flow decrease significantly with aging, reducing clearance and increasing the half-life and bioavailability of medications that undergo extensive first-pass metabolism such as propanolol and labetolol [5]. On the other hand, the bioavailability of several ACE inhibitors, such as enalapril and perindopril, is reduced with advancing age because they require hepatic activation [8]. The activity of the hepatic cytochrome P450 oxidase system diminishes with age, including many Phase I reactions (reduction, oxidation, hydroxylation, and demethylation). Table 1 summarizes important isoenzymes of the P450 cytochrome system and commonly prescribed drugs whose metabolism is affected by them. Of note, grapefruit juice is a known inhibitor of the cytochrome P450 3A4 pathway. Such inhibitors can decrease clearance, increase half-life, and thus increase toxicity of some drugs [9]. Phase II reactions (drug conjugation with glucuronide and sulfate and drug acetylation) are minimally influenced by aging.

Renal Elimination and Clearance

Decreased renal elimination is the most significant pharmacokinetic change seen in the geriatric population. In one study of 10,000 long-term care residents, 40 % had significant renal insufficiency [10]. Renal mass decreases an average of 20 % from the fourth to the eighth decades of life with concomitant age-associated reductions in glomerular filtration rate, renal blood flow, and tubular secretion. Thus drugs that depend upon renal clearance require a dosage reduction [11].

Table 1 Common metabolic effects of P450 cytochrome enzymes (adapted from [9])

P450 enzyme	Common substrate medications	Common inhibitor/ inducer* medications	Problematic drug-drug interactions	Clinical problem
CYP 3A4	Simvastatin Atorvastatin Amiodarone Azithromycin Erythromycin Warfarin Quetiapine Solefenain Losartan Amlodipine Prednisone Omeprazole Sertraline Sitagliptin Oxycontin Vardenafil Mirtazapine	Amiodarone (moderate) Erythromycin (moderate) Ciprofloxacin (moderate) Amlodipine (weak) Rifampin Atripla*	Fat soluble Statin + Amiodarone Fat soluble Statin + Cipro	Increased statin level, which can cause a myopathy
			Azithromycin + Amiodarone Amiodarone + Ciprofloxacin	Leads to QT prolongation, and arrhythmia
			Warfarin + Amiodarone	High INR can lead to bleeding
			Statin + Atripla	Decreases statin levels
			Warfarin + Rifampin	Decreases INR and efficacy
			Rifampin + Atripla	Decreased HAART efficacy
CYP 2D6	Fluoxetine Aripiprazole Metoprolol Sertraline Oxycontin Mirtazapine	Fluoxetine (strong) Sertraline (weak) Amiodarone (weak)	Metoprolol + Fluoxetine	Bradycardia, AV block
CYP 2C9	Losartan Glipizide Vardenafil Warfarin	Fluoxetine (weak) Amiodarone (weak)	Warfarin + Fluoxetine	High INR can lead to bleeding
			Glipizide + Amniodarone	Hypoglycemia
CYP 2C19	Fluoxetine Omeprazole Sertraline Warfarin	Fluoxetine (moderate) Omeprazole (moderate)	Omeprazole + Warfarin	High INR can lead to bleeding

INR international normalized ratio, *HAART* Highly active antiretroviral therapy

With decreased muscle mass in the geriatric population, serum creatinine by itself is not an accurate measure of renal function. Calculators based on equations such as the *Cockcroft–Gault Equation*, that take into account a patient's measured serum creatinine, sex, age, and estimated lean body weight, give a more accurate approximation of creatinine clearance [12]. Another method to estimate creatinine clearance, the *Modification of Diet in Renal Disease (MDRD) equation*, can be used in clinical practice but is not yet recommended for adjustment of medication doses in the elderly nor routinely used in drug information sources and drug labeling on dosage recommendations [13].

Increased response:

- Increased sensitivity to CNS effects of benzodiazepines and alcohol
- Greater analgesic response to opioids
- Increased sensitivity to anticoagulants (warfarin, heparin)
- Increased risk of delirium from anticholinergic medications
- Increased risk of bladder outlet obstruction from anticholinergics
- Increased risk of extrapyramidal side effects and tardive dyskinesia from antipsychotics

Decreased response:

- Reduced sensitivity to beta-adrenergic agonists and antagonists

Adapted from references [4] and [5]

Fig. 2 Age-related changes in pharmacodynamics

Pharmacodynamics

Pharmacodynamics is the interaction between a drug and its effector organ(s) (i.e., receptor) that results in either a therapeutic or adverse response or both. In addition the elderly can exhibit increased sensitivity to the therapeutic as well as the toxic effects of many medications due to comorbid illness such as Alzheimer's disease, Parkinson's disease, strokes, congestive heart failure, and other disorders that increase frailty and reduce the ability of the body to maintain homeostasis. Figure 2 lists some pharmacodynamic changes commonly seen in the elderly.

Preventing Adverse Drug Events

A consensus panel of experts established the Beers' criteria. This is a list of medications best avoided in the elderly due to the high likelihood of *potential* adverse effects that has subsequently been included in State surveys of LTCFs. The Beers' criteria include medications with anticholinergic effects such as antihistamines (diphenhydramine) and antiemetics (promethazine), and other medications with a propensity to cause worsening mental status, (i.e., delirium), falls, urinary retention, orthostatic hypotension, dehydration, and movement disorders such as extrapyramidal signs and tardive dyskinesia. Benzodiazepines are also included because they increase the risk of a change in mental status, sedation, and falls [14].

A more recent screening tool, the *STOPP* (*S*creening *T*ool of *O*lder *P*erson's *P*rescriptions), may be more user-friendly than the Beers' list. A recent systematic review found it to be a more sensitive measure of potentially inappropriate prescribing patterns in community-dwelling, acute and long-term care older patients in Europe, Asia and North America. The STOPP tool was developed as many clinicians considered that certain drugs designated as inappropriate by the Beers' criteria were debatable, and could be prescribed in certain specific clinical situations. The STOPP criteria were designed to incorporate commonly encountered prescribing pitfalls that practitioners often encounter.

Both the Beers' and STOPP criteria do not substitute for thorough clinical assessment and good judgment, as clinicians must first and foremost consider whether medications are the possible cause of signs and symptoms seen in older adults. By optimizing and minimizing medication use in the elderly, unnecessary and potentially harmful adverse side effects and *prescribing cascades* (use of medication to treat the side effects of another) can be lessened or avoided. The STOPP criteria are summarized in Table 2 including examples of potential adverse outcomes due to inappropriate prescribing [15].

Use of Antipsychotic Medication

Older adults are especially vulnerable to adverse effects from atypical antipsychotic medication including delirium, extrapyramidal symptoms, postural hypotension, falls and cardiac arrhythmias. Although these medications have been used *off-label* to manage behavioral and psychological symptoms of dementia, safety concerns have been raised [16]. A population-based retrospective cohort study of older Canadian adults demonstrated an associated increase in the risk of acute kidney injury (AKI) with use of three different atypical antipsychotic medications (quetiapine, risperidone or olanzapine) [17].

In February 2014, the American Geriatrics Society (AGS) recommended as part of their *Choosing Wisely*® guidelines that physicians employ non-pharmacologic strategies as first-line treatment for aggression and disruptive behaviors associated with dementia. Identifying and addressing the underlying cause of the behavior can preclude the use of medication. If other approaches have failed and the clinician feels they need to prescribe an antipsychotic medication, patients and their families should be warned about adverse effects. Many facilities now require the family to sign informed consent prior to their use. Proactive monitoring of blood pressure, as well as serum lipid, glucose and creatinine measurements should all be part of the overall treatment plan for any patient on an atypical antipsychotic medication [18].

Diabetic Medication

Several studies have suggested that older persons with diabetes and high levels of comorbidity receive diminished cardiovascular benefit from intensive blood glucose control (Hgb A1C less than 6.5–7 %), and have an increased risk for hypoglycemia and would *benefit more from improved control of other risk factors* including serum lipids, dietary consumption of sodium, and blood pressure [19, 20]. Certain medications such as metformin are contraindicated in older patients with renal disease, ischemic heart disease, and heart failure (HF), due to the potentially increased risk for lactic acidosis. Thiazolidinediones can exacerbate bone loss and cause fluid retention, which in turn can exacerbate HF. (See Chap. "Common Clinical Conditions in Long-Term Care" on Common Medical Conditions for further discussion on the treatment of diabetes.)

Table 2 STOPP criteria for potentially inappropriate prescriptions[a]

Medication by physiological system	Prescribing pitfall	Potential adverse outcome
Cardiovascular system		
Digoxin	>125 µg per day with impaired renal function	Digoxin toxicity from decreased renal clearance
Thiazide diuretics	With history of gout	Gout attack, nephropathy
β-blockers	With COPD	COPD exacerbation
Diltiazem or verapamil	Class III or IV heart failure	CHF exacerbation
Calcium channel blockers	Chronic constipation	Worsening constipation, impaction
Dipyridamole	As monotherapy for cardiovascular secondary prevention	Orthostatic hypotension
Aspirin	With history of PUD without histamine H2 antagonist or PPI	Gastrointestinal bleeding
	≥150 mg/day	
	With no history of coronary, cerebral, or peripheral vascular symptoms or occlusive event	
Central nervous system		
TCAs	With dementia	CNS adverse effects
	With cardiac conductive abnormalities	Cardiac arrhythmia
	With constipation	Impaction, worsening constipation
	With prostatism or history of urinary retention	Urinary retention
Long-term, long-acting benzodiazepines	Any use	Falls, confusion, lethargy, overdose
Long-term neuroleptics	In those with parkinsonism or dementia	CNS and extrapyramidal adverse effects, cardiovascular events
First generation antihistamines	Prolonged use	Falls, CNS adverse effects
Gastrointestinal system		
Diphenoxylate, loperamide or codeine phosphate	For treatment of diarrhea of unknown cause	Delay in treatment of bacterial/other causes of diarrhea
	For severe infective gastroenteritis, i.e., bloody diarrhea, high fever, or severe systemic toxicity	Bacteremia, sepsis, death
Proton pump inhibitors	For peptic ulcer disease at full therapeutic dosage for >8 weeks	Aspiration pneumonia, B12 deficiency, magnesium deficiency
Respiratory system		
Theophylline	As monotherapy for COPD	Poorly controlled COPD, theophylline toxicity

(continued)

Table 2 (continued)

Medication by physiological system	Prescribing pitfall	Potential adverse outcome
Systemic corticosteroids	Instead of inhaled corticosteroids for maintenance therapy in moderate–severe COPD	Any corticosteroid side affect, especially hyperglycemia, osteoporosis, cataracts, confusion
Musculoskeletal system		
NSAIDs	With history of PUD or gastrointestinal bleeding, unless with concurrent histamine H2 receptor antagonist, PPI or misoprostol (Cytotec)	Gastrointestinal bleeding
	With moderate to severe HTN	Poorly controlled HTN
	With heart failure	Exacerbation of HF
	With warfarin (Coumadin)	Bleeding
	With chronic renal failure	Worsening renal function
	For relief of mild–moderate joint pain in osteoarthritis	Bleeding, exacerbation of renal function, heart failure, hypertension
Long-term corticosteroid	As monotherapy for rheumatoid or osteoarthritis	Corticosteroid adverse effects (see above)
Long-term NSAID or colchicine	For chronic treatment of gout where there is no contraindication to allopurinol	NSAID or colchicine adverse effects
Urogenital system		
Bladder antimuscarinic drugs	With dementia	CNS adverse effects
Antimuscarinic drugs	With chronic prostatism	Urinary retention
Endocrine system		
β-blockers	In those with DM	Unrecognized hypoglycemia
Drugs that adversely affect persons who are at risk to fall		
Benzodiazepines		Fall with or without injury
Neuroleptic drugs		
Vasodilator drugs	With postural hypotension	
Long-acting benzodiazepine		
Long-term opiates	In those with recurrent falls	
Analgesic drugs		
Long-term potent opioids	Use as first-line therapy for mild-moderate pain, e.g., morphine or fentanyl patch	CNS adverse effects, Falls with or without injury, hypotension
Long-term opioids	In those with dementia unless used for palliative care	
Regular scheduled opioids	For more than 2 weeks in those with chronic constipation without concurrent use of laxatives	Impaction, worsening constipation, bowel perforation, and ischemia

[a]Adapted from ref. [15]

Analgesics

The most recent pain treatment guidelines published by the American Geriatric Society (AGS) discourage both the use of *nonselective NSAIDs* (especially those with a long half-life such as naproxen and piroxicam) and *COX-2 selective inhibitors* due to their potential cardiac (fluid and sodium retention), gastrointestinal (inflammation, bleeding), CNS (altered mental status, psychosis), and renal effects (altered blood flow) [21]. Both these classes of medication have significant drug interactions with ACE inhibitors (potential for hyperkalemia), diuretics (diminished diuresis due to changes in renal blood flow), methotrexate (decreased clearance), anticoagulants (potentiated effects), and lithium (decreased renal clearance and increase risk of lithium toxicity). Additionally, there is concern that concomitant use of a NSAID (especially ibuprofen) or a COX-2 inhibitor with a once daily cardio-preventive dose of aspirin *will negate aspirin's cardio-preventive effect* [22].

In 2009, a FDA Advisory Panel recommended sweeping safety restrictions on the use of acetaminophen alone and in combination with opioids such as hydrocodone/acetaminophen and oxycodone/acetaminophen due to the reporting of increased cases of liver damage and acute liver failure associated with acetaminophen overuse. The panel advised that because combination prescription opioid/acetaminophen analgesics increase the possibility of accidental overdose and acute liver failure, that they either should be not used or their drug labeling should contain a black box warning to increase consumer awareness regarding the amount and content of acetaminophen in prescription and over-the-counter formulations. The panel also recommended that the maximal *amount per unit dose of acetaminophen be lowered to 325* mg in lieu of the current 500 and 650 mg tablets currently available on the market and that the maximum daily dosage for osteoarthritis be *less* than 4 g per day [23]. Useful medication guidelines for many drugs can be downloaded from the FDA website. These guidelines provide specific information for patients and caregivers and may help prevent ADEs [24].

Transitions in Care and Medication Errors

"Transitions of care" for patients typically involve changes in location, level of care, and providers. These transitions are common scenarios for potential medication errors and adverse outcomes for patients. Injuries related to medications were the most common adverse event during care transitions [25]. For this reason one of the National Patient Safety goals of the Joint Commission on Accreditation of Hospital Organizations (JCAHO) has been *medication reconciliation* and the transmission of accurate and up-to-date medication information across care settings. Table 3 identifies specific patient characteristics predictive of adverse medication outcomes.

Comprehensive and up-to-date records that accompany the patient through care transitions and a timely evaluation of the patient after care transfers can help alleviate medication errors, diagnose new problems or deteriorating conditions, and avoid adverse outcomes. Until a universally available electronic health care record (EHR) connects all care providers across all settings this will continue to be of the utmost importance [26].

Table 3 Risk factors for adverse events with care transitions

• Polypharmacy (>4 medications)
• Careful monitoring required by the medication: insulin, warfarin
• Chronic complex illness: stroke, cancer, diabetes, COPD, cancer
• Hurried transfers at nonstandard times of day/night/weekend
• Inadequate patient support post-discharge from a care setting

Medication Selection in the Elderly

In LTCFs, the primary responsibility for prescribing, ordering and procuring, initiation, dosing, monitoring, and when appropriate, altering or discontinuing medication therapy involves the triad of prescriber, nursing personnel, and pharmacy provider/consultant. Each has specific responsibilities for ensuring the patient receives the most appropriate medical therapy. Collaborative communications between all three providers is essential. Although studies assessing suboptimal prescribing often focus on identification of overuse and misuse of medications, it is equally important to ensure against the underuse of medication or the omission of a medically indicated drug for treatment or prevention of disease if appropriate to patient's goals of care. Such occurrences are reported in up to 50 % of community dwelling elders. Examples of possible therapy omissions in LTCFs include the lack of GI protection with proton pump inhibitors (PPIs) for those taking prednisone, no ACE inhibitor therapy for diabetics, no vitamin D supplementation for individuals at risk for osteoporosis, and lack of venous thromboembolism (VTE) prophylaxis [27].

The *START* (*S*creening *T*ool to *A*lert *D*octors to *R*ight *T*reatment) is a tool to help identify potentially beneficial medications that may have been omitted from a LTCF resident's treatment regimen. START is similar to STOPP and both have been validated in the elderly, derived from evidence-based prescribing indicators, and arranged according to physiological systems; but unlike STOPP, START identifies *possible prescribing omissions* in older adults, as opposed to medication overuse. Such tools can enable practitioners to better evaluate an older person's prescription drug regimen in the context of their current clinical diagnoses [15].

Special Considerations

Hypertension

The elderly are at high risk for cardiovascular events and thus hypertension should be monitored and treated. New recommendations from the Joint National Commission 8 (JNC-8) published in January 2014 set BP goals for individuals over the age of 60 years at < 150/90. This recommended goal has proven controversial

Table 4 Secondary causes of hypertension and identification clues

Cause	How to identify
Medications	Medication reconciliation: check for nonsteroidal anti-inflammatory (NSAIDS), steroids, venlafaxine, estrogen-containing preparations (found in herbals, over-the-counter meds)
Alcohol abuse	AUDIT-C
Obstructive sleep apnea	Epworth Sleepiness Scale, Sleep Study, Snoring history
Lifestyle	High sodium diet, increased Body Mass Index (BMI), lack of exercise
Primary renal disease	Basic metabolic profile (BMP), urine sediment, urine for microalbumin/creatinine
Renovascular disease	Clinical atherosclerosis: PVD, CAD, CVD. Acute onset/exacerbation of hypertension; +abdominal bruit, deterioration of renal function after angiotensin converting enzyme inhibitor (ACEI) or Angiotensin receptor blocker (ARB)
Primary aldosteronism	Electrolytes (low potassium)

Adapted from ref. [28]

and a minority of clinicians have dissented and advocated a lower blood pressure goal of 140/90 in patients under the age of 80 and the higher goal of 150/90 for those over the age of 80. There also was a change in the recommended BP goals for patients with chronic kidney disease and diabetes from <130/80 to <140/90. The Joint National Commission also recommended that clinicians investigate for secondary causes/contributors to hypertension (see Table 4), assess for end organ damage, and monitor for side effects of antihypertensive medications (including postural hypotension) [28].

If clinically appropriate, it is particularly important in geriatric patients to optimize antihypertensive therapy with lifestyle modifications, including the implementation of the Dietary Approaches to Stop Hypertension (DASH) diet with a sodium restriction of 1500 mg/day (4 g or two-thirds of a teaspoon of table salt) [29]. Restrictive diets are not recommended in the frail elderly because of their potential to cause weight loss. If, however, dietary intervention is insufficient to control the blood pressure, a low-dose thiazide diuretic and long-acting calcium channel blocker can be prescribed unless there are comorbidities that merit the choice of other drugs as reviewed in Fig. 3. (See chap. "Common Clinical Conditions in Long-Term Care" on Common Medical Conditions for further discussion on the treatment of hypertension).

Beta-Blocker Use in Post-Myocardial Infarction

Beta-blockers are important for patients in the early course of acute MI and as secondary prevention to reduce cardiac morbidity, mortality, and MI recurrence. Age greater than 75 has been associated with the *underuse* of beta-blockers. This is concerning given that mortality rate has been reported to be 43 % less among beta-blocker recipients than non-recipients [30].

- **Angina** – Beta-blockers decrease myocardial oxygen consumption and long acting calcium channel blockers (CCBs) improve diastolic dysfunction.

- **Post myocardial infarction** – Beta-blockers decrease risk of recurrent myocardial infarction (MI); angiotensin converting enzyme inhibitors (ACEIs) and angiotensin receptor blockers (ARBs) mitigate congestive heart failure and ventricular remodeling.

- **Diabetes** - Angiotensin Converting Enzyme inhibitors (ACEIs) and ARBs can help preserve normal renal blood flow and function early in the course of kidney disease.

- **Heart Failure** - ACEIs, ARBs, and diuretics improve afterload reduction and beta-blockers improve survival.

- **Gout** - Avoid thiazide diuretics if possible due to elevation in uric acid level. ARBs such as losartan are uricosuric.

- **Chronic Obstructive Lung Disease** - Avoid beta-blockers, which may exacerbate bronchospasm.

*Adapted from [28]

Fig. 3 Clinical situations meriting specific antihypertensive therapy. Adapted from ref. [28]

Anticoagulants in Non-valvular Atrial Fibrillation

Warfarin (vitamin K antagonist (VKA)) is recommended as a first line agent in patients older than age 75 with atrial fibrillation due to the increased rate of stroke. Warfarin is also recommended for patients with atrial fibrillation between the ages of 65 and 75 if other risk factors for stroke are present (i.e., hypertension, diabetes mellitus, CHF, previous history of stroke, transient ischemic attack, or peripheral vascular disease). The CHA2DS2VASc calculator incorporates these risk factors and is a tool recommended by the American Heart Association to predict the yearly stroke risk in patients with chronic non-valvular atrial fibrillation [31]. Patients with a score of 1 (male) or greater than 1 (female) are at high risk for embolic stroke and anticoagulation should be seriously considered if not contraindicated. The INR should be in the recommended range of 2–3 in order to provide the maximal benefit. Although the risk of bleeding during warfarin therapy is of concern, careful patient selection and frequent, regular monitoring of therapy minimizes the risk, particularly with the widespread use of anticoagulant specialty care clinics [32].

Several new oral anticoagulant drugs have been available from two broad classes. The direct thrombin inhibitor (dabigatran) and direct factor Xa inhibitors (rivaroxaban and apixaban) that have comparable efficacy to warfarin, with less risk of intracranial hemorrhage but higher risk of major GI bleeding. They offer the added convenience of needing no anticoagulation monitoring and having less significant food and drug interactions [33, 34]. The anticoagulant effects are not reversible except by dialysis (dabigatran) or a prothrombin complex concentrate (rivaroxaban and apixaban).

Subclinical Hypothyroidism

Subclinical hypothyroidism is identified in up to 18 % of elderly persons, and progression from subclinical to overt hypothyroidism occurs at a rate of 5–18 % per year [35]. Use of medications such as lithium, alpha interferon and amiodarone increase the risk for hypothyroidism. Lithium, amiodarone, propanolol, and glucocorticoids inhibit peripheral conversion of T4 to active T3, whereas alpha interferon and amiodarone can cause thyroiditis. Subclinical hypothyroidism has been associated with subtle cardiac function abnormalities, atherogenic serum lipid profiles, blood pressure dysregulation, impaired endothelial function, alterations in cerebral blood flow, and impairment of memory [36].

Bedtime dosing of thyroid replacement normalizes serum TSH levels more optimally than daily dosing in the morning [37]. Replacement dosing should be increased gradually in geriatric patients as they may have undiagnosed heart disease, and can develop dysrhythmias, angina, or myocardial infarction if started on full replacement dosages or if their dose is increased too rapidly. Treatment of subclinical hypothyroidism, even at TSH levels of 5–10 mIU/L, produces beneficial effects on lipoprotein profiles. However, in elderly patients it is prudent to start with a levothyroxine dose of 25–50 mcg/day, with subsequent dose increments of 25 mcg every 4–6 weeks until target TSH goals are reached. The Clinical Practice Guidelines of the American Association of Clinical Endocrinologists for the management of hypothyroidism are posted on their website [38]. (See Chap. "Common Clinical Conditions in Long-Term Care" on Common Medical Conditions for further discussion of the treatment of thyroid disease).

Gradual Dose Reduction in SNFs/NFs

Federal nursing facility regulations require that gradual dose reductions (GDR) of patients' medication be attempted at least quarterly for all *sedative/hypnotics* and *psychotropics* that are used routinely and taken beyond the manufacturer's recommendations for duration of use.

However, the consultant pharmacist's recommendation for a GDR can be declined on clinical grounds if:

1. Continued use of the medication is in accordance with the current standard of practice and a GDR would likely impair the patient's function or cause psychiatric instability by either exacerbating an underlying medical condition or psychiatric disorder.

   or

2. Patient's target symptoms for which the medication had been prescribed either returned or worsened after the most recent GDR, and further GDR attempts would likely impair the patient's function or psychiatric stability.

Practitioners should note that current State Operations Manual (SOM) guidelines to surveyors state that the medications should be prescribed *only* when necessary and in the lowest effective dose and that each resident's drug regimen be free from *unnecessary* drugs (F-Tag 329). Once symptoms have resolved or stabilized, these guidelines also suggest that attempts be made to either discontinue the medication or reduce the dose through GDR. Previously, efforts to reduce unnecessary medication use focused solely on antipsychotics, benzodiazepines, and other centrally acting drugs. The current guidelines encourage GDR be attempted for *all medications* unless the patient's current condition would be adversely affected. See Appendix A for more detailed information on what defines an unnecessary medication and the intent of their regulation.

Choosing Wisely® and Medication Management

The American Board of Internal Medicine Foundation recently initiated a campaign to discourage medical interventions of no clinical benefit to patient care or that could potentially cause harm to patients. As such many subspecialties and AMDA-The Society for Post-Acute and Long-Term Care Medicine have developed several medication-related recommendations. These are listed in Appendix B and are available for review at the Choosing Wisely® website where the rationale of each recommendation is briefly discussed.

In response to the 2014 GAO report on adverse events in SNF patients, in 2015 AMDA-The Society for PA and LTC Medicine began spearheading the Quality Prescribing Initiative in collaboration with CMS and other long-term care provider organizations.

Pharmacogenomics

Pharmacogenomics is an evolving field of investigation, which explains how the response seen to a drug varies as the individual's genetic makeup varies, because the individual's genetic makeup helps to determine a drug's pharmacodynamics and pharmacokinetics. Information on a person's genome can then help to customize pharmacologic therapy, reducing adverse drug reactions and optimizing drug benefits. Commercial testing for genetic variants of the hepatic cytochrome P-450 isoforms is now available. Although not currently in mainstream clinical practice pharmacogenetic testing may soon be a commonly used tool to guide medication prescribing. The Pharmacogenetics Research Network was established by the National Institutes of Health in 2000 in order to:

- Investigate relationships between genetic variations and variable drug responses.
- Create a base of knowledge available to the public which provides reliable information about genetic makeup and medication responsiveness.
- Facilitate collaboration among investigators.

A central web-enabled repository of known genetic variants that determine drug responses is available at http://www.pharmgkb.org. It is updated regularly and links the results of patient pharmacogenetic tests to specific recommendations on therapeutic dosing for many drugs in current use [39].

Summary

Timely and aggressive pharmacologic intervention for a new or worsening medical condition is essential in the elderly who are relatively healthy and who have a favorable life expectancy. However the intended positive outcomes of any medication must be balanced against the risk of an adverse drug event and a sub-therapeutic response. Efforts to optimize appropriate, effective, and safe medication use in the elderly have become a priority for health care systems, clinicians, and the state and federal agencies. Tools such as the Beers', STOPP, and START criteria can remind practitioners of potentially inappropriate and appropriate medication use. *Quality prescribing* has the potential for primary and secondary prevention and an improved quality of life. It is incumbent upon practitioners to collaborate with pharmacists, nursing personnel, caregivers, and patients. Practitioners must also regularly assess for both negative and positive medication outcomes and decide whether to continue pharmacologic treatment based upon patient goals and preferences for care, prognosis, and time needed to treat in order to obtain the desired therapeutic benefit.

Pearls for the Practitioner

- Polypharmacy (sometimes called "multiple medication use") is characterized by excessive or unnecessary use of medications (often at doses higher than necessary for the clinical situation) or drug combinations that put the elderly at excessive risk due to drug–drug, drug–disease, or drug–nutrient interactions.
- Request elderly patients and their caregivers to bring in all medications, including over-the-counter and herbal medications to each office visit or upon admission from home to an assisted living or nursing facility.
- Regularly review the LTCF resident's medication administration record (i.e., MAR) looking for unnecessary medication use (i.e., no apparent indication, either subtherapeutic or in excessive dose, prolonged duration of action, drug interactions, inappropriate dosage forms, and excessive cost) and adjust accordingly.
- Consider a potential adverse drug event in the differential diagnosis of any change in the clinical status of an elderly patient.

- Gradual up-titration is appropriate when starting a new medication in the elderly, particularly when prescribing thyroid hormone replacement in a patient who may have underlying ischemic heart disease.
- The Beers' and STOPP criteria can be used to help clinicians avoid prescribing potentially inappropriate medication in older adults, especially those with anticholinergic properties or hypotensive effects.
- Dietary and behavioral interventions rather than pharmacotherapy may be more useful, less expensive and have other salutary effects for treating some chronic conditions in the elderly.
- Anticipate decreased renal clearance and hepatic oxidative metabolism and accordingly individualize drug doses when initiating or modifying drug therapy in the elderly.
- Until pharmacogenetic testing is in general use, a personal and family history of medication intolerances and adverse effects may be indicate the presence of genetic variations in CYP-P450 enzymes and suggest alternative medication choices and/or dosing.

Websites

1. GFR Calculator Using Cockcroft–Gault, MDRD equations. http://www.medcalc.com/gfr.html.
2. U.S. Food and Drug Administration. Public health advisory: deaths with antipsychotics in elderly patients with behavioral disturbances. Silver Spring, DM: US Food and Drug Administration; 2005. Accessed at: www.fda.gov/Drugs/DrugSafety/PostmarketDrugSafetyInformationforPatientsandProviders/DrugSafetyInformationforHelathcareProfessionals/PublicHealthAdvisories/ucm053171.htm.
3. AGS Clinical Practice Guidelines for Pharmacological Management of Persistent Pain in Older Persons. Available at: http://www.americangeriatrics.org/files/documents/2009_Guideline.pdf. Accessed on March 30, 2015.
4. US Food and Drug Administration Medication Guides. http://www.fda.gov/Drugs/DrugSafety/ucm085729.htm.
5. FDA Drug Safety Alert. FDA recommends health care professionals discontinue prescribing and dispensing prescription combination products with > 325 mg acetaminophen to protect consumers. http://www.fda.gov/Drugs/DrugSafety/ucm381644.htm.
6. In Brief: Your Guide to Lowering Your Blood Pressure with DASH. The DASH Eating Plan. Available on:http://www.nhlbi.nih.gov/files/docs/public/heart/dash_brief.pdf.

7. MD+CALC. CHA2DS2-VASc Score for Atrial Fibrillation Stroke Risk. Available at: http://www.mdcalc.com/cha2ds2-vasc-score-for-atrial-fibrillation-stroke-risk/
8. Choosing Wisely: An initiative of the American Board of Internal Medicine Foundation.www.choosingwisely.org.
9. Clinical Practice Guidelines of the American Association of Clinical Endocrinologists for management of patients with hypothyroidism and suspected hypothyroidism. 2012 Updates www.aace.com/pub/pdf/guidelines/hypo_hyper.pdf.
10. Pharm GKB. The Pharmacogenomics Knowledgebase. Pharmacogenomics. Knowledge, Implementation. Pharm GB is a comprehensive resource that curates knowledge about the impact of genetic variation on drug response for clinicians and researchers. http://www.pharmgkb.org.

Appendix A. Unnecessary Drugs in the NF/SNF

F-tag #	Regulation	Guidance to surveyors
F329	*Unnecessary drugs* *1. General.* Each resident's drug regimen must be free from unnecessary drugs. An unnecessary drug is any drug when used: (i) In excessive dose (including duplicate therapy); or (ii) For excessive duration; or (iii) Without adequate monitoring; or (iv) Without adequate indications for its use; or (v) In the presence of adverse consequences which indicate the dose should be reduced or discontinued; or (vi) Any combinations of the reasons above.	*Intent: Unnecessary drugs* The intent of this requirement is that each resident's entire drug/medication regimen be managed and monitored to achieve the following goals: The medication regimen helps promote or maintain the resident's highest practicable mental, physical, and psychosocial well-being, as identified by the resident and/or representative(s) in collaboration with the attending physician and facility staff; Each resident receives only those medications, in doses and for the duration clinically indicated to treat the resident's assessed condition(s); Non-pharmacological interventions (such as behavioral interventions) are considered and used when indicated, instead of, or in addition to medication; Clinically significant adverse consequences are minimized; and The potential contribution of the medication regimen to an unanticipated decline or newly emerging or worsening symptom is recognized and evaluated, and the regimen is modified when appropriate. *NOTE*: This guidance applies to all categories of medications including antipsychotic medications.

Source: Code of Federal Regulations 483.25(l)

Appendix B. Choosing Wisely® and Medication Management in PA/LTC

Organization	Recommendation
AMDA-Society for PA/LTC Medicine	Do not use sliding scale insulin for long-term diabetes management for individuals residing in the nursing home.
	Do not routinely prescribe lipid-lowing medication in individuals with limited life expectancy.
	Do not initiate hypertensive treatment in individuals > 60 years of age for SBP <150 mm Hg or DBP < 90 mm Hg.
	Do not prescribe antipsychotic medications for behavioral and psychological symptoms of dementia (BPSD) in individuals with dementia without an assessment for an underlying cause of the behavior.
American Geriatrics Society	Do not prescribe a medication without conducting a drug regimen review.
	Do not prescribe cholinesterase inhibitors for dementia without periodic assessment for perceived cognitive benefits and adverse GI effects.
	Avoid using prescription appetite stimulants or high calorie supplements for treatment of anorexia or cachexia in order adults.
AAHPM	Do not use ABH gel (Ativan, Benadryl, Haldol) for nausea.
American Psychiatric Association	Do not routinely prescribe antipsychotic medication as a first-line intervention for insomnia in adults.
	Do not routinely use antipsychotics as first choice to treat BPSD (see above).
	Do not routinely prescribe two or more antipsychotic medications concurrently.
American Society of Nephrology	Do not administer erythropoiesis-stimulating agents (ESAs) to chronic renal disease patients with hemoglobin levels ≥ 10 g/dl (without symptoms of anemia).
	Avoid NSAIDs in individuals with hypertension or heart failure or chronic kidney disease of all causes including diabetes.

References

1. The State of Aging and Health in America 2013. Available at: http://www.cdc.gov/features/agingandhealth/state_of_aging_and_health_in_america_2013.pdf. Accessed 30 Mar 2015.
2. Cooper JW. Probable adverse drug reactions in a rural geriatric nursing home population: a four year study. J Am Geriatr Soc. 1996;44:194–7.
3. McLean AJ, Le Conteur DG. Aging biology and geriatric clinical pharmacology. Pharmacol Rev. 2004;56:163–84.
4. Heidelbaugh JJ. Proton pump inhibitors and risk of vitamin and mineral deficiencies: evidence and clinical implications. Ther Adv Drug Saf. 2013;4(3):125–33.
5. Roskos KV, Maibach HI, Guy RH. The effect of aging on percutaneous absorption in man. J Pharmacokinet Biopharm. 1989;17:617–30.

6. Parker BM, Cusack BJ, Vestal RE. Pharmacokinetic optimization of drug therapy in elderly patients. Drugs Aging. 1995;7:10–8.
7. Greenblatt DJ, Sellers EM, Shader RI. Drug disposition in old age. N Engl J Med. 1982;306:1081–7.
8. Todd PA, Fitton A. Perindopril. A review of its pharmacological properties and therapeutic use. Drugs. 1991;42:90–114.
9. Oates JA, Wilkinson GR. Principles of drug therapy (Chapter 68). In: Fauci AS, Braunwald E, Isselbacher KJ, et al., editors. Harrison's principles of internal medicine, vol. 1. 14th ed. New York: MGraw-Hill; 1998. p. 411–24.
10. Garg AX, Papaioannou A, Ferko N, et al. Estimating the prevalence of renal insufficiency in long-term care. Kidney Int. 2004;65(2):649–53.
11. Bennett WM. Geriatric pharmacokinetics and the kidney. Am J Kidney Dis. 1990;16:283.
12. Cockcroft DW, Gault MH. Prediction of creatinine clearance from serum creatinine. Nephron. 1976;16:31–41.
13. MedCalc: Glomerular filtration rate estimation. GFR Calculator using Cockcroft-Gault, MDRD equations. http://www.medcalc.com/gfr.html Accessed on 15 Mar 2015.
14. Beers MH. Explicit criteria for determining potentially inappropriate medication use by the elderly. Arch Intern Med. 2001;135:703.
15. Gallagher P, Ryan C, Byrne S. STOPP (Screening Tool of Older Person's Prescriptions) and START (Screening Tool to Alert Doctors to Right Treatment). Consensus Validation. Int J Clin Pharmacol Ther. 2008;46(2):72–83.
16. U.S. Food and Drug Administration. Public health advisory; deaths with antipsychotics in elderly patients with behavioral disturbances. Silver Spring, MD: U.S. Food and Drug Administration. 2005. Accessed at: http://www.fda.gov/Drugs/DrugSafety/PostmarketDrugSafetyInformationforPatientsandProviders/ucm053171.htm. Accessed 30 Mar 2015.
17. Hwang YJ, Dixon SN, Reiss JP, et al. Aypical antipsychotic drugs and the risk for acute kidney injury and other adverse outcomes in older adults. a population-based cohort study. Ann Intern Med. 2014;161(4):242–8.
18. Choosing Wisely: An initiative of the American board of internal medicine foundation). Available at: www.choosingwisely.org. Accessed 26 Mar 2015.
19. Gerstein HC, Miller ME, Byington RP, et al. Action to control cardiovascular risk in diabetes study group. effects of intensive glucose lowering in type 2 diabetes. N Engl J Med. 2008;358:2560–72.
20. Duckworth W, Abraira C, Moritz T, et al. VADT investigators. glucose control and vascular complications n veterans with type 2 diabetes. N Engl J Med. 2009;360:129–39.
21. AGS Clinical Practice Guidelines for Pharmacological Management of Persistent Pain in Older Persons. Available at: http://www.americangeriatrics.org/files/documents/2009_Guideline.pdf. Accessed 30 Mar 2015.
22. McGettigan P, Henry D. Cardiovascular risk and inhibitors of cyclooxygenase: a systemic review of observational studies of selective and non-selective inhibitors of cyclooxygenase-2. JAMA. 2006;296(13):1633–44.
23. Kuehn J. FDA focuses on drugs and liver damage: labeling and other changes for acetaminophen. JAMA. 2009;302:369–71.
24. US Food and Drug Administration Medication Guides. http://www.fda.gov/Drugs/DrugSafety/ucm085729.htm. Accessed 30 Mar 2015.
25. Forster AJ, Murff HJ, Peterson JF, et al. The incidence and severity of adverse events affecting patients after discharge from the hospital. Ann Intern Med. 2003;138:161–7.
26. Joint Commission Center for Transforming Health Care. Project Detail. Hand-off Communications. Available at: http://www.centerfortransforminghealthcare.org/projects/detail.aspx?Project=1. Accessed on 30 Mar 2015.
27. Higashi T, Shekelle PG, Adams JL, et al. The quality of pharmacologic care for vulnerable older patients. Ann Intern Med. 2004;140:714–20.

28. James PA, Oparil S, Carter BL, et al. 2014 evidence-based guideline for the management of high blood pressure in adults: report from the panel members appointed to the Eighth Joint National Committee (JNC 8). JAMA. 2014;311(5):507.
29. Moore TJ, Conlin PR, Ard J, et al. DASH (Dietary Approaches to Stop Hypertension) diet is effective treatment for stage 1 isolated systolic hypertension. Hypertension. 2001;38:155–8.
30. Soumerai SB, McLaughlin TJ, Spiegelman D, et al. Adverse outcomes of underuse of beta-blockers in elderly survivors of acute myocardial infarction. JAMA. 1997;277(2):115–21.
31. MD+CALC. CHA2DS2-VASc Score for atrial fibrillation stroke risk. Available at: http://www.mdcalc.com/cha2ds2-vasc-score-for-atrial-fibrillation-stroke-risk/ Accessed 30 Mar 2015.
32. Dhond AJ, Michaelena HI, Ezekowitz MD. Anticoagulation in the elderly. Am J Geriatr Cardiol. 2003;12(4):243–50.
33. Connally SJ, Ezekowitz MD, Yusuf S, et al. Dabigatran vs warfarin in patients with atrial fibrillation. N Engl J Med. 2009;361:1139–51.
34. Patel MR, Mahaffey KW, Garg J, et al. Rivaroxaban vs warfarin in nonvalvular atrial fibrillation. N Engl J Med. 2011;365:883–91.
35. Hollowell JG, Staehling NW, Flanders WD, et al. Serum TSH T4 and thyroid antibodies in the United States population (1988–94): National Health and Nutrition Examination Survey (NHANES III). J Clin Endocrinol Metab. 2002;87:489–99.
36. Samuels MH, Schuff KG, Carlson NE, et al. Health status, mood and cognition in experimentally induced subclinical hypothyroidism. J Clin Endocrinol Metab. 2007;92:2545–51.
37. Bolk N, Visser TJ, Kalsbeek A, et al. Effects of evening vs morning thyroxine ingestion on serum thyroid hormone profiles in hypothyroid patients. Clin Endocrinol (Oxf). 2007;66:43–8.
38. Clinical practice guidelines of the American association of clinical endocrinologists for management of patients with hypothyroidism and suspected hypothyroidism. 2012. Available at: https://www.aace.com/files/final-file-hypo-guidelines.pdf . Accessed 30 Mar 2015.
39. Roden DM, Altman RB, et al. Pharmacogenomics: challenges and opportunities. Ann Intern Med. 2006;145(10):749–57.

Rehabilitation and Maximizing Function

Thomas Lawrence

Introduction

Federal nursing facility regulations require that necessary care and services be provided for residents to "attain or maintain" the highest practicable level of physical, mental, and psychosocial well-being [1, 2]. Rehabilitation (rehab) services and care to promote maximum function are a fundamental component of nursing facility care.

Providing recuperative and rehabilitative services to patients following hospitalization is among the fastest growing segment of health care spending in the USA. A growing number of elders being discharged from hospitals will spend some time convalescing in the long-term care setting especially in a skilled nursing facility with about 1.5 million American elders receiving rehabilitation in nursing facilities each year [3]. This subset of skilled nursing facility residents represents the largest percentage of short-stay nursing facility admissions.

Background

The decision of *where* to provide rehabilitation therapy following an acute illness is dependent on several factors:

- How many therapy modalities are to be utilized.
- The number and complexity of concurrent medical problems.

T. Lawrence, MD, CMD (✉)
System Medical Director of Geriatric Medicine and Long Term Care,
Main Line Health System, Main Line Health Center, 3855 West Chester Pike, Suite 300,
Newtown Square, PA 19073, USA
e-mail: tomlawrence@comcast.net

© Springer International Publishing Switzerland 2016
P.A. Fenstemacher, P. Winn (eds.), *Post-Acute and Long-Term Medicine*,
Current Clinical Practice, DOI 10.1007/978-3-319-16979-8_19

- The individual's physical ability to participate in therapy:

    - Inpatient rehab facility: requires the patient be able to participate in at least 2–3 h of combined therapies daily.
    - Skilled nursing facility: the patient is able to tolerate less than 2–3 h of combined therapies daily.

- Sites of care:

    - Inpatient Rehabilitation Facility (IRF).
    - Long-term Acute Care Facility (LTAC).
    - Nursing facility and skilled nursing facility.
    - Assisted living facility.
    - Program of All-Inclusive Care of the Elderly (PACE).
    - Home care.

- Rehabilitation services can also be provided to long-stay residents of nursing facilities if physical function deteriorates due to an acute and/or chronic illness.

In all settings successful rehabilitation requires that a variety of therapeutic interventions be delivered in a coordinated and timely fashion with the goal to restore and maximize function [2, 4].

- Goals for rehabilitation in the nursing facility must be established by a interdisciplinary team including therapists (OT, PT, ST), nurses, and the attending physician, and aligned with the preferences of the resident.
- Goals should be realistic, attainable, and aimed at improving resident function and independence, while respecting the individual's quality of life and dignity.
- Overall prognosis of residents often change over time and can result in the therapy plan being temporarily suspended or altered due to acute change in status and changing or competing goals of care. For example, an acute illness can result in the decision to forego rehabilitation goals of care and instead initiate a more palliative approach or admission to hospice.

Types of Therapy Services

Therapy services have evolved into three traditional rehabilitation disciples: *physical therapy, occupational therapy*, and *speech therapy*. Other therapy modalities that are growing in both importance and availability include *respiratory therapy, psychotherapy, cognitive therapy*, and *recreational therapy* (which includes music and pet therapy). Although some of these latter modalities (e.g., psychotherapy) may be covered separately under Medicare or other insurance plans, such supportive therapy services may not be separately reimbursed but be routinely provided as part of the nursing facility care per diem. All rehabilitation professionals must coordinate services as part of the comprehensive assessment and plan of care conducted as part of the Federally mandated nursing facility resident assessment protocols (now called *care area assessments*).

Physical therapy is the discipline that focuses on the restoration of movement and functional ability involving the extremities with particular attention to ambulation and transfer skills.

Occupational therapy as a discipline focuses on promoting the residents ability to participate in activities of daily living such as dressing, grooming, and bathing. While physical therapy focuses on the function of the lower extremities occupational therapy focuses on upper extremity function. Some occupational therapists have acquired expertise in the evaluation of patients with eating and swallowing difficulties.

Speech and language therapy addresses disorders of speech, language, voice, communication, cognition, and swallowing. Speech therapists often provide recommendations for altered consistency diets in residents with dysphagia.

Payment for Rehabilitation Therapy

Under Medicare, the cost of rehabilitation therapy is included in the prospective payment daily rate paid to skilled nursing facilities following hospitalization. (This SNF benefit requires at least a 3-day hospitalization). The daily rate is calculated according to the variety and intensity of rehab and nursing services that are needed and are to be provided. For residents whose nursing facility stay is no longer covered by the Medicare Part A benefit or other private insurance, rehabilitation therapies can then be covered under the Medicare Part B benefit (during an NF or in the community). This coverage is contingent upon the service meeting medical necessity requirements as being reasonable and necessary for the resident's care. Part B therapy services are subject to cap limits on annual payment.

Multi-morbidities and Frailty

In many cases there is a rather small window of opportunity to initiate rehabilitation therapy services. Elders have an increasing number and complexity of both acute and chronic medical problems—medical *multi-morbidities*—that can delay rehab. Common conditions include cardiac, pulmonary, gastrointestinal, renal disease, malnutrition, depression, musculoskeletal and neurological problems (including dementia), and finally muscle deconditioning and generalized weakness. Such conditions can interact in dynamic and complex manner to trigger acute functional decline that will then limit the patient's response to therapy and result in less than optimal rehabilitation outcome.

Prevention During Rehabilitation

Pressure Ulcer Prevention

Residents who are undergoing rehabilitation are often at high risk for pressure ulcer development due to risk factors of immobility, urinary incontinence, and multiple comorbid medical conditions (including diabetes). Aggressive prevention strategies should be implemented. Principles of pressure ulcer prevention that are particularly appropriate include: a frequent turning and positioning schedule (at least every 2 h), managing urinary and fecal incontinence, management of contractures, frequent skin inspection, maintenance of adequate nutrition and hydration, use of offloading or pressure-redistribution devices, and proper transfer and lift techniques [5]. Worsening and delayed healing of pressure ulcers can result in a suboptimal rehabilitation outcome. Prevention and successful management of pressure ulcers will promote the best outcomes (see "Wound Care" chapter for further detail).

Prevention of Venous Thromboembolism (VTE)

Nursing home residents are a frequently overlooked risk group for VTE [6]. Although universal application of VTE prophylaxis to all rehab patients is of unproven benefit, there are circumstances when prophylaxis is essential. VTE prophylaxis has proven benefit for patients who have had surgery for hip fracture or who have had hip or knee arthroplasty. Various agents are approved for use and the duration of treatment for prophylaxis is variable but usually continues for a minimum of 4 weeks. Ongoing research will help determine other high-risk residents who may benefit from VTE prophylaxis. One clinical dichotomy that needs to be balanced as to benefit/risk is the fact that some residents while at high risk for VTE, are also at high risk for bleeding when treated with anticoagulants [7]. Individual patient clinical risk factors and preferences for treatment need to be considered when deciding whom to anticoagulate.

Rehabilitation Approaches for Specific Conditions

Stroke

The goals of rehabilitation for stroke patients include:

- Stabilizing and, if possible, optimizing treatment of comorbid medical and psychologic conditions.
- Implementing stroke prevention strategies to include the treatment of modifiable risk factors.

- Preventing and managing stroke-related sequelae.
- Promoting neurological and physical functional recovery.

The rehabilitation phase is critical as up to 20 % of first-ever stroke patients die within the first 30 days with pneumonia, pulmonary embolism, and cardiac complications (e.g., MI, CHF) being the most common causes of death.

Stroke rehabilitation begins immediately upon medical stabilization. The goal should be to prevent recurrent stroke, avoid medical complications, mobilize the patient, and encourage self-care activities. Complications that require active prevention and management strategies include pressure ulcers, spasticity and contractures, bowel and bladder issues (e.g., incontinence, urinary retention, fecal impaction) and prevention of respiratory complications (e.g., aspiration, pneumonia).

Spasticity occurs in over 60 % of patients following a stroke [8]. This manifests as an increase in muscle tone with exaggerated deep tendon reflexes. Although spasticity can sometimes help ambulation, it is often painful and can be debilitating. Management involves daily stretching exercises and avoidance of stimuli that trigger spasticity. In the elderly oral antispasmodic drugs are poorly tolerated due to the common side effects of sedation and confusion. For more severe cares, focal injections of phenol or botulinum toxin may be effective as is serial casting. Muscle contractures occur when there is permanent shortening of a muscle or tendon due to continuous increased muscle tone, which occurs with spasticity of the extremities. Contractures are difficult to reduce and may require surgical intervention. Managing spasticity and promoting stretching and maintaining range of motion are critical to preventing contractures.

Bowel and bladder dysfunction following stroke occurs in 50–70 % of patients but in many resolves within 3–6 months [8]. Most strokes cause a hyperreflexic bladder and uninhibited bladder contractions resulting in urinary urgency. This is best managed with a timed voiding schedule. Monitoring urine output and post-void residual bladder volume is helpful. Urinary retention and overflow incontinence are less common complications following stroke. Prostate enlargement in men, medication effects on bladder function, and preexisting urinary incontinence can complicate bladder management. Urinary incontinence is one of the major risk factors for pressure ulcer development, so skin protective interventions must be utilized. Bowel incontinence is less common and less chronic but can be complicated by fecal impaction. Here risk factors include inactivity, poor nutrition, and inadequate fluid intake. A high fiber diet and adequate fluid intake can usually achieve bowel continence.

Respiratory complications are often precipitated by stroke-related dysphagia. Aspiration usually occurs during the pharyngeal phase of swallowing and significant dysphagia can often occur without clinical evidence of aspiration. Up to one-third of patients with dysphagia have episodes of aspiration [8]. Formal evaluation of swallowing function by a speech therapist is often needed and a video fluoroscopic swallowing study can be both diagnostic and helpful with selecting the most appropriate diet consistency for the patient.

The incidence of pulmonary embolism after stroke is 10–15 %, so VTE prophylaxis should be considered. Attaining ambulation of at least 50 feet per day reduces the risk of DVT and pulmonary embolism [8].

Therapy interventions can begin once neurological deficits are no longer progressing, usually within 48 h after a stroke. Initially, when the affected extremities are more flaccid, interventions involve passive range of motion and bed positioning exercises with progressively increasing intensity. In the past the approach to the older stroke patient was mostly supportive and focused on preventing complications while allowing spontaneous recovery to occur. Modern approaches now involve the use of more aggressive treatment, which include compensation strategies, neurophysiologic training techniques, task-oriented retraining, as well as strengthening exercises [8].

Compensation refers to using alternate approaches to task completion such as using the *unaffected* extremity to perform a specific task or using a wheelchair to improve mobility and functional recovery. *Neurophysiologic training* involves using the *affected* side to perform tasks and relearn normal movement. This also minimizes spasticity. *Task-oriented retraining* involves intensive practice with the affected extremity preformed for relatively long time periods. This technique sometimes includes restraining the *unaffected* extremity in order to force greater use of the affected extremity. *Strengthening exercises* utilizing progressive resistance target both general fitness and extremity strengthening. *Aerobic exercise* has been shown to improve outcomes such as gait speed and decreased fall risk.

Fracture Care

Hip fracture occurring in the community or a nursing facility is a common reason for admission to a skilled nursing facility. The annual mortality rate in the elderly following a hip fracture is extremely high (up to 36 %) and optimal outcomes require successful management of comorbidities. Up to 50 % of patients do not regain their previous ambulatory function while up to 20 % may become nonambulatory [9]. Rehabilitation should start as soon as possible after surgery. The most important issue is early mobilization. This is considered essential in order to prevent complications such as pneumonia, deep venous thrombosis, pulmonary embolism, urinary tract infection, and pressure ulcers. Other common complications include delirium, depression, anorexia, weight loss, and unsuccessful healing (nonunion, instability, and dislocation) of the hip fracture.

An early goal of therapy following hip surgery is retaining strength and preventing muscle atrophy on the unaffected lower extremity while isometric exercise of the limb that recently had surgery is performed to full extension. The speed of rehabilitation usually depends on the type of surgery performed, with prosthetic joint replacement progressing more quickly than after pinning. Full weight bearing can begin as soon as day 2 after surgery if the joint is replaced, followed by balance retraining and ambulation exercises beginning within 4–8 days. Stair-climbing exercises are the final stage of rehabilitation that usually can begin after 10 days. Strengthening of the trunk and quadriceps muscles are performed daily and taught to patients. Occasionally, in cases of high surgical risk, *rehabilitation without surgery* may be the best treatment approach. Here secondary disabilities such as pressure ulcers, muscle atrophy, and joint contractures, and general deconditioning are quite common and usually limit the functional outcome. *Effective pain management is essential.*

Pelvic fractures involving the pubic rami and ischium are less common than hip fractures. These are the most common sites of pelvic fracture, not the ilium. Because the ilium provides most of the weight bearing strength of the pelvis, weight bearing can usually be achieved as soon as pain eases. Isolated pubic ramus fractures often heal without causing significant long-term functional disability, with many patients able to walk short distances with a walker within a week. Early mobilization reduces similar complications as has been discussed with hip fractures.

Thoracic and lumbar vertebral compression fractures are often nontraumatic and occur spontaneously during ordinary activity in the setting of preexisting osteoporosis. In thoracic fractures the vertebrae are frequently deformed into a wedge shape causing kyphosis and subsequent impairment in respiratory function. In lumbar fractures the deformity is usually narrowing of the vertebral plates. With multiple vertebral fractures, spinal deformity can result in chronic pain and a permanent gait abnormality. The goals of therapy are to control pain and restore function. Use of a brace may help in pain management but will not prevent deformity. Newer techniques aimed at vertebral fracture repair, including kyphoplasty, may help to relieve pain and prevent deformity in selected patients.

Joint Replacement

Rehabilitation following total hip and knee joint replacement surgery is increasingly being carried out in the nursing facility setting. This is especially true in recent years since Medicare has limited financial payment for total joint replacement care in acute inpatient rehabilitation facilities. In contrast to hip fracture surgery, rehabilitation following total joint replacement must carefully balance therapy aimed at preventing deconditioning while avoiding overuse of the new joint. Typically, patients with cemented joints can weight bear as tolerated immediately after surgery, whereas patients with cementless joints are initially put on partial weight bearing to allow bony in-growth to occur. Due to the relative uniformity of joint replacements, rehabilitation can often take place according to a highly structured therapy protocol. Pain management is usually a greater challenge in elderly patients than other rehab conditions.

Amputation and Orthotics

The higher incidence of amputation, especially of the lower extremity, among the elderly relates to the higher prevalence of peripheral arterial disease and diabetes. In this age group trauma and tumor are less common causes. These patients present additional challenges to therapists due to presence of medical comorbidities that include decreased cardiopulmonary capacity, neuromuscular disease, muscle weakness, poor nutrition, and visual impairment. In addition, preexisting and functional decline makes high intensity prosthetic training more difficult and challenging.

Common amputation sites in the lower limb include below the knee (transtibial), and above the knee (transfemoral) [10]. The rehab time immediately following an amputation is referred to as the *pre-prosthetic period*. During this time the rehabilitation focus is on good wound healing and initiation of the therapy process. Specific clinical issues include: wound management, pain control, edema control, strengthening, functional training and maintenance of range of motion to prevent contracture.

Pain management addresses both surgical procedure-related pain and phantom limb pain. Phantom limb sensation is a perception that all or part of the amputated limb is still present. This sensation can be quite disturbing. It often improves over time and can be responsive to desensitization treatments. Edema of the residual limb is common. Reducing edema helps to promote healing and control pain. Management includes elastic wraps and elastic shrinker socks.

Once good healing is achieved (which can take weeks), the prosthesis can be fabricated. The components of the prosthesis include: *the socket* (interface between the residual limb and the prosthesis), the *suspension* (secures the prosthesis to the body), *joint* (such as the knee in a transtibial amputation), and *terminal device* (such as a foot) [11]. Collaboration between the patient, therapist, prosthetist, and prescribing physician is critical to successful fabrication of the prosthesis. Fit and comfort of the socket is a special challenge. Optimal fit in the socket is accomplished by placing residual limb socks in multiple layers in the socket till fit is achieved. Weight shifts and edema can lead to changes in fit and may necessitate refitting the socket.

Prosthetic training often involves significant cardiopulmonary stress as oxygen demand increases by about a third in a transtibial amputee and nearly doubles for a transfemoral amputee [10]. Thus, cardiac or respiratory compromise can limit an individual's ability to attain independent function with the prosthesis. Psychological issues often surface during this phase of rehabilitation and the services of a psychologist or counselor can be helpful.

Deconditioned State

It is very common for nursing facility residents admitted from hospital following an acute illness to suffer generalized weakness. This condition is often referred to as *deconditioning and results in generalized debility*. It is also an extremely common complication of long-stay nursing facility residents when either an acute problem or exacerbation of a chronic condition results in weakness and functional decline. Rehabilitation interventions, often combined with other therapy modalities, can be implemented in order to restore strength and function. As mentioned previously, for long-stay residents whose stay is not covered under the Medicare Part A benefit, this rehab therapy is covered under the Medicare Part B benefit. Most assisted living facilities can also arrange for therapy services covered under the Medicare Part B or other private insurance either on-site with a contracted therapy provider or at an out-patient therapy center.

Other Issues in Rehab

Maximizing Function

Federal nursing facility regulations require facilities to provide services to support and maintain a resident functioning at the highest practicable and achievable level of well–being. For residents with acute weakness, neurological deficits, or who are convalescing from an acute illness or surgery, therapy services are provided in a highly coordinated manner to achieve individual treatment goals. For those with sub-acute or chronic decline, the variety of services may be less complex and intense, and the frequency of treatments less often, but the goals of rehabilitation still apply.

There is another arm of long-term rehabilitation that focuses on maintaining function. This intervention is often referred to as *restorative care*. Restorative care is a program of ongoing exercise and activities of daily living training that is individually developed for each resident by the therapy team. It is usually then carried out by the nursing staff of the facility, including nursing assistants who provide most of the daily care in the nursing home or by a specially designated *restorative therapy aide*. Maintaining the improvement in physical function gained by rehabilitation is an important goal in the overall care of the resident.

Pain Management

Adequate analgesia for patients is a key priority in rehabilitation. Many elders receiving therapy have underlying conditions that cause pain, such as hip fracture or spasticity related to stroke, and experience pain during therapy exercises. The administration of analgesics should be provided around the clock (not only as needed) for patients with continuous pain and additional medication (as needed) should be given for breakthrough pain. Because of the intensity of therapy it has become common practice for patients to receive pain medication prior to the start of a therapy session to prevent excessive pain that may limit performance during therapy. As physical function improves, or surgical sites heal, pain frequently lessens so that reevaluation of the analgesic regimen should occur.

Depression

Depression is an extremely common condition among residents of long-term care facilities with prevalence in excess of 50 %. Similar high rates of depression occur among those who are undergoing rehabilitation for conditions such as stroke and hip fracture. Depression among rehabilitation patients may involve several factors including multiple medications, medical comorbidities, neuroendocrine imbalance related to the primary illness, or reactive features related to psychological stress or disability. Depressed patients are at risk for slower rehabilitation progress, longer length of stay, achieving worse outcomes, and not completing the therapy program designed for them. Practitioners should be vigilant in diagnosing depression and treatment should be timely and comprehensive to include both psychotherapy and pharmacotherapy (see Chap. "Dementia, Delirium and Depression" for further discussion of depression).

Care Transitions

Therapy services are available to residents in all settings. Often residents will transition from one level or site of care to another, and therapy services need to transition as well. Ensuring that progress notes are available to the therapists assuming care is an important step in care transitions. This is especially important in the transition from facility-based services to the home or outpatient setting, as well as across multiple levels of care during one period of illness. An example of this is a patient with a hip fracture who is admitted to the hospital for surgery and then transitions to a skilled nursing facility for rehab therapy, and is then discharged to home with therapy provided by a home care agency. Engaging family members in their understanding and support of the goals of care at each transition is a high priority.

Outcomes Related to Site of Rehab Care

There is emerging evidence from the research literature that there may be differences in outcomes based on the site of rehabilitation in various post-acute settings [12, 13]. Evidence suggests that rehab at an inpatient rehabilitation facility may predict better functional outcomes with shorter lengths of stay, though at higher cost. This is an area of health care spending that is currently being intensively studied.

Summary

Rehabilitation is a critically important part of health care delivery services in long-term care and ultimately serves all residents at some time during their nursing facility stay and many elderly in other long-term care settings. Preserving and restoring function is an essential element of quality long-term care. Two challenges that must be addressed are:

- First, impairment in cognition common among nursing facility residents often makes reaching optimal rehabilitation goals difficult.
- Second, resident treatment goals and the likelihood for achieving them are often continually changing so the approach to care must be frequently revised.

For long-stay nursing facility residents, who proceed toward progressive irreversible functional decline at the end of life, treatment priorities centered on maintaining the quality of life and dignity will replace traditional rehabilitation goals.

Pearls for the Practitioner

- A skilled nursing facility is the most appropriate location for patients who are unable to tolerate the 2–3 h of daily intensive rehab therapy as required for an impatient rehabilitation facility.
- Physical therapy focuses on lower extremity function and ambulation while occupational therapy focuses on upper extremity tasks.
- Concomitant medical conditions, referred to as medical comorbidities or multimorbidities can interact in dynamic and complex ways to impact both the outcome and complications that can occur during rehabilitation.
- Pressure ulcers that are poorly healing can adversely affect rehab therapy.
- Stroke rehabilitation begins immediately upon medical stabilization of the patient—often within 48 h.
- Up to 50 % of hip fracture patients do not regain their previous level of ambulation and up to 20 % become nonambulatory.
- Generalized weakness following acute illness in the elderly, referred to as deconditioning, is an extremely common complication of either a hospitalization or a stay in a long-term care facility.
- Restorative care is the provision of exercises and training in activities of daily living at a nursing facility following an episode of acute rehabilitation.
- Depression among rehabilitation patients is extremely common and may involve several mechanisms including: medication side effects, medical comorbidities, neuroendocrine imbalance, as well as a psychological reaction to disability.
- Short-term and long-term prognosis are constantly changing such that treatment goals in rehab must be periodically revised.

Websites

American Geriatrics Society http://www.americangeriatrics.org
American Academy of Physical Medicine and Rehabilitation http://www.aapmr.org
Centers for Medicare and Medicaid Services http://www.cms.hhs.gov
Cochrane Collaboration, Cochrane Reviews http://www.cochrane.org/reviews/
National Institute of Neurological Disorders and Stroke, Post-Stroke Rehabilitation
    Fact Sheet http://www.ninds.nih.gov/disorders/stroke/poststrokerehab.htm

References

1. Centers for Medicare & Medicaid. State operations manual, Appendix PP – Guidance to sur-veyors for long term care facilities, Rev. 55 12-2-09. http://www.cms.hhs.gov/manuals/down-loads/som107ap_pp_guidelines_ltcf.pdf.
2. Kochersberger G, Hielema F, Westlund R. Rehabilitation in the nursing home: how much, why, and with what results. Public Health Rep. 1994;109:372–6.
3. Quinn CQ, Port CL, Zimmerman S, Gurber-Baldini AL, Kasper JD, Fleshner I, et al. Short-stay nursing home rehabilitation patients: transitional care problems pose research challenges. J Am Geriatr Soc. 2008;56:1940–5.
4. Cruise CM, Sasson N, Lee MH. Rehabilitation outcomes in the older adult. Clin Geriatr Med. 2006;22:257–67.
5. American Medical Directors Association. Pressure ulcers in the long-term care setting clinical practice guideline. Columbia, MD: AMDA; 2008.
6. The surgeon general's call to action to prevent deep vein thrombosis and pulmonary embolism. 2008. http://www.surgeongeneral.gov/topics/deepvein/.
7. Jaffer AK, Brotman DJ. Prevention of venous thromboembolism in the geriatric patient. Clin Geriatr Med. 2006;22:93–111.
8. Shah MV. Rehabilitation of the older adult with stroke. Clin Geriatr Med. 2006;22:469–89.
9. Zuckerman JD. Hip fracture. N Engl J Med. 1996;334:1519–25.
10. Pomeranz B, Adler U, Shenoy N, Macaluso C, Parikh S. Prosthetics and orthotics for the older adult with a physical disability. Clin Geriatr Med. 2006;22:377–94.
11. Cristian A. The assessment of the older adult with a physical disability: a guide for clinicians. Clin Geriatr Med. 2006;22:221–38.
12. Herbold JA, Bonistall K, Walsh MB. Rehabilitation following total knee replacement, total hip replacement, and hip fracture: a case-controlled comparison. J Geriatr Phys Ther. 2011;34:155–60.
13. Leighton C, Sandel ME, Jette AM, Apelman J, Brandt DE, Cheng P, et al. Does postacute care site matter? a longitudinal study assessing functional recovery after a stroke. Arch Phys Med Rehabil. 2013;94:622–9.

Index

A

ACA. *See* Affordable Care Act (ACA)
Accountable Care Organizations (ACOs), 27, 66, 67, 149–150
Acute care hospital (ACH), 64–65
ACIP. *See* Advisory Committee on Immunization Practices (ACIP)
Active euthanasia, 273
Acute kidney injury (AKI), 312
Acute/chronic immune activation (ACI), 108
ADEs. *See* Adverse drug events (ADEs)
ADL, 8, 37, 57
Adult Protective Services, 264, 266, 268
Adverse drug events (ADEs), 84
Advisory Committee on Immunization Practices (ACIP), 136, 169
Affordable Care Act (ACA), 6, 26
Agency for Health Care Policy and Research (AHCPR), 223
Agency home care
  background information, 6
  face-to-face encounter, 6
  "homebound" status, 5
  multiple medical providers, 6
  transition in care, 6
AGS. *See* American Geriatrics Society (AGS)
AHCPR. *See* Agency for Health Care Policy and Research (AHCPR)
Aide and attendance program, 49
AL. *See* Assisted living (AL)
AL Communities (ALCs). *See* Assisted living (AL)
ALC. *See* Assisted living care (ALC)
ALF. *See* Assisted living facility (ALF)
Alzheimer's disease, 237, 241–242

American Academy of Physician Assistants, 96
American Association of Nurse Practitioners, 96
American Geriatric Society (AGS), 52, 312, 315
American Heart Association, 318
American Medical Association, 273
American Medical Association's Committee on Aging, 79
American Medical Directors Association. *See* Society for Post-Acute and Long-Term Care Medicine
Analgesics, 315
Anorexia
  African Americans, 182
  definition, 181
  management of, 181
  treating primary symptoms, 182
Ansak, Marie-Louise, 38
Antihypertensive therapy, 317, 318
Antipsychotic medication, 312
Appetite stimulants, 182, 208, 210–211
Artificial feeding, 211
Assisted living (AL)
  assisted living care (*see* Assisted living care (ALC))
  CEAL, 14
  change in, 27
  core values, 14
  cost variation, 19
  definition, 15
  facility characteristics
    dementia prevalence, 16
    documentation and charting, 16
    rooms, 16
    staffing, 16

© Springer International Publishing Switzerland 2016
P.A. Fenstemacher, P. Winn (eds.), *Post-Acute and Long-Term Medicine*,
Current Clinical Practice, DOI 10.1007/978-3-319-16979-8

Made in United States
North Haven, CT
03 January 2022